Perioperative Pain Ma

Edited by

Felicia Cox MSc (ECP), PGDip, RN
Senior Nurse, Pain Management
Royal Brompton & Harefield NHS Trust

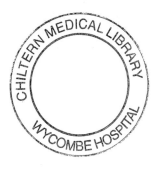
WILEY-BLACKWELL

A John Wiley & Sons, Ltd., Publication

Library of Congress Cataloging-in-Publication Data

Perioperative pain management / edited by Felicia Cox.
     p. ; cm.
  Includes bibliographical references and index.
  ISBN 978-1-4051-8077-1 (pbk. : alk. paper)
  1. Postoperative pain. 2. Analgesia. I. Cox, Felicia.
  [DNLM: 1. Pain–therapy. 2. Analgesia–methods. 3. Analgesics–therapeutic use.
  4. Anesthesia–methods. 5. Anesthetics–therapeutic use. 6. Perioperative Care–methods.
  WL 704 P445 2008]
  RD98.4.P47 2008
  617'.9195–dc22

                                     2008015231

A catalogue record for this book is available from the British Library.

Set in 10/12.5 pt Palatino by Aptara® Inc., New Delhi, India
Printed in Singapore by Markono Print Media Pte Ltd

1 2009

Contents

Contents

Contents

Contents

Contents

Contents

Contents

Dedication

With my heartfelt thanks to Cruisaid Ward staff at St Mary's Hospital, Paddington, and the haematology team at University College Hospital, London, for the care that I received. Special thanks to my stem cell donor for the gift of life.

List of Contributors

Dr Elizabeth M.C. Ashley, BSc, FRCA
Consultant Anaesthetist, Department of Anaesthesia, University College
Hospitals NHS Trust, The Heart Hospital, London

Joanne Bagley, MSc, RN
Clinical Nurse Specialist Team Manager, Department of Anaesthetics, Leeds
General Infirmary, Leeds

Dr Brigitta Brandner, FRCA
Consultant Anaesthetist, Department of Anaesthesia, University College
Hospitals NHS Trust, London

Dr Lesley Bromley, MBBS, FRCA
Consultant Anaesthetist, Department of Anaesthesia, University College
Hospital NHS Trust, London

Dr Donna Brown, PhD, MA, PGDip (HP), PGCert (LLL), RN
Senior Acute Pain Nurse, Acute Pain Service Royal Hospitals, Belfast Trust,
Belfast

Dr Dee Burrows, PhD, BSc (Hons), RGN, RNT
Independent Consultant Nurse and Director of Pain Consultants Limited,
Painconsultants, Great Missenden, Buckinghamshire

Julia Cambitzi, BSc, RN, CNS
Pain Management, University College Hospitals NHS Trust, London

Dr Eloise Carr, PhD, MSc, BSc, RN
Reader in Pain Management and Research, Bournemouth University,
Bournemouth

Dr Gillian Chumbley, PhD, BSc (Hons), RN
Nurse Consultant Pain Service, Imperial College Healthcare NHS Trust,
London

Angela Cousins, RN
CNS, Pain Management Service, Royal Brompton & Harefield NHS Trust,
Royal Brompton Hospital, London

Felicia Cox, MSc (ECP), PGDip, RN
Senior Nurse, Pain Management, Royal Brompton & Harefield NHS Trust,
Harefield, Middlesex

Dr Shane George, FRCP, FRCA
Consultant Anaesthetist & Intensivist, Department of Anaesthesia, Royal
Brompton & Harefield NHS Trust, Harefield, Middlesex

Dr Rachel Hagger-Holt, MA (Cantab), ClinPsychD
Clinical Psychologist, Buckinghamshire Primary Care Trust,
Buckinghamshire Hospitals NHS Trust, Buckinghamshire

Dr Joan Hester, MBBS, FRCA, LRCP, MRCS
Consultant in Pain Medicine, King's College Hospital, London, President,
The British Pain Society, London

Dr Siân Jaggar, MBBS, FRCA, MD
Consultant Anaesthetist, Royal Brompton & Harefield NHS Trust Royal
Brompton Hospital, London

Dr Mark I. Johnson, PhD, BSc, PGCHE
Professor of Pain and Analgesia, Faculty of Health, Leeds Metropolitan
University, Leeds

Dr Rohit Juneja
Specialist Registrar in Anaesthesia, Royal Brompton & Harefield NHS Trust
Royal Brompton Hospital, London

Dr Ian McGovern, FRCA
Consultant Anaesthetist, Harefield Hospital, Royal Brompton & Harefield
NHS Trust, Middlesex

Dr Jeremy Mitchell, FRCA, MSc
Consultant Anaesthetist & Lead Clinician Clinical Risk, Harefield Hospital
Royal Brompton & Harefield NHS Trust, Harefield, Middlesex

Dr Barbora Parizkova, MUDr
Consultant Anaesthetist, Department of Anaesthesia, Papworth Hospital,
Cambridge

Dr Jane Quinlan, MB, BS, FRCA
Consultant Anaesthetist, Nuffield Department of Anaesthetics, John Radcliffe Hospital, Oxford

Kirsty Scott, MRPharmS, Dip Clin Pharm, IP
Lead Directorate Pharmacist, Critical Care & Accident & Emergency, West Hertfordshire Hospitals NHS Trust, Hemel Hempstead General Hospital, Hertfordshire

Elaine Taylor, MSc, RN
Pain Service Manager, Stoke Mandeville Hospital, Aylesbury, Bucks

Foreword

The National Health Service celebrated its 60th birthday in 2008, and the relief of pain during and after surgery is a fine example of successful and sophisticated advances in patient care that have taken place over those 60 years. Gone are the days of the heavy premedication with a barbiturate, followed by oblivion for a few hours to awaken with vomiting and immense pain, unrelieved by an opioid because of the fear of respiratory depression.

Postoperative pain management is measured as a hallmark of the quality of care that is given to hospital patients, and rightly so. Not only does it relieve suffering but lessens anxiety, aids early mobilisation, lessens respiratory complications and, we now know, lessens the chance of the development of persistent pain after surgery.

There have been advances in anaesthesia, too, and the anaesthetist's skill also makes an enormous impact on postoperative recovery, well-being and number of days spent in hospital. Operations are now performed as day cases that would have been considered unbelievable 60 years ago. The role of the nurse in managing and educating others about postoperative pain relief is pivotal, and will expand further.

This is a detailed textbook that portrays the state of the art of perioperative pain management in the latter part of the first decade of the new millennium. It is a comprehensive, evidence-based account that examines psychological and physical methods of pain management as well as the well-established role of opioids. Patient-controlled analgesia, nerve blocks and continuous epidural infusions have a well-established place, but there is always scope for further advances.

Perhaps in another 60 years it will be possible to decide in advance, for each individual, exactly which medicines to use, and in what dose, by genetic testing. At the present time, pain management remains an art, but an art informed by science and technology.

This is an authoritative book, well-written and -presented. I hope you will enjoy reading it.

Joan Hester
Consultant in Pain Medicine, King's College Hospital, London
President of the British Pain Society

Preface

Pain is always a subjective experience; therefore, it cannot be quantified by any objective means. The management of pain is considered to be a fundamental human right, yet remains deficient, with the focus on the medical model (Brennan *et al*. 2007) rather than a biopsychosocial one. Reactions to pain vary due to previous experiences and the emotional response to this current pain. Sex also plays a role as women have lower pain thresholds and tolerance to a range of painful stimuli as compared to men (International Association for the Study of Pain 2007). Sex differences in pain and analgesia are present on the day of birth.

Comfort after surgery and fear of unrelieved pain remain major concerns for patients (Royston & Cox 2003). Poorly managed acute pain can impact negatively on the patient's recovery from surgery – discouraging the patient from mobilising and performing physiotherapy exercises (so-called dynamic analgesia) due to discomfort. This unrelieved pain may lead to an increase in morbidity and extend the length of hospital stay.

The evidence base for acute pain management is expanding and access to this information is improving through a combination of Open Access publishing of full-text articles (e.g. Biomed Central), electronic information for professionals (e.g. Bandolier) and patients and databases of peer-reviewed publications.

Perioperative Pain Management is an up-to-date evidence-based guide to the effective management of perioperative pain even in the most challenging situations. The level of evidence for interventions (National Health and Medical Research Council 1999) is provided, where appropriate, within the brackets next to the reference. The evidence for acute perioperative pain management and an explanation of the levels of evidence are provided in Chapter 7.

This text is aimed at all nurses from undergraduate students to experienced clinical nurse specialists and lecturers as well as pharmacists, operating department practitioners, physiotherapists, psychologists and trainee doctors. It provides readers with an understanding of the physiology, pharmacology and psychology of acute pain together with key messages for best practice. Examples of assessment documentation and guidelines for specific patient subgroups are reproduced throughout the text.

The authors of the stand-alone chapters are widely published and are recognised as clinical and research experts in their specialist fields. Barriers to effective acute pain management are explored and suggestions for improving practices and removing obstructions are given. The psychosocial impact of acute pain and personal coping strategies are reviewed in an easy-to-read and -understand format.

This text also tackles questions that are frequently addressed, but in insufficient depth in more general texts. How different medicines produce pain relief (analgesia) and what evidence exists to support different choices of pain-relieving strategies will be addressed. Common routes of administration of analgesia are described in detail; regional techniques including epidural, intravenous patient-controlled analgesia together with less frequent routes and the management of side effects.

Managing pain in special circumstances describes the diverse challenges faced by members of the multidisciplinary team and pain management service. Specific sections focus on managing perioperative pain in:

- Paediatrics
- The older patient
- Patients taking opioids for chronic painful conditions
- The known or suspected drug misuser
- The patient with renal dysfunction
- Day-case surgery

The use of transcutaneous electrical nerve stimulation in perioperative settings is explored. Examples of specific analgesia-related risks (such as epidural haematoma and abscess formation) are explored alongside in depth. Examples of the varied approaches to enhancing patient and staff education are provided.

I hope this new text provides you with sufficient details for all aspects of perioperative pain management and provides suggestions and motivates you to improve your practice.

Felicia Cox

References

Brennan, F., Carr, D.B. & Cousins, M. (2007) Pain management: a fundamental human right. *Anesthesia and Analgesia*, **105** (1), 205–221.

International Association for the Study of Pain (2007) *Differences in Pain Between Women and Men*. International Association for the Study of Pain, Seattle. www.iasp-pain.org. Accessed 23 May 2008.

National Health and Medical Research Council (1999) *A Guide to the Development, Implementation and Evaluation of Clinical Practice Guidelines*. National Health and Medical Research Council, Canberra.

Royston, D. & Cox, F. (2003) Anaesthesia: the patient's point of view. *The Lancet*, **362**, 1648–1658.

1 The Physiology of Pain

Rohit Juneja and Siân Jaggar

Key Messages

- Pain is still underdiagnosed and undertreated.
- Pain is a subjective experience and may even be present in the absence of any painful stimulus.
- Pain is multifactorial in nature and its management involves pharmacological, behavioural and psychosocial approaches.
- Transmission of nociceptive impulses depends on a balance of inhibitory and excitatory influences.
- With so many and diverse signalling mechanisms, there are numerous potential targets for analgesic therapies.

Introduction

Pain is an elaborate interaction between sensory, behavioural and emotional aspects, and past experiences of pain can dictate an individual's future response. In evolutionary terms, pain as a sensation serves to prevent ongoing trauma and to protect the injured area from harm whilst it is healing. However, there are situations where the painful experience far outlasts any tissue damage and does not convey any survival value but does prolong the suffering of the individual.

Definitions

There are many terms which require clarification in order to fully understand the processes involved when experiencing pain:

- *Nociception*
  The sensory process of detecting tissue damage. Nociceptors are the diverse group of receptors stimulated in this process.

- *Pain*

  The International Association for the Study of Pain defines this as 'an unpleasant sensory and emotional experience associated with actual or potential tissue damage' (Merskey & Bogduk 1994, p. 209).

  Thus, pain and nociception are not, despite common belief, the same. It is quite possible to experience pain without nociception and vice versa; nociception can occur without any pain being experienced.

- *Transduction*

  This is the conversion of one form of energy into another. This occurs at many stages in the pain pathway.

- *Transmission*

  Nociceptor excitation is conducted to its target via a combination of electrical and chemical transmitters.

- *Modulation*

  At all stages along the pain pathway, the transmitted signal is liable to amplification (upregulation) or dampening (downregulation).

In the example shown in Figure 1.1, the above terms are illustrated at various points along the pain pathway.

Nociceptors are excited not only by the physical trauma (such as pressure energy) to the tissue, but also by the consequent release of a multitude of chemical mediators (transduction). This information is further transduced into an electrical signal, which is transmitted along the primary afferent neurone to the dorsal horn of the spinal cord. The signal is transduced into quantal release of chemical neurotransmitters, which transmits the signal across the synaptic cleft to the second-order neurone. These events may be subject to presynaptic or postsynaptic modulation. Modulating influences may arise from primary afferent neurones, interneurones or descending pathways.

The majority of second-order neurones decussate at this point, crossing to the contralateral side of the spinal cord where they synapse again on third-order neurones, in anterolateral tracts, which ascend to the brainstem and sensory cortex.

Peripheral mechanisms

Peripheral receptors

It was once believed that painful stimuli were detected by the 'hyperstimulation' of receptors for other sensory modalities. We now know that in somatic tissues at least, this is not the case and painful stimuli are detected by specific receptors, called nociceptors. There is even a distinction between the fast 'sharp' pain transmitted along myelinated Aδ fibres and the slow 'dull' ache transmitted along non-myelinated C fibres.

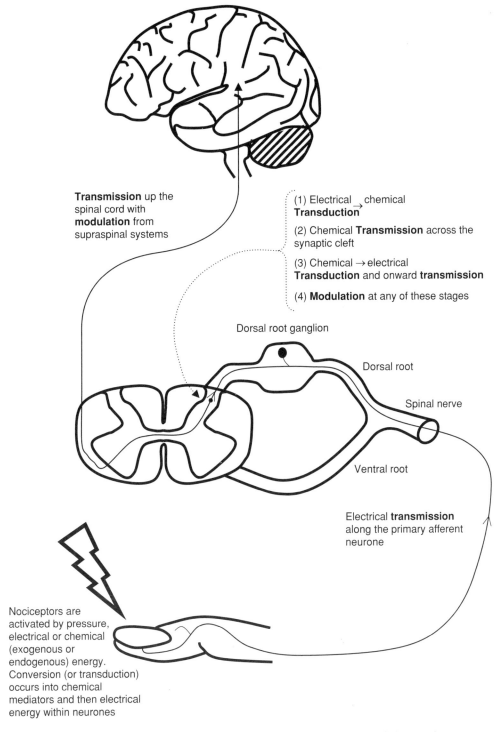

Transmission up the spinal cord with **modulation** from supraspinal systems

(1) Electrical → chemical **Transduction**

(2) Chemical **Transmission** across the synaptic cleft

(3) Chemical → electrical **Transduction** and onward **transmission**

(4) **Modulation** at any of these stages

Dorsal root ganglion

Dorsal root

Spinal nerve

Ventral root

Electrical **transmission** along the primary afferent neurone

Nociceptors are activated by pressure, electrical or chemical (exogenous or endogenous) energy. Conversion (or transduction) occurs into chemical mediators and then electrical energy within neurones

Figure 1.1   Transduction, transmission and modulation of a painful stimulus.

- *Cutaneous nociceptors*
  These are unlike other sensory receptors in that they are free nerve endings and respond to highly intense stimuli, i.e. those likely to cause injury to the tissue. The stimuli detected may be chemical, thermal or mechanical, hence their full title *polymodal* nociceptors. Information from cutaneous nociceptors (transmitted along C-fibre neurones) is responsible for the burning sensation in response to sufficient thermal stimulation (threshold usually about 44°C in humans).
- *Deep-tissue nociceptors*
  These are located in the deep structures such as joints, bones, muscles and viscera. Compared to their cutaneous counterparts, their receptive fields are much larger and pain experienced is more diffuse in nature. Moreover, visceral pain can also be referred to distant parts of the body, as is the case with cardiac pain referred to the left arm. This may be due to the primary afferent neurones from the heart entering the dorsal root entry zone at the same level as those cutaneous nociceptors which serve the left arm. As the brain can make no distinction between the two, it interprets the pain as coming from the superficial structure. The same mechanism is behind diaphragmatic pain being experienced in the shoulder tip.

Sensory neurones (primary afferent neurones)

There are numerous types of sensory neurones which are involved in conveying the information of the peripheral milieu to the central nervous system (CNS). A common classification is according to axon diameter, myelination and conduction velocity (Table 1.1).

A fibres differ grossly from C fibres in that they are of much larger diameter and are myelinated, hence their faster conduction velocities. Aβ fibres have a low threshold for activation, are cutaneous mechanoreceptors involved in

Table 1.1 Properties of different nerve fibres.

Fibre type	Function	Fibre diameter (mm)	Conduction velocity (m/sec)	Myelination
Aα	Motor	12–20	70–120	Yes
Aβ	Touch, pressure via cutaneous mechanoreceptors	5–12	30–70	Yes
Aγ	Muscle spindle afferents	3–6	15–30	Yes
Aδ	'Fast' pain, temperature	2–5	12–30	Yes
B	Autonomic preganglionic	<3	3–15	Yes
C	'Slow' pain	0.4–1.2	0.5–2.0	No

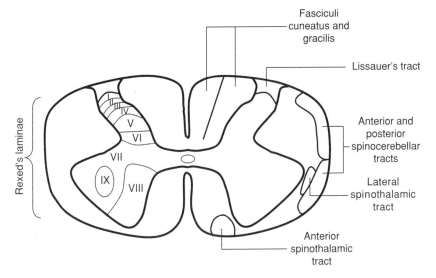

Figure 1.2 A cross section of the spinal cord, illustrating Rexed's laminae and the ascending tracts.

conveying the sensation of touch from somatic tissues and do not contribute directly to the sensation of pain.

Aδ fibres in somatic tissues (e.g. skin) transmit the action potentials from excited high-threshold thermo/mechanoreceptors which respond to more noxious stimuli; i.e. they are thermal and mechanical *nociceptors*. However, in visceral tissues there are no Aβ fibres and small C and Aδ fibres must respond to all stimuli. Aδ fibres terminate in laminae I and V of the dorsal horn of the spinal cord and, by virtue of their myelination and diameter (compared to C fibres), are responsible for the 'first' or 'fast' pain that occurs following injury. It allows rapid and fine localisation of the stimulus so that it can be removed swiftly, thus limiting further damage.

C fibres are non-myelinated and relatively thin neurones which convey information from high-threshold polymodal nociceptors. These receptors are free nerve endings which respond to chemical, mechanical and thermal stimuli and are responsible for the 'second' or 'slow' pain, which is the main area of interest in postoperative pain management. C fibres terminate in laminae I and II (the *substantia gelatinosa*) (see Figure 1.2) but are subject to many modulating systems. It is also worth noting that approximately 15% of C-fibre nociceptors are 'silent' and can become active under inflammatory conditions.

Mechanisms of inflammatory pain

The degree of activation of nociceptors in a dynamic state is dependent on the degree of tissue injury and modulatory factors. For example, in areas of overt trauma or inflammation, nociceptor activity is heightened; i.e. the *threshold* for nociceptor excitation and action potential generation is reduced. This results in a situation in which nociceptors are excited both in greater numbers and at a greater frequency for a given degree of stimulation. This phenomenon is referred to as *hyperalgesia*.

This reduced threshold for mechanical and thermal stimuli in the area of damage, *primary hyperalgesia*, manifests as tenderness and ongoing pain. When the reduced threshold extends beyond the area of damage (usually only to mechanical stimuli) and affects undamaged tissue, it is known as *secondary hyperalgesia*.

The mechanisms underlying each pathology are different.

* *Primary hyperalgesia*
  This results in part from the natural tissue-healing process. Inflammatory mediators are released from damaged cells and can act directly on nociceptors themselves. Examples of these include protons (H^+ ions), K^+ ions, adenosine triphosphate and bradykinin, which itself recruits mast cells and basophils to the damaged area.

  Mast cell degranulation results in the release of mediators including histamine and attracts platelets to the site of injury. Platelets are a rich source of serotonin (5-hydroxytryptamine, 5-HT), which is known to sensitise nociceptors to further activation via 5-HT_{2A} receptors present on the primary afferent terminal.

  The chemical mediators described are responsible for the classical signs of inflammation, namely:

  * Calor (warmth)
  * Tumour (swelling)
  * Rubor (redness)
  * Dolor (pain)

  Inflammation also brings about the breakdown of the membrane phospholipid, arachidonic acid, via the enzymes cyclooxygenase (COX) and lipoxygenase (LOX). The COX metabolites are the numerous prostaglandins, of which PGE_2 and PGI_2 have been identified as causing *peripheral sensitisation* of nociceptors afferents. The LOX pathway also produces nociceptor 'sensitisers', an area of current investigation. Inhibition of the COX enzyme is the target for *non-steroidal anti-inflammatory drugs* (NSAIDs), in a bid to reduce the production of prostaglandin metabolites.

  It is because of the huge number of chemical mediators (including those yet to be identified) involved in the inflammatory process that the term 'inflammatory soup' has been coined to collectively refer to these factors.

  A multitude of different receptors exist on the surface of nociceptive neurones. They include gamma aminobutyric acid (GABA), tachykinin, serotonin, histamine, prostaglandins, substance P (SP), H^+ ion, K^+ ion opioid and cannabinoid receptors, to name just a few. These receptors are intimately involved in the modulation of activity in the peripheral portion of pain pathways.

- *Secondary hyperalgesia*
  This is the phenomenon of reduced nociceptor threshold to mechanical stimuli in the *undamaged* tissue surrounding the area of injury.

  Unlike primary hyperalgesia, which results from peripheral sensitisation of nociceptor afferents by the 'inflammatory soup', secondary hyperalgesia is thought to be mediated by a central mechanism, i.e. *central sensitisation*.

  Peripheral sensitisation, with increased primary afferent activity, results in increased frequency of dorsal horn activity in the spinal cord. This is liable to *modulation* – either amplification or inhibition of the signal before onward transmission up the spinal cord to the higher centres of the midbrain and cortex.

  Ongoing injury and inflammation will present the dorsal horn with unrelenting stimulation and can result in the phenomenon called *wind-up*, which leads to a state of spinal hyperexcitability. This reduces the threshold of nociceptors in surrounding undamaged tissue, by antidromic activation, and increases their receptive field. These nociceptors may now be excited by usually innocuous stimuli in areas adjacent to the area of injury.

- *Neurogenic inflammation*
  Stimulation of peripheral C fibres results in retrograde transport and local release of the neuropeptides calcitonin gene-related peptide (CGRP) and substance P (SP), which act on the surrounding vasculature to cause vasodilatation, mast cell degranulation and increased capillary permeability, which manifests as 'flare'.

Central mechanisms

Spinal cord modulation

Having established the receptors and neurones involved in the transmission of noxious stimuli to the spinal cord, we can now explore the routes which this information takes from entry into the spinal cord to being perceived as a painful experience in the higher centres of the brain. The cell body of the first-order neurone (primary afferent neurone) lies within the dorsal root and is called the dorsal root ganglion. A neurone projects from this cell body to the periphery and another projects to the dorsal horn where it synapses with a second-order neurone (see Figure 1.2). These second-order neurones then decussate to the contralateral side of the spinal cord and ascend in one of two main pathways/ tracts. Depending on the ascending pathway, the second-order neurone synapses once more either in the midbrain or in the thalamus on a third-order neurone which will project onto higher cortical centres (see Figure 1.3). Each of these stages shall now be addressed individually.

The ascending pain pathways display evolutionary differences in that the 'older' *spinoreticulodiencephalic tract* (see Figure 1.4) is primarily involved in the

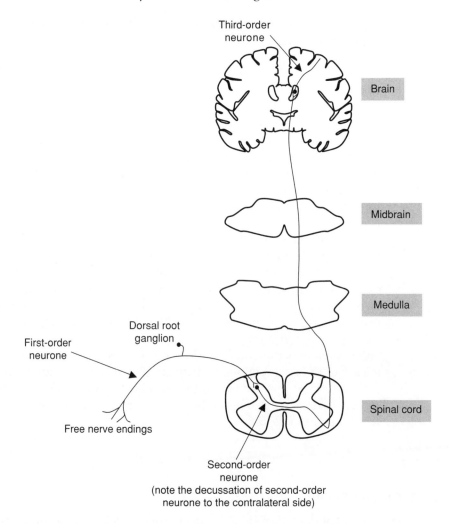

Third-order
neurone

Brain

Midbrain

Medulla

Dorsal root
ganglion

First-order
neurone

Spinal cord

Free nerve endings

Second-order
neurone
(note the decussation of second-order
neurone to the contralateral side)

Figure 1.3 Schematic showing first-, second- and third-order neurones.

affective component of pain perception. Its fibres pass via the reticular formation, medial thalamic nuclei, and onto the secondary sensory cortex (S2), anterior cingulate gyrus, insula and limbic system.

In comparison, the phylogenetically advanced *spinothalamic tract* is responsible for the localisation of pain. Its fibres are highly organised and pass via the lateral thalamic nuclei onto the primary sensory cortex (S1), with specific areas of the body corresponding to specific areas of S1 cortex – the brain *homunculus*. In essence, the fibres of the spinoreticulodiencephalic tract convey the sensation that something is 'painful', whereas the spinothalamic tract conveys the exact location and the discriminatory quality of the painful stimulus.

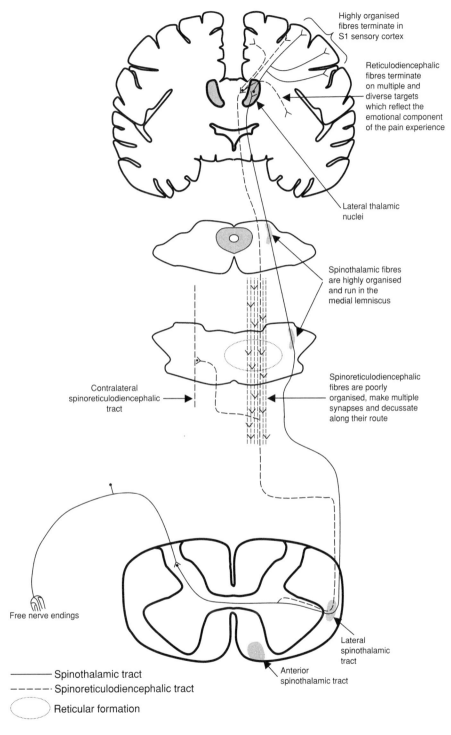

Highly organised
fibres terminate in
S1 sensory cortex

Reticulodiencephalic
fibres terminate
on multiple and
diverse targets
which reflect the
emotional component
of the pain experience

Lateral thalamic
nuclei

Spinothalamic fibres
are highly organised
and run in the
medial lemniscus

Spinoreticulodiencephalic
fibres are poorly
organised, make multiple
synapses and decussate
along their route

Contralateral
spinoreticulodiencephalic
tract

Free nerve endings

Lateral
spinothalamic
tract

Anterior
spinothalamic tract

——— Spinothalamic tract

------- Spinoreticulodiencephalic tract

Reticular formation

Figure 1.4   Ascending pain pathways.

Steps to consider include:

- Initial spinal connections
- Local spinal interneurones
- Ascending pathways
- Descending pathway – discussed later

The dorsal horn of the spinal cord plays a crucial role in integrating the many excitatory and inhibitory neurones, including interneurones and descending inhibitory pathways. Aδ- and C-fibre primary afferent neurones enter the dorsal horn and immediately ascend or descend one or two levels in a thin tract called Lissauer's tract, before synapsing with second-order neurones in the grey matter. The grey matter of the spinal cord contains the neuronal cell bodies and is highly organised into ten *laminae*.

The important laminae with reference to pain transmission are:

- *Laminae I and V*
  Many Aδ fibres terminate here.
- *Laminae I–V*
  Non-myelinated C fibres terminate here.
- *Laminae II and III* – substantia gelatinosa
  Many interneurones are present in these laminae and are involved in modulation of the pain signal. In fact, the majority of Aδ and C fibres synapse in this area.
- *Gate control theory*
  In 1965, Ron Melzack (a psychologist) and Pat Wall (a neuroscientist) postulated that perception of pain was influenced by the *pattern* of neuronal activity and proposed two classes of second-order neurones. The first class respond to non-noxious stimuli (e.g. touch carried via large-diameter, fast, myelinated Aβ fibres) and intense noxious stimuli (e.g. pain carried via small-diameter, slow, non-myelinated C fibres) – they are termed *wide dynamic range* (WDR) neurones. The second class respond solely to noxious stimuli and are termed nociceptive-specific neurones.

  They suggested that stimulation of low-threshold, myelinated Aβ afferent fibres would result in activation of an inhibitory interneurone in the substantia gelatinosa synapsing on the WDR second-order neurone, thus decreasing the output from the WDR neurone up the spinal cord. Smaller, non-myelinated C fibres would inhibit the inhibitory interneurone, thus allowing onward transmission of the 'pain signal' by the WDR neurone.

  They named this the gate control theory because stimulation of Aβ fibres in the painful area activated inhibitory interneurones and *closure of the gate* to C-fibre transmission (Figure 1.5). It explains the phenomenon of 'rubbing it better', as fast Aβ touch fibres are stimulated and block WDR neuronal transmission of the slower C-fibre input. It is also the principle behind *transcutaneous electrical nerve stimulation*, which utilises high-frequency, low-amplitude current to stimulate large peripheral Aβ fibres.

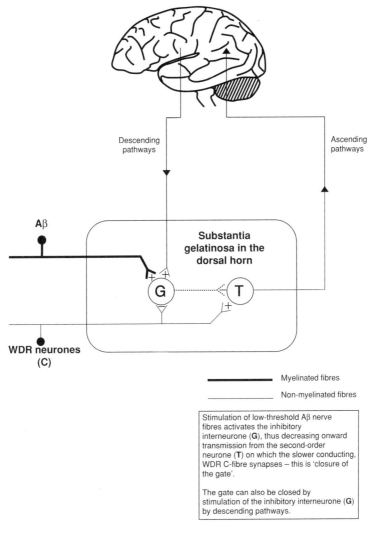

Figure 1.5 Gate control theory of pain. (© R. Melzack, reproduced with permission.)

- *Dorsal horn inhibitory mechanisms*
  Descending inhibitory pathways (see Figure 1.6) from higher centres in the brain can also close the gate. Descending neurones synapse on the dorsal horn inhibitory interneurones releasing excitatory neurotransmitters, including norepinephrine and serotonin. The excited inhibitory interneurones secrete opioid peptides, in particular enkephalins, which inhibit the transmission of pain signals by blocking the release of SP (an excitatory neurotransmitter) from the primary afferent neurone and by blocking SP receptors on WDR neurones.

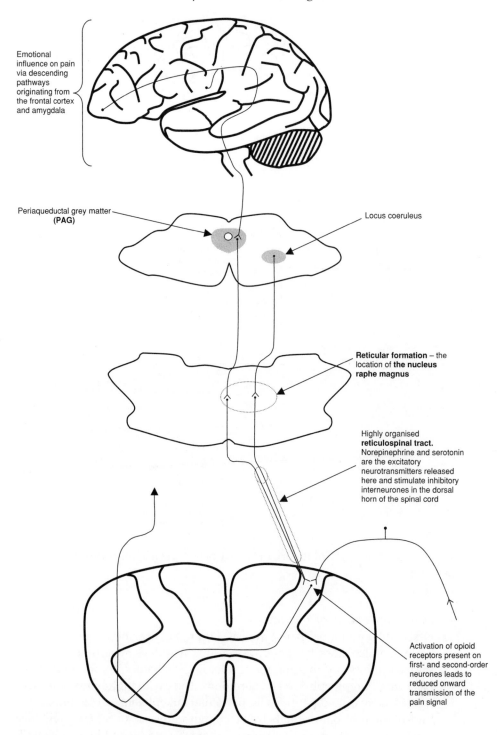

Figure 1.6 Descending pain pathways.

There are an abundance of opioid receptors in the superficial dorsal horn on both presynaptic primary afferent neurone terminals and postsynaptic second-order neurones. Activation of these receptors results in the opening of K^+ ion channels leading to hyperpolarisation of the neurone and consequent increased activation threshold. Thus, it is more difficult for nociceptive activity to be transmitted.

- *Central sensitisation and wind-up*

Pain signals are subject to modulation (augmentation or inhibition) both peripherally and centrally. When peripheral sensitisation occurs, pain signals arriving in the CNS are of greater amplitude and frequency. This increased barrage of *high-frequency* afferent activity can result in a state of *central sensitisation* in which the threshold of central neurones is decreased; allowing ordinary sensory information, such as innocuous touch and pressure, is perceived as painful.

Glutamate is the primary excitatory neurotransmitter involved in pain transmission and it exerts its effects on the *NMDA* (*N*-methyl-D-aspartate) and *AMPA* (α-amino-3-hydroxy-5-methyly-4-isoxazolepropionic acid) receptors. It is the NMDA receptor which is of great interest with regard to the phenomenon of *wind-up*.

Wind-up describes the situation in which dorsal horn second-order neurones are sensitised, increasing their output in response to *repeated* stimulation. Thus, although the strength of the repeated stimulation remains the same, the dorsal horn output increases.

Both low- and high-threshold, sensory, afferent fibres release glutamate when stimulated. This binds to both AMPA and NMDA receptors, although at different levels of activity. Normal noxious stimuli cause glutamate to bind to AMPA receptors and open a fast voltage-gated Na^+ ion channel, which results in short-lived postsynaptic depolarisations. When glutamate binds to NMDA receptors, a large Ca^{2+} channel is opened, allowing a large Ca^{2+} influx. Such large amounts of Ca^{2+} influx can be detrimental to cells and for this reason the channel is 'guarded' by Mg^{2+} ions while 'resting'. Only in the presence of continuous, unrelenting noxious stimuli is the 'Mg^{2+} block' from the Ca^{2+} channel of the NMDA glutamate receptor removed.

Continuous noxious stimulation results in dorsal horn release of the neuropeptides SP and CGRP. SP acts on neurokinin$_1$ (NK_1) receptors, which are abundant in the dorsal horn of the spinal cord. Activity of these receptors is essential for central sensitisation to occur but not for the normal transmission of painful stimuli. The key elements in the establishment of wind-up are the activation of the NMDA receptor, successful depolarisation and subsequent generation of increased levels of intracellular Ca^{2+}. A cascade of events then follows, which include activation of many Ca^{2+}-dependent second-messenger systems, such as protein kinases, and consequent phosphorylation of the AMPA receptor, which increases NMDA receptor sensitivity to released glutamate and the probability of NMDA receptor channel opening.

The increased strength of the chemical synapse following NMDA activation can last from minutes to days, and is referred to as *long-term potentiation*. It is postulated to be one of the mechanisms involved in forming memories, including those of pain.

Supraspinal modulation

Descending pathways can close the 'gate' in the dorsal horn, as described above. In addition, they can inhibit pain transmission independently of the dorsal horn 'gate'. They originate from three main areas:

- Cortex
- Thalamus
- Brainstem – especially the *periaqueductal grey* (PAG) area

and descend in the dorsolateral columns of the spinal cord to terminate in dorsal horn regions. Release of norepinephrine, 5-HT and enkephalin opioids results in antinociceptive effects.

The PAG is crucial in integrating information from higher centres such as the frontal cortex and amygdala (both of which are involved in emotion) and from ascending afferent activity from the dorsal horn of the spinal cord.

Neurones pass from the PAG to the *reticular formation* of the *rostroventromedial* (RVM) medulla. The reticular formation is the collective term for the many nuclei that lie in the RVM and make synapses with descending fibres from the PAG. The most important of these nuclei is the *nucleus raphe magnus* (NRM).

The descending neurones from the PAG to the NRM are serotonergic in nature and fibres pass on to the dorsal horn via the *reticulospinal tract*. Activation of this pathway causes inhibition of ascending pain impulses by releasing enkephalins, which hyperpolarise the postsynaptic membrane of second-order ascending neurones, reducing the amount of SP released by the presynaptic neurone.

A second pathway utilising norepinephrine runs from the *locus coeruleus* in the pons to the spinal cord, via the brainstem. As with fibres in the reticulospinal tract, they act to modulate afferent impulses in the spinal cord and enhance the action of endogenous opioids. This is the principle behind the use of the exogenous α_2-agonist clonidine, which acts in a similar way to norepinephrine although is limited by its side effects, which include hypotension and sedation.

The abundance of opioid peptide transmitters and receptors in all aspects of the descending pathways is of particular interest. Enkephalinergic neurones are prevalent in the PAG, NRM, locus coeruleus and dorsal horn and in part explain the analgesic mechanisms of opioid drugs such as morphine and codeine.

These descending pathways are under tonic GABAergic inhibition and opioids not only reduce this inhibitory tone but also increase the synthesis and release of norepinephrine and 5-HT along the pathways, which in turn augment the action of opioids.

Pain perception

All of the stages in the pain pathway which have been explained so far are part of the process of nociception. The final stage of the ascending pathway is the conscious experience and perception of the noxious stimulus as being painful. This experience will vary between individuals and depend on the context in which the injuries occur. A given degree of noxious stimulation does not equate with a predetermined pain response. For example injuries sustained in the battlefield or those during competitive sport may go unnoticed at the time they occur. In evolutionary terms, this has obvious survival benefits, and descending inhibitory pathways utilising norepinephrine may also play a role in these scenarios.

Recent functional imaging studies of the brain have illustrated the numerous and diverse areas which are involved in pain processing – areas such as the thalamus, S1 and S2 sensory cortex, primary motor and supplementary motor cortex, anterior cingulate gyrus, insula and the limbic system. The anterior cingulate gyrus, insula and limbic system are all known to be involved in emotion and explain why psychological factors such as arousal, attention, past experience and expectation can influence CNS circuits involved in modulation. Areas of the brain involved in processing emotion project down to the PAG and activate descending inhibitory pathways, such as the spinoreticular tract. The manipulation of these psychological factors is the basis behind the placebo effect, hypnosis and the Lamaze technique for pain during labour. It is also the reason why psychotherapy and cognitive behavioural therapy can play a crucial role in the multidisciplinary treatment of pain.

Finally, pain may be experienced in the absence of nociception. An example is the 'thalamic syndrome' which can occur following a stroke, where pain is experienced despite any injury, probably due to the loss of descending inhibitory signals from the thalamus.

Summary

Pain is a complex interaction between sensory, behavioural and emotional aspects of the experiencing person, yet it can occur in the absence of a stimulus. Past experiences of pain can dictate an individual's future response. Effective pain management requires the use of appropriate pharmacological, behavioural and psychosocial approaches.

Further reading

Cross, S.A. (1994) Pathophysiology of pain. *Mayo Clinic Proceedings*, **69** (4), 375–383.
Holdcroft, A. & Jaggar, S. (eds) (2005) *Core Topics in Pain*. Cambridge University Press, Cambridge.

Merskey, H. & Bogduk, M. (eds) (1994) *Classification of Chronic Pain*, 2nd edn. International Association for the Study of Pain Task Force on Taxonomy, IASP Press, Seattle, WA, pp. 209–214.

Prithvi Raj, P. (2000) *Practical Management of Pain*, 3rd edn. Mosby, St Louis.

Sandkühler, J. (2007) Understanding LTP in pain pathways. *Molecular Pain*, **3**, 9.

Wall, P.D. & Melzack, R. (eds) (1999) *Textbook of Pain*, 4th edn. Churchill Livingstone, Oxford.

Useful websites

The Digital Anatomist: *http://sig.biostr.washington.edu/projects/da/*.
The Whole Brain Atlas: *http://www.med.harvard.edu/AANLIB/home.html*.
International Association for the Study of Pain: *http://www.iasp-pain.org*.

2 Principles of Acute Pain Assessment

Donna Brown

Key Messages

A pain assessment tool should be used. The selected tool should:

- Be easily understood by patients and staff.
- Be quick to apply.
- Be consistently applied and evaluated with patient input.
- Be used with consideration to context and behavioural signs.
- Offer a sensitive, reliable and valid measure.

Introduction

The phenomenon of pain is difficult to define largely because it is influenced by psychosocial factors, an individual's perception of pain and how the brain deals with the messages it is receiving (Carr & Mann 2000). While there are a variety of definitions of pain (Carr & Goudas 1999, Francis & Munjas 1975, Katz & Melzack 1999, Mountcastle 1980, Nightingale 1859/1992, Sternbach 1968, Sullivan 1953), most fall short of being acceptable to all, as pain signifies a 'multitude of different, unique experiences having different causes, and characterised by different qualities varying along a number of sensory, affective and evaluative dimensions' (Melzack & Wall 1982, p. 46).

The most widely adopted definition of pain describes it as 'an unpleasant sensory and emotional experience associated with actual or potential tissue damage, or described in terms of such damage' (International Association for the Study of Pain 1979, p. 250). This definition recognises the complex multifaceted nature of pain and encompasses physical, psychological, social, cultural and environmental factors that interconnect and affect how pain is perceived, managed and evaluated (International Association for the Study of Pain 2003). Nurses have also embraced a second definition, proposed by Margo McCaffery (1968), who asserts that 'pain is whatever the experiencing person says it is, existing whenever he says it does' (p. 95). Central to this definition of pain is the tenet that the patient's self-report of pain is the most reliable indicator of their pain experience; thus, the importance of belief in what the patient says is fundamental to enhanced pain management practices. Both definitions emphasise the subjective nature of pain and provide practitioners with a guideline towards the diversity of pain experiences they will face.

However, it is the very subjectivity of pain that poses difficulties and challenges for the practitioner as a report of pain requires the caregiver to try and develop some understanding of the intensity, quality, location, duration, pattern and emotional impact of the pain being described and treat it appropriately. Social attitudes and cultural beliefs, of both the person in pain and practitioners, prevail and can limit effective assessment and management of pain (McCaffery & Pasero 1999). It is, therefore, imperative that formal pain assessment tools are utilised to facilitate effective communication and reduce the chance of error or bias (Carr & Mann 2000).

Measurement of acute pain

While assessing, relieving and evaluating pain are the responsibility of all members of the health care team who care for patients, nurses have a pivotal role. The Agency for Health Care Policy and Research (1994) proposes that failure to conduct adequate pain assessment is an important indication of undertreatment of pain. Many studies have concentrated on the complexities of pain assessment and have shown that the correlations between self-reported pain and objective perception of pain by others are poor (McKinley & Botti 1991, Zalon 1993). The literature supports the notion that pain can only be assessed on an individual basis using self-report, careful pain histories and external indicators (McCaffery & Pasero 1999), although, due to the 'busyness' of the general ward, external indicators and histories are frequently dismissed. Therefore, it is necessary to ensure that appropriate pain assessment tools that encourage communication (De Rond *et al.* 2001), enhance therapeutic relationships and formally document the efficacy of interventions are embedded into daily clinical practice. Health care professionals are encouraged to document the patient's pain alongside regular patient observations (Harmer & Davies, 1998) as the fifth vital sign (Joint Commission on the Accreditation of Healthcare Organisations 2001, Rutledge 1999).

The use of tools not only offers patients an opportunity to make a largely subjective experience, objective, by describing pain in a way that is meaningful to them, but may also facilitate continuity of care (Bouvette *et al.* 2002). Bucknall *et al.* (2001) argue that pain assessment tools should accommodate the patient's age, language and educational and cognitive status. However, applying the appropriate pain assessment tool accurately is only one part of pain management. Of equal importance is accepting the patient's self-report of pain and planning pain management interventions on the basis of that which is reported. This is not without its difficulties as researchers have repeatedly highlighted the inconsistencies that exist between nurses' and patients' interpretations of pain (Level IV: Carr *et al.* 2005, Level III-3: Dahlman *et al.* 1999, Level IV: Harmer & Davies 1998, Idvall 2004, Level IV: Sjöström *et al.* 2000). Arguably, discrepancies may be due, in part, to the fact that the parameters being compared by patients and nurses are not necessarily measuring the same pain experience. That is, the patient's report of pain is based on their perception of whether their pain has been relieved, increased or stayed the same, while nursing staff's record of pain describes an actual level of pain and its acceptability (Brown *et al.* 2007).

To further assist our understanding of the patient's pain experience, it is necessary to develop some clarity around pain threshold and pain tolerance. When individuals discuss pain, they frequently refer to having either a high or low threshold for pain. 'Pain threshold' is considered to be the point at which an individual (or group of people) considers a stimulus to be 'painful' or intolerable. In contrast, pain tolerance is measured by the amount of time a person can or will tolerate a certain level of pain (McClean & Cunningham 2007). It is useful to bear in mind the differences between threshold and tolerance when assessing, discussing and evaluating pain with patients. Ultimately, issues surrounding threshold and tolerance offer only one aspect of pain, as Manias *et al.* (Level IV: 2002, 2005) propose that the differences between patients' and nurses' estimates of pain are likely to be the consequence of multiple influences that are difficult to quantify.

Presented below are some pain assessment tools which may be used in a variety of clinical settings to promote the patient's self-report of pain and assist teams in pain management planning. A critique of their advantages and disadvantages is also offered to aid decision making for applying the most appropriate tool for individual patients.

Unilateral pain-rating scales

Single indicators of pain are arguably the most straightforward tools to apply and are primarily used to determine 'how much a person hurts' (McCaffery & Pasero 1999, p. 62). The verbal rating scale (VRS), numerical rating scale (NRS), visual analogue scale (VAS) and faces of pain scale (FPS) are all useful to interpret the intensity of pain and may be easily integrated into documentation processes.

Verbal rating scale

Known also as the verbal descriptor scale (VDS) or simple descriptor scale (SDS), this tool offers a choice of four adjectives to describe increasing levels of pain experienced by an individual. The scale may be assigned numbers (ranging from 0 to 3) or letters (ranging from A to D) to assist recording as shown in Table 2.1. For acute pain, VRS provides a quick and simple method of pain assessment in the surgical ward and can be easily integrated

Table 2.1 Verbal rating scale.

0	Or	A	No pain
1	Or	B	Mild pain
2	Or	C	Moderate pain
3	Or	D	Severe pain

into routine observation charts. Additionally, their simplicity may be more appropriate for older people or those with mild cognitive impairment (Lawler 1997), as VAS or NRS for pain can be conceptually difficult for older people to use (Level IV: Closs 1996). While offering a limited choice of words could be deemed prescriptive (Schofield 1995), extending the word choice makes the VDS time-consuming and more complicated for patients (Level IV: Jensen & Karoly 1992). A significant difficulty of employing a VRS is that it can be difficult to ascertain small changes in pain, as the VRS intervals are less sensitive than those of the NRS and VAS (Level IV: Williamson & Hoggart 2005). Nevertheless, Lara-Munoz *et al.* (Level II: 2004) propose that the VRS can provide reliable scientific information.

Visual analogue scale

This tool comprises a 10-cm line with 'no pain' located at the point of 0 and 'worst imaginable pain' located at the opposite end. The patient is asked to place or move the marker to a level that best indicates the intensity of their pain. The VAS (Figure 2.1) may be administered using a plastic ruler with a sliding marker or by paper. It is largely presented to the patient horizontally (Level IV: Ogon *et al.* 1996), but as pain may be considered as something that 'rises', it may also be used vertically (Level III-1: Aun *et al.* 1986, Level III-2: Stephenson & Herman 2000).

There are variations of the VAS available with numbers (from 0 to 10 or 0 to 100) or words (no pain, moderate pain or severe pain) being added (Figure 2.2).

Williamson & Hoggart (2005) suggest that the more levels a pain tool has, the more sensitive it is to detecting changes in pain. Therefore, employing a VAS with numerical ratings can enhance the practitioner's ability to discuss pain-rating goals with patients. Studies have consistently reported the VAS to be reliable, valid and sensitive (Level III-2: Gallagher *et al.* 2002, Lara-Munoz

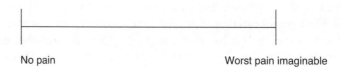

No pain   Worst pain imaginable

Figure 2.1 Visual analogue scale.

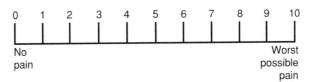

Figure 2.2 Example of a VAS with numbers or intensity descriptors. (Reprinted from McCaffery & Pasero (1999, p. 63), copyright (1999), with permission from Elsevier.)

et al. 2004, Stephenson & Herman 2000, Williamson & Hoggart 2005). Nevertheless, Jensen & Karoly (1992) have urged caution in its use due to patients experiencing difficulty in understanding and using the VAS compared to other scales. Thus, educating patients on its use is vital.

Numerical rating scale

The NRS is an interval-level tool that is typically administered verbally by the practitioner who asks the patient to rate their pain intensity from 0 to 5 or 10. In some studies, NRS is presented as increasing from 0 to 5, 10, 20 or 100 (Williamson & Hoggart 2005). As with the VAS, the end point 0 signifies no pain and 5 (10, 20 or 100) represents the worst pain possible. As an alternative, this scale (Figure 2.3) may also be presented graphically, with the numbers enclosed in boxes (Williamson & Hoggart 2005).

As many patients understand the concept of rating their pain from 0 to 10 with minimal explanation, this method of pain assessment can be useful when trying to determine the degree of pain an individual is experiencing in situations where they will not or cannot tolerate lengthy questioning. Thus, NRS may be useful for patients recovering from anaesthesia, those admitted under stressful or traumatic conditions, the less well educated, the visually impaired or in instances when visual contact is not possible (e.g. telephone conversation), (McCaffery & Pasero 1999). Ferrell (1995) suggests that applying an NRS from 0 to 5 may be the most appropriate pain-rating scale for cognitively impaired patients.

The validity of the NRS has been well established (Jensen & Karoly 1992). Additionally, its sensitivity to small changes in pain and its correlation to the VAS are robust (Level III-2: Jensen *et al.* 1986). Its ease of understanding and application makes it a useful tool for daily practice, research and audit purposes. However, practitioners need to remain mindful that not all patients have the ability to perceive their pain numerically (Bird 2003, Level III-3: Carpenter & Brockopp 1995). The main consideration in applying this tool is that the

| 0 | 1 | 2 | 3 | 4 | 5 | 6 | 7 | 8 | 9 | 10 |

Figure 2.3 Numerical rating scale.

end-point number (5, 10, 20 or 100) is agreed on and applied consistently in order for meaningful pain assessment to be achieved.

The faces of pain scale

The FPS employs six facial expressions that range from a smile through to a grimace. The smiling face at the 0 end point signifies that the individual has no pain and as they progress through the faces, the expressions change, indicating that the pain is gaining in intensity. On the reverse or below the faces scale, there is an NRS ranging from 0 to 5. (Zero to ten versions are also available.) The patient is asked to choose the face that best represents their pain, which in turn corresponds to the appropriate number. The incorporation of an NRS permits the patient's pain to be documented.

The Wong-Baker FACES pain scale

A popular variation of the FPS, the Wong-Baker FACES pain scale (FPS) (Figure 2.4), comprises a series of six facial expressions (ranging from a smile through neutral to a sad crying face). The smiling face at the 0 end point signifies that the person feels happy because they have no hurt or pain. In face 1, the person has just a little bit of hurt and progression through the faces and numbers signifies that the hurt is getting worse. Face 5 hurts as much as the person can imagine. When educating the patient in the use of this tool, it is important to emphasise that while the individual may not actually be crying, they feel this bad. The patient is asked to choose the face that best describes how they are feeling. Hurt and pain can be used interchangeably, depending on the age of the person who is using the tool.

In a modification of the Wong-Baker scale, a VAS has been added to the faces (McCaffery & Pasero 1999). This amended tool has been recommended as the choice for most clinical settings because of its popularity among children from 3 years (McCaffery & Beebe 1994) through to adult patients and because it has been translated into several different languages (p. 66). The FPS and Wong-Baker scale also have the advantage of avoiding the bias that can be associated with some interpretations of the FPS (e.g. Oucher scale (Beyer & Wells 1989)

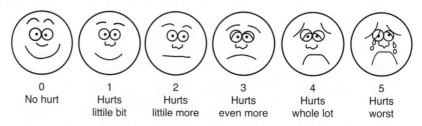

| 0 | 1 | 2 | 3 | 4 | 5 |
| No hurt | Hurts little bit | Hurts littile more | Hurts even more | Hurts whole lot | Hurts worst |

Figure 2.4 Wong-Baker FACES pain scale. (Reprinted from Hockenberry *et al.* (2005), copyright (2005), with permission from Elsevier.)

for children and adolescents), because the faces do not depict one particular age, culture or sex. However, a primary drawback of this tool is that it can be a barrier for the visually impaired.

Several studies (Level III-2: Herr *et al.* 1998, Level III-3: Jowers Ware *et al.* 2006, Level III-3: Kaasalainen & Crook 2004, Level III-2: Keck *et al.* 1996) have confirmed the validity, reliability and sensitivity of the faces scale. Questions have been raised as to whether the FPS may measure overall well-being or fear as opposed to the construct of pain. While Stein (1996) presented that in preschool children, ratings of anxiety were not related to pain scores, Jowers Ware *et al.* (2006) argued that the FPS added an affective component to the scale in their study of older patients. However, Jowers Ware *et al.* ultimately concluded that ease of use and the reliability and validity of the FPS made it a useful tool for evaluating pain intensity.

Limitations

Although useful for encouraging practitioners to apply a pain scale in busy environments, limitations of all these rating scales exist in that:

(i)   They offer a unilateral approach to pain assessment.
(ii) They focus primarily on the intensity of pain (Bruera & Watanabe 1994, Flaherty 1996).
(iii) They fail to take account of the context of pain (Williamson & Hoggart 2005).

Other important factors such as location, quality, duration, emotional impact and type of pain along with things that may exacerbate or reduce pain are omitted. In addition, they fail to take into account cognitive and/or behavioural changes, which may be significant when caring for cognitively impaired patients across the age spectrum.

Multidimensional pain-rating scales

Increasingly, patients admitted to hospital have an underlying chronic pain condition for which they are already receiving treatment. For such patients unilateral pain-rating scales may be of limited use, as it is necessary to develop some understanding of their previous pain experience and treatment as well as considering their acute pain episode.

Multidimensional pain scales assess the location, intensity, quality, duration, pattern and/or effects of pain.

The McGill Pain Questionnaire

Melzack & Torgerson (1971) developed the McGill Pain Questionnaire (MPQ) to obtain quantifiable measures of the sensory, affective and intensity dimensions of pain. The questionnaire attempts to enhance communication between the patient and the practitioner in an effort to develop the correct diagnosis and effect the best treatment. This multidimensional pain assessment tool includes an extensive range of descriptive words to establish details such as location, quality, duration and factors that affect pain. Additionally, it has a genderless figure to plot pain sites.

Utilising an assessment tool that identifies all areas of pain is particularly useful for research purposes. The extensively tested MPQ offers a more precise measure of persistent pain (Herr & Mobily 1991) and, arguably, might be an appropriate tool to utilise for some older people with acute pain (Brown 2004). However, the MPQ is complex and takes, on average, 30 min to complete. Its degree of complexity along with the time constraint may be a significant influencing factor, as health care organisations may fail to provide staff with sufficient time or chart space to document pain information (Gordon *et al.* 2000). Therefore, despite its validity, reliability and sensitivity as a pain assessment tool, the MPQ may be considered unsuitable to use on a routine basis in the acute surgical setting.

The Short-Form McGill Pain Questionnaire

Descriptive words offer important clues to the cause and intensity of pain, but overburdening patients and staff with long questionnaires, even for research purposes, is not desirable. Thus, the Short-Form McGill Pain Questionnaire (SF-MPQ) (Figure 2.5) may be more appropriate to use in circumstances where practitioners need in-depth information on the patient's pain or for research or audit purposes.

The SF-MPQ is composed of 15 pain descriptors, the first 11 are concerned with sensory dimensions of pain and the last 4 are affective dimensions of pain. The descriptors are scored on a scale of intensity from 0 to 3. Three intensity ratings for (i) pain sensation, (ii) pain affect and (iii) total pain score are derived from the scale. In addition, the SF-MPQ includes the present pain intensity index found in the original MPQ.

Melzack (1987) conducted a series of studies to ascertain the validity of the SF-MPQ with patients in surgical and obstetric wards and those with musculoskeletal and dental pain (Level II). His findings revealed high correlations between the standard and short-form MPQ. More recent studies have also shown the SF-MPQ to be a sensitive and valid tool for use in the postoperative setting (Grindley & Van den Dolder 2001, Level IV: McDonald & Weiskopf 2001).

Royal Brompton and Harefield NHS Trust pain assessment tool

The guiding principles of the MPQ and SF-MPQ have been incorporated and adapted, by those working within the clinical pain management environment, into a variety of pain assessment tools. For the acute pain setting, ease and speed of administration of a pain tool are fundamental if pain assessment is to be applied as the fifth vital sign. With this in mind, the Royal Brompton

Patient's Name:_____   Date:_____

	NONE	MILD	MODERATE	SEVERE
THROBBING	0)____	1)____	2)____	3)____
SHOOTING	0)____	1)____	2)____	3)____
STABBING	0)____	1)____	2)____	3)____
SHARP	0)____	1)____	2)____	3)____
CRAMPING	0)____	1)____	2)____	3)____
GNAWING	0)____	1)____	2)____	3)____
HOT-BURNING	0)____	1)____	2)____	3)____
ACHING	0)____	1)____	2)____	3)____
HEAVY	0)____	1)____	2)____	3)____
TENDER	0)____	1)____	2)____	3)____
SPLITTING	0)____	1)____	2)____	3)____
TIRING-EXHAUSTING	0)____	1)____	2)____	3)____
SICKENING	0)____	1)____	2)____	3)____
FEARFUL	0)____	1)____	2)____	3)____
PUNISHING-CRUEL	0)____	1)____	2)____	3)____

NO PAIN |—————————————————————| WORST POSSIBLE PAIN

PPI
0 NO PAIN
1 MILD
2 DISCOMFORTING
3 DISTRESSING
4 HORRIBLE
5 EXCRUCIATING

Figure 2.5 The Short-Form McGill Pain Questionnaire (SF-MPQ). (© Dr R. Melzack (1970, 1975, reprinted with permission from Dr R. Melzack.)

and Harefield Hospital pain assessment tool (Figure 2.6) provides a valuable multidimensional pain assessment tool that can be readily applied in the acute pain setting. This pain assessment tool is based on the MPQ (Melzack 1975) and Bourbonnais pain assessment tool (1981). Pain is assessed through the use of a genderless figure, a modified VAS, pain descriptors and the pattern of pain.

The ability to localise pain is important for patients and nurses, making body charts particularly useful for pinpointing the source of pain (Latham 1990). Generally, body charts are presented as genderless drawings of the front and back of the body on which a patient can plot the source(s) of their pain. Many body charts also incorporate numerical pain-scoring systems (e.g. Bourbonnais 1981, Bouvette *et al.* 2002, Carr 1997) along with pain descriptors. Within their pain assessment chart, Bouvette *et al.* (2002) also included symptoms that

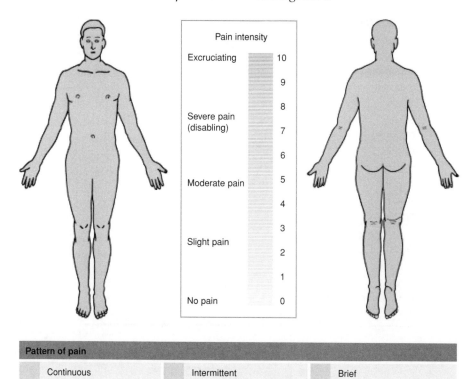

Pattern of pain		
Continuous	Intermittent	Brief

Description			
Tender	Pressure	Aching	Cramping
Gnawing	Dull	Burning	Electric shock
Throbbing	Sharp	Stabbling	Like a weight
Squeezing	Crushing	Discomfort	Sore

Graphic guide and descriptors based on the McGill Pain Questionnaire:

Melzack, R. (1975) The McGill Pain Questionnaire: major properties and scoring methods. *Pain*, **1**, 277–299.

Supplementary analogue guide:

Bourbonnais, F. (1981) Pain assessment: development of a tool for the nurse and the patient. *Journal of Advanced Nursing*, **6**, 277–282.

Figure 2.6 The Royal Brompton and Harefield NHS Trust pain assessment tool. (© Royal Brompton and Harefield NHS Trust (2005), reprinted with permission.)

were considered to distress patients with palliative pain (pain and symptom assessment record, PSAR) in an attempt to achieve holistic patient assessment.

Brief Pain Inventory

The Brief Pain Inventory (BPI) focuses on the pain the patient has experienced over a 24-hr period. It is divided into a series of questions that not only assess the patient's pain but also consider their suffering (McCaffery & Pasero 1999). Taking approximately 15 min to complete, either by the patient or by the practitioner, the BPI has been applied in a variety of clinical settings (Cleeland *et al.* 1994, Larue *et al.* 1995, Saxena *et al.* 1999, Wang *et al.* 1996 (all Level III-2)). This tool is based on a series of questions:

> Question 1 asks if the patient has experienced pain other than common everyday kinds of pain.
>
> Question 2 asks the patient to identify the location of that pain in the figure drawing.
>
> Questions 3 through to 6 ask the patient to use a pain-rating scale of 0–10 to rate their pain at its worst and least over the past 24 hr and its intensity on average and at this moment.
>
> Question 7 asks about treatment or medication the patient is receiving for pain.
>
> Question 8 asks the percentage of pain relief provided by these treatments.
>
> Question 9 is divided into seven parts that try to identify how much pain has interfered with the patient's life. It includes general activity, relations with other people and sleep.
>
> (McCaffery & Pasero 1999, p. 62)

It is argued that utilising a 24-h tool may more accurately reflect a patient's pain history (Mazanec *et al.* 2002) and more appropriately set the patient's pain in context. This in turn can lead to enhanced pain management, particularly for those patients who present practitioners with a challenge (e.g. those with palliative pain or underlying painful conditions). The BPI has been widely used in research where its reliability and validity have been found to be creditable (Level III-3: Daut *et al.* 1983, Level III-3: Keller *et al.* 2004). It also has the advantage of having been translated into several different languages, including French (Larue *et al.* 1995), Chinese (Wang *et al.* 1996), German (Level III-2: Radbruch *et al.* 1999) and Hindi (Saxena *et al.* 1999).

Considerations

Due to pressures of time, the MPQ, SF-MPQ and BPI need not be used on all patients. However, they are particularly applicable for (i) patients who have underlying pain conditions that are not well controlled (e.g. chronic, palliative, pain in older people), (ii) acute pain patients whose pain is proving difficult to manage, (iii) patients with a potential underlying neuropathic pain that has been undiagnosed, or (iv) practitioners wishing to conduct research (Caraceni *et al.* 2002). Should a multidimensional tool be applied for initial pain assessment, it ought to be followed up by using a unidimensional tool to assess the effect of any intervention (Bird 2003).

Leeds Assessment of Neuropathic Symptom and Signs Pain Score

There are a limited number of pain scales developed specifically for neuropathic pain (Level IV: Galer & Jensen 1997). As patients may not initially experience neuropathic pain, it has the potential to go unnoticed or undiagnosed until the patient becomes dissatisfied with their pain management treatment or until the pain becomes unbearable for the sufferer. Patients experiencing neuropathic pain may describe pain as sharp, hot, burning, cold or tingly, to give but a few examples. Regardless of how they describe their pain, it remains that it is distinctive from acute everyday-type pain and often resistant to standard analgesia.

The Leeds Assessment of Neuropathic Symptom and Signs Pain Score (S-LANSS) has been designed predominantly to identify the unique aspects of neuropathic pain (Level II: Bennett *et al.* 2005). This pain scale (Figure 2.7) is based on analysis of sensory description and bedside examination of sensory dysfunction, and provides immediate information in clinical settings (Bennett 2001). Utilising a genderless figure, VAS and seven questions requiring yes or no responses, the questionnaire scores the patient's pain. A score of 12 or more indicates that pain is of a neuropathic origin.

Although a number of studies have been conducted using the S-LANSS questionnaire (Level III-2: Kaki *et al.* 2005, Level III-2: Martinez-Lavin *et al.* 2003, Level III-2: Yucel *et al.* 2004), there is limited research available on neuropathic pain scales in general. However, early identification of neuropathic pain may facilitate diagnosis and treatment for patients (McCaffery & Pasero 1999). For this reason it is essential that researchers evaluate the effectiveness of those tools that are available to determine their reliability, validity and sensitivity.

Assessing pain in patients across the age spectrum

Paediatric pain assessment tools

It is essential that pain assessment in children is appropriate for the individual child and his or her family (Twycross *et al.* 1998). As culture, belief, cognitive level (including those with developmental disability), perceptions and the tolerance of pain differ in all children, determining the level of pain experienced can offer a significant challenge. Thus, there are a number of pain assessment tools, ranging from assessing preverbal to adolescent patients, available. As a rule of thumb, pain in paediatric patients can be measured by:

(i)   What children do (behaviour)?
(ii) How their bodies react (biological)?
(iii) What children say (self-report) (Twycross *et al.* 1998)?

A number of studies have been conducted to ascertain the reliability and validity of the tools. Meinhart & McCaffery (1983) have concluded that no tool is superior to any other. However, Twycross *et al.* (1998) have offered some guidance to practitioners in terms of which pain assessment tool should be used when (Table 2.2).

THE S-LANSS PAIN SCORE

Leeds Assessment of Neuropathic Symptoms and Signs (self-complete)

NAME _____   DATE _____

- This questionnaire can tell us about the type of pain that you may be experiencing. This can help in deciding how best to treat it.

- Please draw on the diagram below where you feel your pain. If you have pain in more than one area, **only shade in the one main area where your worst pain is.**

- On the scale below, please indicate how bad your pain (that you have shown on the above diagram) has been in the last week where:
  '0' means no pain and '10' means pain as severe as it could be.

NONE 0   1   2   3   4   5   6   7   8   9   10 SEVERE PAIN

- On the other side of the page are 7 questions about your pain (the one in the diagram).

- Think about how your pain that you showed in the diagram has felt **over the last week.** Put a tick against the descriptions that best match your pain. These descriptions may, or may not, match your pain no matter how severe it feels.

- Only circle the responses that describe your pain. **Please turn over.**

S-LANSS

Figure 2.7 (*continued*)

1. **In the area where you have pain, do you also have 'pins and needles', tingling or prickling sensations?**

    a)   NO – Idon't get these sensations   (0)

    b)   YES – I get these sensations often   (5)

2. **Does the painful area change colour (perhaps looks mottled or more red) when the pain is particularly bad?**

    a)   NO – The pain does not affect the colour of my skin   (0)

    b)   YES – I have noticed that the pain does make my skin look different from normal   (5)

3. **Does your pain make the affected skin abnormally sensitive to touch? Getting unpleasant sensations or pain when lightly stroking the skin might describe this.**

    a)   NO – The pain does not make my skin in that area abnormally sensitive to touch   (0)

    b)   YES – My skin in that area is particularly sensitive to touch   (3)

4. **Does your pain come on suddenly and in bursts for no apparent reason when you are completely still? Words like 'electric shocks', jumping and bursting might describe this.**

    a)   NO – My pain doesn't really feel like this   (0)

    b)   YES – I get these sensations often   (2)

5. **In the area where you have pain, does your skin feel unusually hot like a burning pain?**

    a)   NO – I don't have burning pain   (0)

    b)   YES – I get burning pain often   (1)

6. **Gently <u>rub</u> the painful area with your index finger and then rub a non-painful area (for example, an area of skin further away or on the opposite side from the painful area). How does this rubbing feel in the painful area?**

    a)   The painful area feels no different from the non-painful area   (0)

    b)   I feel discomfort, like pins and needles, tingling or burning in the painful
         area that is different from the non-painful area   (5)

7. **Gently <u>press</u> on the painful area with your finger tip then gently press in the same way onto a non-painful area (the same non-painful area that you chose in the last question). How does this feel in the painful area?**

    a)   The painful area does not feel different from the non-painful area   (0)

    b)   I feel numbness or tenderness in the painful area that is different from
         the non-painful area   (3)

Scoring: a score of 12 or more suggests pain of predominantly neuropathic origin

Figure 2.7   (*continued*) The S-LANSS pain score (© Dr M. Bennett *et al.* (2005), reprinted with permission from Dr M. Bennett.)

Table 2.2   Paediatric pain assessment tools and age suitability.

Which tool should be used when?	
Tool	**Age group**
Faces	From 3 years
Poker chips	4–8 years
Eland colour scale	4–10 years
Numerical rating scale	From 9 to 10 years
Verbal rating scale	9–15
Oucher scale	3–12 years (useful for young children and those with language difficulties)

Reproduced with permission of Twycross *et al.* (1998).

Older people (65 years and over)

Pain in older people is frequently underrecognised and unrelieved in comparison to that of younger patients (Level III-2: Feldt *et al.* 1998, Melzack 1987, National Confidential Enquiry into Perioperative Deaths 1999). Since two-thirds of beds, in the National Health Service (UK), are occupied by older people (Department of Health 2000) and inadequately managed pain is associated with many adverse consequences (Joint Commission on the Accreditation of Healthcare Organisations 2001), the need for appropriate pain management is crucial (Brown 2004). However, older people present practitioners with unique challenges (Table 2.3) and it is necessary to develop some understanding of what these challenges are if practitioners are to enhance their practices.

Herr & Mobily (1991) suggest that a reliable assessment of the older persons' pain can be best obtained if they are offered privacy, rather than asked to discuss pain in a public location. Whilst this can be difficult to achieve in a ward environment, measures such as drawing the curtains or moving closer to the patient may afford some improved degree of enhanced communication and privacy for pain assessment. Thus, the successful assessment and control of pain in older people depend on the development of the nurse/patient relationship and the ability to communicate effectively with older people (Brown & Draper 2003, McClean & Cunningham 2007, Level IV: Van Cott 1993).

Applying pain assessment tools

None-to-mild cognitive impairment

Improved pain assessment is fundamental to improved pain management in older people. The principles for assessing pain in older patients with no or mild/early cognitive impairment (including dementia) are the same as those

31

Table 2.3   The challenges of assessing and managing pain in the older person.

Research findings suggest that	
Pain sensitivity	May differ in people of advanced age (Fine 2001, Helme & Gibson 2001), with subsequent management of pain being complicated by multiple, non-concomitant causes and locations of pain (Closs 1994, Epps 2001, Herr & Mobily 1991, Horgas 2003). However, it is incorrect to assume that 'differ' means that pain reduces or becomes absent. Rather it implies that there is a variation in the experience of pain, with some possible increase in patients' pain tolerance (McClean & Cunningham 2007)
Analgesic intake	Older people receive less analgesia than their younger counterparts with the same degree of pain (Level III-2: Morrison & Sui 2000). This may be due in part to psychological or physical changes associated with age or the dominant ageist belief that it is usual for older people to experience pain daily and they 'simply have to put up with it' (Gloth 2000, Harkins *et al.* 1990, Level IV: Yates *et al.* 1995). However, Owen *et al.* (Level II: 1989) found that older patients, using patient-controlled analgesia as a form of postoperative pain relief, did not self-administer less medication
Cognitive impairment	Cognitively impaired people receive much less analgesia than their cognitively intact peers (Feldt *et al.* 1998, Morrison & Sui 2000). Ferrell & Ferrell (1992) argue that it is dangerous to assume that older people with cognitive impairment perceive pain differently, as there is no available evidence to suggest that individuals with cognitive impairment overstate or invent the pain they report (Bruce & Kopp 2001)
	A major predictor of mental status decline is pain and not analgesic intake, as so often inferred (Level IV: Duggleby & Lander 1994). Additionally, they propose that reduced mental status subsequently influences reduced analgesic intake, thus exacerbating all postoperative complications for this group of people
Perceptions	The older persons' perception of staff being 'too busy' (Yates *et al.* 1995) or fear of being regarded as a nuisance influences the older patients' willingness to communicate their pain concerns (Brown & McCormack 2005, Level IV: Carr & Thomas 1997, Level III-2: Herr & Mobily 1991)

(continued)

Table 2.3   The challenges of assessing and managing pain in the older person. *(Cont.)*

Research findings suggest that	
	Older people may further be disempowered because of negative stereotypical attitudes, which assume that growing older inevitably results in reduced capacity for involvement (McCormack 2003). Thus, complex pain management needs remain unaddressed (Helme & Gibson 2001, Horgas 2003) or discussed with family members, who may themselves not be sufficiently knowledgeable to best advise the older person (Level IV: Brown & McCormack 2006)
Practices	Task-orientated practices in the hospital setting, a lack of awareness of older peoples' needs and wishes and inadequate communication affect pain assessment and management with older people (Brown & McCormack 2006)
Communication	It has been well recognised that older people may experience difficulties in communicating their analgesic needs to others (Sengstaken & King 1993, Level III-1: Simons & Malabar 1995)
	Brockopp *et al.* (Level IV: 1996) found that although 92% of 125 older people understood that the person who is experiencing pain is the authority on their pain, only 66% believed that their pain would not be taken seriously when discussed with others
	Ferrell (1995) highlights that poor memory, depression and sensory impairment may contribute to the challenges of achieving accurate pain assessment
	The practicalities of older people experiencing hearing difficulties make it possible that patients do not respond to questions concerning their pain because they misunderstand or simply did not hear what they were being asked (Brown & McCormack 2006)

for a person with no memory problems (McClean & Cunningham 2007). The evidence suggests that older people can report pain as accurately as their younger counterparts, using the pain-rating scales mentioned earlier. Nevertheless, it may be necessary to consider adopting words other than pain in order to elicit a forthright response (e.g. ache or discomfort). For patients with mild cognitive impairment, it is also helpful to clearly ask if they have pain at present and how big a problem it is and to give them sufficient time to answer (McClean & Cunningham 2007, McCaffery & Pasero 1999). A pain-rating scale should be used until patients are no longer considered to be able to respond to the scale for themselves. They may well be significantly cognitively impaired before this occurs (McClean & Cunningham 2007).

While multidimensional pain scales may be considered useful to develop a full picture of concurrent locations of pain, they might be significantly labour intensive to apply in patients with mild-to-severe cognitive impairment. As patients might experience difficulty in remembering information about their pain history, family members or carers can also be helpful to enhance practitioners' understanding of the patient's preferences and history.

Moderate-to-severe cognitive impairment

As cognitive impairment progresses, it becomes more difficult for patients to accurately describe their pain and practitioners become reliant on other sources of information about the patient's pain. Assessing pain using behavioural indicators can assist practitioners at this stage (Level III-1: Hurley *et al.* 1992, Level III-1: Simons & Malabar 1995). Behavioural indicator pain scales place the practitioner's observation of the patient into a framework that usually consists of:

- Physiological changes – colour, vital signs, sleep pattern, guarding, sweating and loss of appetite
- Body-language changes – agitation, aggression, weeping reaction to touch and increased or decreased movement
- Behavioural changes – facial expression, withdrawal or assuming a fetal position

There are a number of behavioural indicator pain assessment scales available (Level II: Abbey *et al.* 2004, Level III-2: Feldt 2000, Hurley *et al.* 1992, Level IV: Kovach *et al.* 1999, Level III-2: Warden *et al.* 2003) that include observation of some or all of the behaviours mentioned above.

Debate concerning the reliability and validity of observational pain scales is ongoing. In support of behavioural indicators being applied, Simons & Malabar's (1995) pilot study, ascertaining the validity of the discomfort scale – dementia of the Alzheimer's type (DS-DAT) (Hurley *et al.* 1992) behavioural pain assessment tool, indicated that when staff interpreted pain behaviour and administered analgesia in response to this, the exhibited pain behaviours changed in a positive way. Thus, Simons & Malabar concluded that for the cognitively impaired patient, a behavioural pain scale could be used to interpret and treat pain successfully. However, Chapman & Marshall (1993) argue that behavioural pain scales rely heavily on the experience of the nurse, a point refuted by Simons & Malabar. Additionally, behavioural pain scales do not necessarily indicate the nature or location of pain being experienced.

The American Geriatrics Society (AGS) (2002) has also examined the reliability of practitioners utilising observations to make a diagnosis of pain in patients with severe cognitive impairment. Consequently, they have suggested six areas that should be incorporated into behavioural pain assessment charts. They are:

Facial expression
Negative vocalisation
Body language
Changes in activity patterns or routine
Changes in interpersonal interactions
Mental status changes

Currently, the only two behavioural pain assessment scales that take account of all six areas identified by the AGS are the Assessment of Discomfort in Dementia Protocol (Kovach *et al.* 1999) and the Abbey Pain Scale (Abbey *et al.* 2004). This is an area that requires further research.

When should pain be measured?

All patients should have their pain assessed if/when they attend a preassessment clinic or when they are admitted to hospital setting. In day-case surgery, patients frequently are 'healthy' and may present with no pain. Regardless of how or why a patient has been admitted to hospital, it is necessary to obtain a baseline pain assessment in order to ensure appropriate pain management planning following medical intervention. As part of the nursing admission assessment there are a number of core questions that are worthy of consideration, which are outlined in Table 2.4.

Interaction is a two-way process and is characterised by acting on or influencing each other (*The Concise Oxford English Dictionary* 1997). Assessing pain on admission opens communication channels between the nurse and the patient, signifying to patients that practitioners are interested in and willing to discuss their pain. This is important as even assertive individuals may experience depersonalising effects while in hospital. Thus, patients with underlying pain problems may be reluctant to communicate their pain concerns for fear of being regarded as a nuisance (Carr & Thomas 1997). Older people may be further disempowered because of negative stereotypical attitudes, which assume that growing older inevitably results in reduced capacity for involvement (McCormack 2003). In addition to improving communication, nurses can develop knowledge of the individual patient and use the opportunity to select the correct pain assessment tool, taking account of the patient's age range, socio-economic status and educational level (Coll *et al.* 2004).

Recovery ward

Immediately postoperatively patients can be disorientated, nauseated, dizzy and in pain, making this a challenging time for patients and practitioners alike. Field (1996) suggests that recovery-ward nurses have a special and significant

Table 2.4 Guidelines for pain assessment.

Core questions for consideration on admission	Further considerations
Does the patient have acute pain or ongoing pain problems?	Which tool best fits the patient? Do they understand the concept of using a VDS, VAS or NRS best? Do patients have visual or cognitive impairment, making the application of some pain scales difficult?
Where do they have pain?	If there is more than one site, consider using a body figure, BPI, SF-MPQ
Is there more than one type of pain?	Consider using S-LANSS
How much pain do they usually experience?	Everyday or intermittently
How much pain do they have at present?	If there is an underlying pain problem that is not under control, it will be necessary to complete a more comprehensive pain assessment and notify the appropriate medical staff or pain team to ensure that there is a programme of treatment in place
What treatment do they use or receive on a routine basis?	This should include the use of herbal remedies

VDS, verbal descriptor scale; VAS, visual analogue scale; BPI, Brief Pain Inventory; SF-MPQ, Short-Form McGill Pain Questionnaire.

role in assessing and relieving postoperative pain. Postoperative pain assessment should focus on the needs of the individual patient rather than on preconceived ideas of how much pain a certain type of surgery may elicit (Level IV: Sjöström *et al.* 2000). The only way to achieve this is to apply a valid pain assessment tool that the patient has been educated in using preoperatively. Thus consistency between the ward and recovery is vital. As discussed previously, a unilateral pain assessment tool may be best in the initial period, with the recovery-ward nurse taking an active part in asking the patient to rate their pain and documenting the reported pain for the patient. As the patient's presence of mind returns, it becomes easier to apply more multidimensional approaches to pain assessment. Evaluation of effects and side effects linked to pain management interventions should also be conducted and documented at regular intervals. Prior to returning patients to the ward, the recovery-ward nurse should conduct a pain assessment to ensure that patients are as 'pain free' as possible. All necessary information is subsequently documented and communicated to the ward nurse.

Pain assessment at ward level

On return to the ward, pain is required to be reassessed as frequently in transition (from one area to another) patients report an increase in pain. Thereafter, all hospitals have their own guidelines on how frequently pain assessment should be conducted, depending on the type of analgesic technique being employed. De Rond *et al.* (Level IV: 1999) argue that twice daily assessment is sufficient, while Macintyre & Ready (2001) suggest that reassessment should occur as frequently as necessary when pain is not well controlled or changing in nature. Irrespective of how frequently pain assessment is conducted, it should not cease following the discontinuation of sophisticated pain management techniques. Rather it should continue for as long as patients require or receive any form of analgesia and should always be re-evaluated following analgesic administration. Continued pain assessment and evaluation of management strategies will also indicate those patients whose pain has changed or who may be developing neuropathic pain.

Summary

Pain assessment tools enhance communication between patients and practitioners and between the multidisciplinary team by making a subjective experience measurable. However, for successful interventions to be applied, it is imperative that pain assessment tools and charts are:

(1) *Easily understood by patients and staff*

Appropriate for the patient population they are to be used with.

Everyone in the environment should adopt the same language with uniformity in assessment and documentation when using a rating scale (Pasero 1997).

Patient education is an important factor in completing successful pain assessment (Bouvette *et al.* 2002).

Accommodate the patient's age, language, education and cognitive status (Bucknall *et al.* 2001).

(2) *Quick to apply*

Integrated into observation charts.

Documentation of pain assessment is necessary for legal and professional reasons and as a mechanism of formalising pain assessment processes.

(3) *Consistently applied and evaluated with patient input*

Regardless of which pain assessment tool is applied, all require the nurse and patient to be working towards shared goals and they need to be applied conscientiously (Bird 2003, McCaffery & Pasero 1999).

(4) *Consideration needs to be given to context and behavioural signs*

Patients with an underlying pain problem may require a comprehensive and detailed pain assessment to be completed.

In older patients, non-verbal cues may more accurately signify the presence of pain. These may include changes in sleeping or eating patterns, increased frustration, agitated or aggressive behaviours, withdrawal from family and friends or avoidance of activity (American Geriatrics Society 2002).

(5) *Offer sensitive, reliable and valid measures*

Despite many pain assessment tools having been available for some time, their reliability and validity cannot be presumed, because none holds psychometric stability in every environment (Bird 2003).

Carr (1997) argues that the use of a pain assessment tool does not necessarily guarantee that appropriate pain management will occur unless suitable interventions are linked with evaluation. Therefore, it is imperative that patients, nurses, doctors and services dedicated to enhancing pain management practices work in collaboration to bring about effective pain management decisions.

References

Abbey, J.A., Piller, N., DeBellis, A., *et al.* (2004) The Abbey Pain Scale. A 1-minute numerical indicator for people with late-stage dementia. *International Journal of Palliative Nursing*, **10** (1), 6–13.

Agency for Health Care Policy and Research (1994) *Management of Cancer Pain: Clinical Practice Guidelines, no. 9* (AHCPR publication 94-0592). Department of Health and Human Services, Rockville.

American Geriatrics Society (AGS) Panel on Persistent Pain in Older Persons (2002) The management of persistent pain in older persons. *Journal of the American Geriatrics Society*, **50** (Suppl.), 205–224.

Aun, C., Lam, Y.M. & Collett, B. (1986) Evaluation of the use of visual analogue scale in Chinese patients. *Pain*, **25** (2), 215–221.

Bennett, M. (2001) The LANSS pain scale: the Leeds Assessment of Neuropathic Symptoms and Signs. *Pain*, **92** (1–2), 147–157.

Bennett, M.I., Smith, B.H., Torrance, N. & Potter, J. (2005) The S-LANSS score for identifying pain of predominantly neuropathic origin: validation for use in clinical and postal research. *Journal of Pain*, **6** (3), 149–158.

Beyer, J.E. & Wells, N. (1989) The assessment of pain in children. *Pediatric Clinics of North America*, **36** (4), 837–854.

Bird, J. (2003) Selection of pain measurement tools. *Nursing Standard*, **18** (13), 33–39.

Bourbonnais, F. (1981) Pain assessment: development of a tool for the nurse and the patient. *Journal of Advanced Nursing*, **6** (4), 277–282.

Bouvette, M., Fothergill-Bourbonnais, F. & Perreault, A. (2002) Implementation of the pain and symptom assessment record (PSAR). *Journal of Advanced Nursing*, **40** (6), 685–700.

Brockopp, D.Y., Warden, S., Colclough, G. & Brockopp, G. (1996) Elderly people's knowledge of and attitudes to pain management. *British Journal of Nursing*, **5** (9), 556–562.

Brown, A. & Draper, P. (2003) Accommodative speech and terms of endearment: elements of a language mode often experienced by older adults. *Journal of Advanced Nursing*, **41** (1), 15–21.

Brown, D. (2004) A literature review exploring how healthcare professionals contribute to the assessment and control of pain in older patients. *International Journal of Older People Nursing [in association with Journal of Clinical Nursing]*, **13** (6b), 74–90.

Brown, D. & McCormack, B. (2005) *Determining Factors That Impact upon Effective Evidence Based Pain Management with Older People, Following Colorectal Surgery: An Ethnographic Study*. Report. The Royal Hospitals, Belfast.

Brown, D. & McCormack, B. (2006) Determining factors that impact upon effective evidence based pain management with older people, following colorectal surgery: an ethnographic study. *Journal of Clinical Nursing*, **15** (10), 1287–1298.

Brown, D., O'Neill, O. & Beck, A. (2007) Transition from epidural to oral analgesia. *Nursing Standard*, **21** (21), 35–40.

Bruce, A. & Kopp, P. (2001) Pain experienced by older people. *Professional Nurse*, **16** (11), 1481–1485.

Bruera, E. & Watanabe, S. (1994) New developments in the assessment of pain in cancer patients. *Supportive Care Cancer*, **2** (5), 312–318.

Bucknall, T., Manias, E. & Botti, M. (2001) Acute pain management: implications of scientific evidence for nursing practice in the postoperative context. *International Journal of Nursing Practice*, **7** (4), 266–273.

Caraceni, M.D., Cherney, N., Fainsinger, R., *et al.* (2002) Pain measurement tools and methods in palliative care: recommendations of an expert working group of the European Association of Palliative Care. *Journal of Pain and Symptom Management*, **23** (3), 239–255.

Carpenter, J. & Brockopp, D. (1995) Comparison of patients' ratings and examination of nurses' responses to pain. *Cancer Nursing*, **18** (4), 292–298.

Carr, D. & Goudas, L.C. (1999) Acute pain. *The Lancet*, **353** (9169), 2051–2058.

Carr, E.C.J. (1997) Evaluating the use of a pain assessment tool and care plan: a pilot study. *Journal of Advanced Nursing*, **26** (6), 1073–1079.

Carr, E.C.J. & Mann, E.M. (2000) *Pain: Creative Approaches to Effective Management*. Palgrave Macmillan, London.

Carr, E.C.J. & Thomas, V.J. (1997) Anticipating and experiencing postoperative pain: the patients' perspective. *Journal of Clinical Nursing*, **6** (3), 191–201.

Carr, E.C.J., Thomas, V.J. & Wilson-Barnet, J. (2005) Patient experiences of anxiety and depression and acute pain after surgery: a longitudinal perspective. *International Journal of Nursing Studies*, **42** (5), 521–530.

Chapman, A. & Marshall, M. (1993) *Dementia: New Skills for Social Workers*. Jessica Kinsley, London.

Cleeland, C.S., Gonin, R., Hatfield, A.K., Edmonson, H., Blum, R.H., Stewart, A. & Pandya, K.J. (1994) Pain and its treatment in outpatients with metastatic cancer. *New England Journal of Medicine*, **330** (9), 592–596.

Closs, S.J. (1994) Pain and elderly patients: a neglected phenomenon. *Journal of Advanced Nursing*, **19** (6), 1072–1081.

Closs, S.J. (1996) Pain and elderly patients: a survey of nurses' knowledge and experiences. *Journal of Advanced Nursing*, **23** (2), 237–242.

Coll, A.M., Ameen, J.R.M. & Mead, D. (2004) Postoperative pain assessment tools in day surgery: literature review. *Journal of Advanced Nursing*, **46** (2), 124–133.

Dahlman, G.B., Dykes, A.K. & Elander, G. (1999) Patients' evaluation of pain and nurses' management of analgesics after surgery. The effect of a study day on the subject of pain for nurses working at the thorax surgery department. *Journal of Advanced Nursing,* **30** (4), 866–874.

Daut, R.L., Cleeland, C.S. & Flannery, R.C. (1983) Development of the Wisconsin Brief Pain Questionnaire to assess pain in cancer and other diseases. *Pain,* **17** (2), 197–210.

De Rond, M., de Wit, R. & van Dam, F., *et al.* (1999) Daily pain assessment: value for nurses and patients. *Journal of Advanced Nursing,* **29** (2), 436–444.

De Rond, M., de Wit, R. & van Dam, F. (2001) The implementation of a pain monitoring programme for nurses in daily clinical practice: results of a follow up study in five hospitals. *Journal of Advanced Nursing,* **35** (4), 590–598.

Department of Health (2000) *The National Health Service Plan: A Plan for Investment. A Plan for Reform.* The Stationery Office, London.

Duggleby, W. & Lander, J. (1994) Cognitive status and post operative pain: older adults. *Journal of Pain and Symptom Management,* **9** (1), 19–27.

Epps, C. (2001) Recognising pain in the institutionalised elder with dementia. *Geriatric Nursing,* **22** (2), 71–79.

Feldt, K.S. (2000) The checklist of nonverbal pain indicators (CNPI). *Pain Management Nursing,* **1** (1), 13–21.

Feldt, K.S., Ryden, M.B. & Miles, S. (1998) Treatment of pain in cognitively impaired compared with cognitively intact older patients with hip fracture. *Journal of American Geriatrics Society,* **46** (9), 1079–1085.

Ferrell, B. & Ferrell, B. (1992) Pain in the elderly. In: *Pain Management: Nursing Perspective* (eds J. Watt-Watson & M. Donovan). Mosby, Philadelphia, PA.

Ferrell, B.A. (1995) Pain evaluation and management in the nursing home. *Annals of Internal Medicine,* **123** (9), 681–687.

Field, L. (1996) Factors influencing nurses analgesia decisions. *British Journal of Nursing,* **5** (14), 838–844.

Fine, P.G. (2001) Opioid analgesic drugs in older people. *Clinics in Geriatric Medicine,* **17** (3), 479–487.

Flaherty, S. (1996) Pain measurement tools for clinical practice and research. *Journal of the American Association of Nurse Anesthetists,* **64** (2), 133–140.

Francis, G.M. & Munjas, B. (1975) *Promoting Psychological Comfort.* Wm C Brown Company Publishers, Dubuque, IA.

Galer, B.S. & Jensen, M.P. (1997) Development and preliminary validation of a pain measure specific to neuropathic pain: the neuropathic pain scale. *Neurology,* **48** (2), 332–338.

Gallagher, E.J., Bijur, P.E., Latimer, C. & Silver, W. (2002) Reliability and validity of a visual analogue scale for acute abdominal pain in the emergency department. *American Journal of Emergency Medicine,* **20** (4), 287–290.

Gloth, F.M. (2000) Geriatric pain: factors that limit pain relief and increase complications. *Geriatrics* **55** (10), 46–54.

Gordon, D.B., Dahl, J.L. & Stevenson, K.K. (2000) Introduction. In: *Building an Institutional Commitment to Pain Management. The Wisconsin Resource Manual,* 2nd edn (eds D.B. Gordon, J.L. Dahl & K.K Stevenson). University of Wisconsin – Madison Board of Regents, Madison.

Grindley, L. & Van Den Dolder, P.A. (2001) The percentage improvement in pain scale as a measure of physiotherapy treatment effect. *Australian Journal of Physiotherapy,* **47,** 133–138.

Harkins, S.W., Kwentus, J. & Price, D.D. (1990) Pain and suffering in the elderly. In: *The Management of Pain*, 2nd edn (ed. J.J. Bonica). Lea and Febiger, Philadelphia, pp. 552–559.

Harmer, M. & Davies, K.A. (1998) The effect of education, assessment and a standardised prescription on postoperative pain management. *Anaesthesia*, **53** (5), 424–430.

Helme, R.D. & Gibson, S.J. (2001) The epidemiology of pain in elderly people. *Clinics in Geriatric Medicine*, **17** (3), 417–431.

Herr, K. & Mobily, P. (1991) Complexities of pain assessment in the elderly: clinical considerations. *Journal of Gerontological Nursing*, **17** (4), 12–19.

Herr, K.A., Mobily, P.R., Kohort, F.J. & Wagenaar, D. (1998) Evaluation of the Faces of Pain Scale for use with the elderly. *Clinical Journal of Pain*, **14** (1), 29–38.

Hockenberry, M.J., Wilson, D. & Winkelstein, M.L. (2005) *Wong's Essentials of Pediatric Nursing*, 7th edn. Mosby, St Louis, p. 1259

Horgas, A.L. (2003) Pain Management in elderly adults. *Journal of infusion Nursing*, **26**, 161–165.

Hurley, A.C., Volicer, B.J., Hanrahan, P.A., *et al.* (1992) Assessment of discomfort in advanced Alzheimer patients. *Research in Nursing and Health*, **15** (5), 369–377.

Idvall, E. (2004) Quality of care in postoperative pain management: what is realistic in clinical practice? *Journal of Nursing Management*, **12** (3), 162–166.

International Association for the Study of Pain (1979) International Association for the Study of Pain sub-committee on taxonomy, pain terms: a list of definitions and notes on usage. *Pain*, **6** (3), 249–252.

International Association for the Study of Pain (2003) *International Association for the Study of Pain (IASP) Pain Terminology*. http://www.iasp-pain.org/terms-p.html. Accessed 12 July 2007.

Jensen, M.P., Karoly, P. & Braver, S. (1986) The measurement of clinical pain intensity: a comparison of six methods. *Pain*, **27** (1), 117–126.

Jensen, T.S. & Karoly, P. (1992) Self-report scales and procedures for assessing pain in adults. In: *The Handbook of Pain Assessment* (eds D.C. Turk & R. Melzack). The Guildford Press, New York, pp. 135–151.

Joint Commission on the Accreditation of Healthcare Organisations (2001) *Implementing the New Pain Management Standards*. Joint Commission on the Accreditation of Healthcare Organisations, Oakbrook, IL.

Jowers Ware, L., Epps, C.D., Herr, K. & Packard, A. (2006) Evaluation of the revised faces of pain scale, verbal descriptor scale, numeric rating scale, and Iowa pain thermometer in older minority adults. *Pain Management Nursing*, **7** (3), 117–125.

Kaasalainen, S. & Crook, J. (2004) An exploration of seniors' ability to report pain. *Clinical Nursing Research*, **13** (3), 199–215.

Kaki, A.M., El-Yaski, A.Z. & Youseif, E. (2005) Identifying neuropathic pain among patients with chronic low-back pain: use of the Leeds assessment of neuropathic symptoms and signs pain scale. *Regional Anesthesia and Pain Medicine*, **30** (5), 417–421.

Katz, J. & Melzack, R. (1999) Measurement of pain. *Surgical Clinics of North America*, **79** (2), 231–252.

Keck, J.F., Joyce, B.A. & Schade, J.G. (1996) Reliability and validity of the faces and word descriptor scales to measure procedural pain. *Journal of Paediatric Nursing*, **11** (6), 368–374.

Keller, S., Bann, C., Dodd, S., *et al.* (2004) Validity of the brief pain inventory for use in documenting the outcomes of patients with non cancer pain. *Clinical Journal of Pain*, **20** (5), 309–318.

Kovach, C.R., Weissman, D.E., Griffie, J., *et al.* (1999) Assessment and treatment of discomfort for people with late-stage dementia. *Journal of Pain and Symptom Management,* **18** (6), 412–419.

Lara-Munoz, C., De Leon, S.P., Feinstein, A.R., *et al.* (2004) Comparison of three rating scales for measuring subjective phenomena in clinical research. I. Use of experimentally controlled auditory stimuli. *Archives of Medical Research,* **35** (1), 43–48.

Larue, F., Colleau, S.M., Brasseur, L. & Cleeland, C.S. (1995) Multicentre study of cancer pain and its treatment in France. *British Medical Journal,* **310** (6986), 1034–1037.

Latham, J. (1990) *Pain Control.* Austen Cornish, London.

Lawler, K. (1997) Pain assessment (Supplement). *Professional Nurse,* **13** (1), 55–58.

Macintyre, P. & Ready, L.B. (2001) *Acute Pain Management: A Practical Guide,* 2nd edn. Harcourt Publishers, Edinburgh, London, New York, Oxford, Philadelphia, Sydney, Toronto.

Manias, E., Botti, M. & Bucknall, T. (2002) Observation of pain assessment and management – the complexities of clinical practice. *Journal of Clinical Nursing,* **11** (6), 724–733.

Manias, E., Bucknall, T. & Botti, M. (2005) Nurses' strategies for managing pain in the postoperative setting. *Pain Management Nursing,* **6** (1), 18–29.

Martinez-Lavin, M., Lopez, S., Medina, M. & Nava, A. (2003) Use of the Leeds Assessment of Neuropathic Symptoms and Signs Questionnaire in patients with fibromyalgia. *Seminars in Arthritis and Rheumatism,* **32** (6), 407–411.

Mazanec, P., Bartel, J., Buras, D., *et al.* (2002) Transdisciplinary pain management: a holistic approach. *Journal of Hospice and Palliative Nursing,* **4** (4), 228–234.

Meinhart, N.T. & McCaffery, M. (1983) *Pain: A Nursing Approach to Assessment and Evaluation.* Appleton and Lange, East Norwalk, CT.

McCaffery, M. (1968) *Nursing Practice Theories Related to Cognition, Bodily Pain and Man-Environment Interactions.* University of California at Los Angeles Students' Store, Los Angeles.

McCaffery, M. & Beebe, A. (1994) Assessment. In: *Pain Management and Nursing Care* (ed J. Latham). Mosby, London.

McCaffery, M. & Pasero, C. (1999) *Pain: Clinical Manual,* 2nd edn. Mosby, MO.

McClean, W. & Cunningham, C. (2007) *Pain in Older People and People with Dementia: A Practical Guide.* The Dementia Services Development Centre Publications, University of Sterling.

McCormack, B. (2003) A Conceptual framework for person-centred practice with older people. *International Journal of Nursing Practice,* **9** (3), 202–209.

McDonald, D.D. & Weiskopf, C.S. (2001) Adult patients' postoperative pain descriptors and responses to the Short-Form McGill Pain Questionnaire. *Clinical Nursing Research,* **10** (4), 442–445.

McKinley, S. & Botti, M. (1991) Nurses' assessment of pain in hospitalised patients. *Australian Journal of Advanced Nursing,* **9** (1), 8–14.

Melzack, R. (1987) The Short-Form McGill Pain Questionnaire. *Pain,* **30**, 191–197.

Melzack, R. (1975) The McGill Pain Questionnaire: major properties and scoring methods. *Pain,* **1** (3), 277–299.

Melzack, R. & Torgerson, W.S. (1971) On the language of pain. *Anesthesiology,* **34** (1), 50–59.

Melzack, R. & Wall, P.D. (1982) *The Challenge of Pain.* Penguin, London.

Morrison, R. & Sui, A. (2000) A comparison of pain and its treatment in advanced dementia and cognitively intact patients with hip fracture. *Journal of Pain and Symptom Management*, **19** (4), 240–248.

Mountcastle, V.B. (1980) *Medical Physiology.* CV Mosby, St Louis.

National Confidential Enquiry into Perioperative Deaths (1999) *Extremes of Age.* National Confidential Enquiry into Perioperative Deaths, London.

Nightingale, F. (1859/1992) *Notes on Nursing: What It Is and Is Not* (Commemorative edn.). Lippincott Company, Philadelphia, pp. 34–35.

Ogon, M., Krismer, M., Sollner, W., *et al.* (1996) Chronic low back pain measurement with visual analogue scales in different settings. *Pain*, **64** (3), 425–428.

Owen, H., Szekely, J., Plummer, J., Cushnie, J. & Mather, L. (1989) Variables of patient controlled analgesia 2: concurrent infusion. *Anaesthesia*, **44** (1), 11–13.

Pasero, C. (1997) Using the faces scale to assess pain. *American Journal of Nursing*, **97** (7), 19–20.

Radbruch, L., Loick, G., Kiencke, P., *et al.* (1999) Validation of the German version of the Brief Pain Inventory. *Journal of Pain and Symptom Management*, **18** (3), 180–187.

Rutledge, D. (1999) Vital signs: manage pain proactively. *American Journal of Nursing*, **99** (3), 88.

Saxena, A., Mendoza, T. & Cleeland, C.S. (1999) The assessment of cancer pain in north India: the validation of the Hindi Brief Pain Inventory – BPI-H. *Journal of Pain and Symptom Management*, **17** (1), 27–41.

Schofield, P. (1995) Using assessment tools to help patients in pain. *Professional Nurse*, **10** (11), 703–706.

Sengstaken, E.A. & King, S.A. (1993) The problems of pain and its detection among geriatric nursing home residents. *Journal of the American Geriatric Society*, **41** (5), 541–544.

Simons, W. & Malabar, R. (1995) Assessing pain in elderly patients who cannot respond verbally. *Journal of Advanced Nursing*, **22** (4), 663–669.

Sjöström, B., Dahlgren, L.O. & Halijamäe, H. (2000) Strategies used in postoperative pain assessment and their clinical accuracy. *Journal of Clinical Nursing*, **9** (1), 111–118.

Stein, W.M. (1996) Cancer pain in the elderly. In: *Pain in the Elderly: Taskforce on Pain in the Elderly* (eds B.R. Ferrell & B.A. Farrell). IASP Press, Seattle.

Stephenson, N.L. & Herman, J.A. (2000) Pain measurement: a comparison using horizontal and vertical analogue scales. *Applied Nursing Research*, **13**, 157–158.

Sternbach, R.A. (1968) *Pain: A Psychophysiological Analysis.* Academic Press, New York.

Sullivan, H.S. (1953) *The Interpersonal Theory of Psychiatry.* W.W. Norton and Company, New York.

The Concise Oxford English Dictionary (1997), 9th edn. Oxford University Press, Oxford, p. 709.

Twycross, A., Moriarty, A. & Betts, T. (1998) *Paediatric Pain Management.* Radcliffe Medical Press Ltd, Oxon.

Van Cott, M.L. (1993) Communicative competence during nursing admission interviews of elderly patients in acute care settings. *Qualitative Health Research*, **3** (2), 184–208.

Wang, X.S., Mendoza, T.R., Goa, S.Z. & Cleeland, C.S. (1996) The Chinese version of the Brief Pain Inventory (BPI-C): its development and use in a study of cancer pain. *Pain*, **67** (2–3), 407–416.

Warden, V., Hurley, A.C. & Volicer, L. (2003) Development and psychometric evaluation of the pain assessment in advanced dementia (PAINAD) scale. *Journal of the American Medical Directors Association*, **4** (1), 9–15.

Williamson, A. & Hoggart, B. (2005) Pain: a review of three commonly used pain rating scales. *Journal of Clinical Nursing*, **14** (7), 798–804.

Wong, D. & Baker, C. (1995) *Reference manual for the Wong-Baker FACES pain rating scale.* Tulsa, Wong & Baker.

Yates, P., Dewar, A. & Fentiman, B. (1995) Pain: the views of elderly people living in long-term residential care settings. *Journal of Advance Nursing*, **21** (4), 667–674.

Yucel, A., Senocak, M., Kocasoy Orhan, E., *et al.* (2004) Results of the Leeds assessment of neuropathic symptoms and signs pain scale in Turkey: a validation study. *Journal of Pain*, **5** (8), 427–432.

Zalon, M.L. (1993) Nurses' assessment of post operative patients' pain. *Pain*, **54** (3), 329–334.

Useful websites

American Geriatrics Society: *http://www.americangeriatrics.org/.*

British Pain Society: *http://www.britishpainsociety.org/.*

GOS Hospital for Children NHS Trust: *http://www.ich.ucl.ac.uk/cpap/protocols_guidelines/ gos/indexgos_files/index.htm.*

International Association for the Study of Pain: *http://www.iasp-pain.org//AM/Template. cfm?Section=Home.*

National Cancer Institute: *http://www.cancer.gov/cancertopics/pdq/supportivecare/pain/ HealthProfessional/page3.*

UCLA: *http://www.anes.ucla.edu/pain/assessment_tools.html.*

3 Barriers to Effective Pain Management

Eloise Carr

Key Messages

- Patients often have poor understanding regarding pain management, which results in low expectations of pain relief and satisfaction with inadequate pain control.
- The experience of pain has long been accepted as an inevitable part of surgical intervention, but new understanding reveals a dynamic and complex nervous system which can change in response to unrelieved pain, potentially leaving permanent damage and chronic pain.
- Health care professionals often lack appropriate knowledge, attitudes and skills to effectively manage pain due to inadequate education.
- Local hospital regulations and policies may inadvertently inhibit the effective management of pain by causing unnecessary delays to the timely administration of analgesics.
- Globally, many people are denied good pain relief due to some countries' inability to effectively import and distribute morphine for medical reasons.

Introduction

The management of pain is almost one and the same as perioperative care as it has been reported as the second most common nursing intervention (Junttilla *et al.* 2005). Pain after surgery has been reported to be a consistent problem, which has spanned several decades (Marks & Sachar 1973, Seers 1987, Svensson *et al.* 2000, Wu *et al.* 2002). Nearly half (*n* = 67) of 145 patients admitted to a post-anaesthesia care unit experienced severe pain within a 30-min postoperative period (Ekstein *et al.* 2006). The reasons for this are well documented and include patient barriers, inadequate knowledge of health care professionals, lack of assessment and organisational practices which frequently impede the administration of analgesics and non-pharmacological interventions. Despite this knowledge, the changes required in practice are not necessarily forthcoming.

45

This chapter explores how patient as well as professional and organisational barriers affect the optimal management of pain in the perioperative period and provides some practical solutions to reduce these challenges and manage pain more effectively.

Patient barriers

These can be organised into two important areas. The first relates to anxiety and its relationship to the experience of pain and the second are factors that prevent patients reporting their pain.

In a study investigating patients' knowledge of common medical terms and their surgical care, findings revealed that many held misconceptions about pain management and a significant number were unaware that the anaesthetist was medically qualified (Laffey 2000). It is important to recognise how familiar we may be with our hospital world, but for many it remains a frightening mystery.

Anxiety and pain

The period prior to surgery can be an extremely anxious time, with concerns regarding the availability of a bed on admission to hospital, the fear of dying under the anaesthesia, fear of pain and for some the possibility of cancer. High levels of anxiety are known to influence the level of pain (Martin 1996, Shi *et al.* 2003). Many patients come into hospital for surgery expecting pain and often have low expectations about pain relief (Carr & Thomas 1997, Wickstrom *et al.* 2005). Previous experiences and stories from family and friends can further elevate anxiety. These raised levels of anxiety often continue in hospital and are exacerbated by rituals such as wearing night clothes during the daytime and lying on trolleys to go to theatre (Carr *et al.* 2006). Preoperative visits offer an ideal opportunity to explore previous pain experiences, expectations about pain and concerns. Patients who have previously experienced poor pain management in hospital or who are highly anxious will benefit from proactive strategies, such as reassurance, teaching of simple relaxation techniques and being prescribed an anxiolytic agent and analgesics prior to surgery. A Cochrane systematic review on the administration of anxiolytic agents prior to day-case surgery found that they did not delay discharge (Level I: Walker *et al.* 2003). The inclusion of a rest period prior to and after surgery, which includes soothing music, has been found to be beneficial on patients' anxiety (Level II: Ikonomidou *et al.* 2004). The acceptance of anxiety in the perioperative period is not helpful and strategies which reduce this unpleasant feeling can have dramatic effects on the reduction of pain following surgery.

Anxious patients may not communicate their feelings openly and may require a recognition that anxiety whilst normal is unpleasant and there are ways of reducing it. Similarly, many patients do not report their pain despite nurses asking them to do so and a range of factors are known to prevent the patient from reporting his or her pain even when explicitly asked about. The reasons are many but can include thinking the health care professional is the authority on their pain, distracting the surgeon or anaesthetists from his or her job in treating the problem, a fear of injections, worried about being 'unpopular' and that pain is not actually harmful and can be endured. Pain associated with surgery has frequently been thought to be a relatively short event, which passes, gets better and disappears. Indeed, many patients put up with acute pain, knowing that it is an unpleasant short-term experience but one which will get better – a belief which is often endorsed by those caring for them. Yet emerging knowledge in neurobiology indicates that acute pain may have long-lasting effects on the central nervous system.

Acute pain can be harmful in two ways: by causing a sensitisation to the central nervous system often called 'wind-up' and by causing permanent changes in the way the body perceives pain in future situations.

Inflammatory pain from tissue damage, such as surgery, is conveyed through nerves called nociceptors which send volleys of impulses up the spinal cord to the brain where it is interpreted as pain. Repeated volleys of pain travelling up the spinal cord from surgical intervention can result in sensitivity – the nervous system adapts to the repeated impulses, which results in a sensitisation or 'wind-up'. In the clinical setting you have a patient whose pain is very difficult to control and the normal prescription for analgesics may be insufficient. In pain we often refer to the plasticity of the nervous system, which captures an image of a system which is not static but one which adapts and changes – not always for the better. Those patients who have been depressed or highly anxious appear to have an increased risk of wind-up occurring (Haythornthwaite *et al.* 1998).

Acute pain which is not relieved can leave an 'imprint' on the central nervous system, which can make patients' pain difficult to control in future situations. It would seem that the nervous system has been changed and cannot forget the previous pain and those volleys of impulses. Research around the use of pre-emptive analgesia has been one of the major areas of interest in recent years (Gottschalk & Smith 2001), but the evidence continues to be insufficient (Level I: Moiniche *et al.* 2002). Asking patients about their previous pain experience and recognising that the role of mood can help identify those who are at risk, coupled with increased vigilance in the perioperative period, can hopefully reduce the potential harm that pain can evoke.

Sometimes small noxious stimuli may result in amplification of the incoming nociceptive impulses also known as 'hyperalgesia'. This can lead to 'allodynia', where gently stroking of a certain area of skin can produce immense pain out of all proportion to the stimuli. You may remember a patient who has woken up in agony and quickly becomes frightened and distressed. Their pain is difficult to control and they may require large amount of opioids to gain comfort. This state of affairs has been called 'central sensitisation' and is a state of hyperactivity of the central nervous system. The beliefs of patients (and professionals) that pain, especially acute pain, is short term and will eventually go away without

Table 3.1   Surgical intervention and its association with the development of chronic or persistent pain.

Incidence of chronic pain following surgery (%)
• 30–85% amputation
• 11–57% mastectomy
• 13–38% breast augmentation
• 0–63% inguinal hernia repair
• 5–67% thoracotomy

Visser (2006).

harming them is a myth. This needs to be dispelled as pain is harmful and can leave long-term damage. We are beginning to see a nervous system which has 'plasticity' or the ability to change its response depending on the stimulus.

The development of a second type of pain following a surgical intervention may be 'neuropathic' pain and is related to nerve damage during surgery. Whilst pre-emptive analgesics have had variable success in trials, recent research suggests that the period of nerve blockade should be extended to reduce the likelihood of these changes occurring (Xie *et al.* 2006). The use of a preoperative neuropathic analgesic, such as pregabalin, is likely to be helpful for some surgical patients. There are many examples where acute, poorly controlled pain can develop into chronic or persistent pain (Visser 2006) (see Table 3.1 for the associated incidence of chronic/persistent pain following different surgical procedures).

It is important that patients are told that pain can be harmful and a simple explanation of how it can change the way the brain perceives pain. Many patients in pain lie still to avoid the pain and discomfort associated with coughing, deep breathing and moving around, which can contribute to complications postoperatively, such as deep vein thrombosis, chest infection, increased anxiety and even depression. Information for patients should include advice about *why* it is important to take analgesics to relieve pain enough for them to participate in simple mobilisation and take comfortable deep breaths. This knowledge will motivate them to report pain and not underplay their discomfort.

In summary, patients entering hospital are likely to be very anxious and this may affect their pain. Proactive measures, such as preoperative visits, which explore such anxieties and offer simple relaxation strategies can be helpful. It is important to educate patients that pain is not harmless and should be reported rather than endured. Unrelieved pain can leave permanent changes in the central nervous system, which may precipitate the development of chronic pain.

Professional barriers

The management of pain in clinical practice has been problematic for many years. For nearly 30 years there have been studies highlighting the inadequacies of acute pain management in hospitals and pointing fingers at professionals who lack the knowledge and harbour unhelpful attitudes. Particular deficits have been identified around inadequate knowledge, lack of assessment and documentation, and an unwillingness to raise the priority of pain. These then become 'professional barriers' to good pain management. Some of these are potentially exacerbated further in the perioperative period where patients may not be able to communicate easily; thus, the assessment of pain has become a major concern. Woven into the arena is the nature of the work and especially the need to communicate effectively with other health professions. In the next section, these are the two aspects focused on, in particular what can be done to reduce these barriers.

Assessing pain

Pain assessment is the cornerstone of pain management as it forms the basis for decisions about interventions and their evaluation. Yet, in clinical practice, the evidence that pain continues to be problematic continues. The development of tools suitable for patients in the perioperative period as important but the integration of these tools into clinical algorithms which both recognise the complexity of decision-making and permit flexibility in analgesic administration are essential components.

Despite the importance of pain assessment, several authors have written detailed papers considering the management of acute pain and why it continues to be problematic (Schafheutle *et al.* 2001, Sloman *et al.* 2005, Twycross 2002). As well as surgery, routine actions during the delivery of care may elicit intense pain, also known as procedural pain, for many patients. A large multicentre study supported by the American Association of Critical Care Nurses, with a sample of 6000 acutely or critically ill patients, identified six common procedures that elicited pain and distress (Puntillo *et al.* 2001). Table 3.2 illustrates that pain is very prevalent.

In addition to the likelihood that perioperative patients will experience pain, surveys of health professionals continue to find poor knowledge levels

Table 3.2 Six of the most common procedures eliciting pain and distress for acute or critically ill patients.

Turning
Wound drain removal
Tracheal suctioning
Femoral catheter removal
Placement of central venous catheter
Changing of non-burn wound dressings

Puntillo *et al.* (2001).

(Chiu *et al*. 2003, Coulling 2005) and studies concerning beliefs about pain continue to highlight misconceptions, such as neurologically impaired infants feeling less pain (Breu McGrath 2006). Knowledge, beliefs and attitudes comprise a dominant combination which can impede the delivery of good interventions. In addition to the knowledge and attitudes held by professionals is the 'culture' of a particular clinical area. If, for example, practitioners are not encouraged to give opioids intravenously or staff hold rigid or inappropriate views about pain, it is unlikely that effective pain management will occur. In addition to these factors is that assessing pain in people who are not able to communicate easily is notoriously difficult. Whilst reliance on observation and behaviour are important, the utilisation of a reliable and valid pain assessment tool is essential.

As previously discussed (Chapter 2), pain assessment tools which have been specifically designed for the patient population using them should be used. For example a pain assessment tool which has been developed for use in people who are unable to communicate a verbal response is the pain assessment and intervention notation (PAIN) tool, which has been developed and used in critical care nursing (Puntillo *et al*. 2002).

The uniqueness of this assessment tool is that it specifically seeks to address the barriers which may inhibit the effective management of pain in patients being cared for in the critical care unit. In the first section, the assessment focuses on pain behaviours which might be observed and the associated physiological pain indicators, such as movement, facial cues, posture and guarding. Based on these observations, the nurse then makes an overall assessment of how *intense* they think the patient's pain is. If able, the patient is asked to rate their current pain on a scale of 0–10. The following section is particularly important as it assesses for potential problems of administering an opioid (blood pressure, heart rate, respirations etc.) and then asks for an 'analgesic treatment decision'. This facilitates the nurse to assess and make a decision about analgesic administration. The nurse caring for a patient recovering from surgery is often in a difficult position as decisions to give further analgesics are often compromised by concerns about the haemodynamic status and sedation level. By explicitly recognising these patient factors, which the nurse takes into account, the final session of the sheet prompts the nurse to consider various treatment options. It is an excellent example of an assessment tool which recognises the complexity and challenges of pain management in clinical practice and addresses this through a practical tool which is educationally supportive.

The assessment of pain and incorporation of treatment decisions can be integrated into a clinical algorithm, which can be very useful in pain management. Such algorithms may include analgesic interventions through the use of patient group directions (PGDs).

PGDs are written instructions, signed by a doctor and a pharmacist, and authorised by the organisation in which they are to used. These include the supply and administration of named medicines (including some controlled drugs) by specified health professionals in an identified clinical situation. In

Box 3.1 Department of Health consultation document on controlled drugs (March 2007).

22 March 2007: Pain relief made easier: publication of consultations on improving patients' access to medicines

The Government is today launching two consultations that aim to make it easier for patients to get the medicines they need by allowing the prescribing of controlled drugs by nurse independent prescribers and pharmacist independent prescribers; and the supply and/or administration of morphine and diamorphine under Patient Group Directions by nurses and pharmacists for the immediate necessary treatment of sick or injured persons.

Department of Health. http:/www.dh.gov.uk/en/Policyandguidance/ Medicinespharmacyandindustry/Prescriptions/TheNon-Medical PrescribingProgramme/index.htm. Accessed 27 July 2007.

March 2007, the Department of Health published a consultation documentation which proposed several changes which would bring pain relief more quickly to patients (see Box 3.1). Widening the scope of prescribing, and in particular the ability of nurses to prescribe opioids, is welcome as it is likely to facilitate effective pain management. The contribution of such initiatives is discussed later on in this chapter when organisational aspects are considered.

Communication with other health care professionals

The development and implementation of clinical algorithms usually entail several different professionals working together. The outcome of such work integrates good practice and provides a document which permits the practitioner to assess and manage pain more effectively. One of the major barriers to good pain management is the effective communication between the different professionals. Interesting research has identified what has been happening in practice.

Margo McCaffery and Betty Ferrell are two nurses with a passion to improve pain education. They conducted a range of studies in the 1980s and revisited their original questions to ask 'how much improvement have we made?' (McCaffery & Ferrell 1997). Whilst several studies revealed that knowledge levels had improved, the actual practice or management showed less development. This was demonstrated by observational studies in the clinical setting, which gave a better understanding of what is actually happening (Dihle *et al.* 2006). Elizabeth Manias and her colleagues in Australia have conducted a series of observational studies in practice. Their observational studies found a complex environment which impeded nurses delivering good pain management, constant interruptions and nurses' reliance on assessing pain only whilst taking observations and competing demands, e.g. the doctor's requirement for the patient to be in an uncomfortable position whilst having a drain removed.

Other studies have pointed to insufficient cooperation by doctors and inadequate prescription of analgesic medications (Titler *et al.* 2003, Van Niekerk & Martin 2003). The clinical arena is complex and the relationships with colleagues are crucial as decisions concerning a patient are rarely reliant on one person's judgement and actions. The processes are frequently woven between different professionals, especially when pain begins to escalate.

These difficulties can be partly overcome by ensuring that nurses are confident to communicate with medical staff on the pain management of their patient. I recently heard of the difficulties facing recovery staff when a particular anaesthetist was reluctant to prescribe adequate pain relief for his patients, resulting in many waking from anaesthesia in pain and distress. Despite requests he would not reconsider his prescribing, a major barrier for effective pain relief. There may be many reasons for this; a survey of anaesthesia clinicians concerning their use of regional analgesia revealed that many overrated the risk of complication, and whilst 100% said they used or would allow this technique, in practice only 6% actually did (Boyd *et al.* 2006). So an audit was undertaken over a 1-month period. All anaesthetists were assigned a letter to ensure that anonymity and pain scores on 'waking' from anaesthesia and at 10-min intervals were recorded for all patients for the first hour. These were transferred to simple graphs and hung in a prominent place. Interestingly, a great deal of interest in the scores emerged and discussion began as to 'how did B manage his list so well' and 'what does P do that makes them all so sick?' It was an excellent way of illuminating difficulties and also facilitating discussion and the identification of good practices. Too often complaints of poor practice are not handled well as people may feel intimidated or lack the evidence to support their concerns. Quite often the 'evidence' is readily available and can be used to start helpful conversations about how to work together to improve care.

More junior members of the team may struggle to communicate the needs of their patients confidently. A technique which can be helpful is using role-play (see Box 3.2). It is an invaluable teaching approach which, if used well, can help practitioners feel more confident.

Interprofessional education has been espoused as a way of helping different professionals learn together and improve their collaborative skills, but early research in the field was poor, which meant little could be concluded from the studies published (Level II: Zwarenstein *et al.* 2001). More recent work has suggested a growing amount of evidence with outcomes from interprofessional education, including improved teamwork, better communication and collaboration (Level I: Barr *et al.* 2005). Short meetings, may be at the end of a clinical round, using a patient's case study can be a great way of learning together. Study days, which include a range of professionals, invariably allow new understanding of each other's role and clarification of new knowledge and understanding.

This section has considered how assessment and communication with other health care professionals contribute to the barriers evident in managing pain. In concluding this section, I am left with an uncomfortable question – why

Box 3.2 Role-play for communicating inadequate pain management.

Set the scene

You take the part of a junior anaesthetist on a busy recovery unit and ask your junior colleague or student to role-play him- or herself. They have been looking after a young man who is just waking up following extraction of wisdom teeth. His pain is not well controlled and despite having had the maximum dose of I.V. morphine prescribed (15 mg), he still has pain, is restless and calling out with a BP of 145/85 mm Hg.

What usually happens

Student: Dr . . . Mr Thomas is in a great deal of pain. Can he have something more?

Doctor: Well he's had the maximum prescription. See how he goes and let me know if it doesn't settle.

Student: Reluctantly returns to the patient . . . .

The crux of the problem is that the doctor doesn't have enough information to be able to make a decision. The nurse is also blocked – having to go back to the poor patient without any more analgesic.

How to get more analgesics prescribed

Student: Dr . . . Mr Thomas woke up 10 min ago following extraction of four wisdom teeth. He was very anxious and gave a verbal pain score of 8/10. I gave 15 mg I.V. morphine but he says his pain score is still 8/10. His respirations are 26 and regular and oxygen saturation 98%. Could you prescribe a further 15 mg I.V. I can titrate in 5-mg increments against his pain? I'd like him to be comfortable and have a score of 2–3/10 before going back to the ward.

Dr: That seems a good idea.

---

has education and the professional preparation of practitioners failed to equip health care professionals with good knowledge about pain management? I pose some responses. For one reason it is not mandatory to include any education on pain in pre-registration training and education. There have been numerous studies highlighting the inadequacies of pain content in the nursing curricula (Coulling 2005, McCaffery & Ferrell 1997), as well as other health professionals including medicine pharmacy (Lebovitz *et al.* 1997), occupational therapy (Strong *et al.* 1999) and physiotherapy (Scudds & Solomon 1995) across a variety of countries. A review of 50 nursing textbooks concluded that pain content was limited (Ferrell *et al.* 2000).

In Coulling's study she found when questioning nurses about where they gained their pain knowledge from, the majority stated that it was attained following registration (through journals, professional updates etc.). This suggests that qualified practitioners rely on their professional journals for information and knowledge about pain management. It is surprising then that a

Table 3.3 Most frequently covered clinical topics in *AORN*, July 2006–June 2007 (9 issues).

Topic	Number of articles
Patient safety	10
Infection control	8
Surgical techniques	8
Health promotion/public health	5
Medicine administration	4
Deep vein thrombosis	3
Managing complications	2
Preoperative anxiety	2
Hypothermia	2
Instruments	2
Resuscitation	1
Laboratory diagnostics	1
Continuous infusion local anaesthetics	1
Screening techniques	1
Septic shock	1
Total	52

recent scan of clinical articles in the *American Journal of Operating Room Nursing* (AORN) from July 2006 to June 2007, given an average of 6 per issue, resulted in 52 opportunities, but just 2 were published on pain management (Banks 2007, Vaughn *et al.* 2007) (see Box 3.2). The paucity of articles dedicated to pain management in the perioperative setting seems at odds with the study by Junttilla *et al.* (2005), who found that 'performing pain management' was the second most important nursing intervention in the perioperative area (see Table 3.4). Comparing Box 3.2 and Table 3.3 reveals a strong congruence with the activities performed by nurses and the articles published in a professional journal. However, the notable exception appears to be those articles related to pain management, given how many perioperative nurses perform this activity. Clearly, the activity and the theory are at odds and one of the 'barriers' appears to be a lack of publication in pain management. Perhaps, this book will stimulate an avalanche of interest and publications will increase exponentially.

Organisational barriers

The organisation within which pain management takes places often imposes a number of restrictions which may inadvertently hinder the effective management of pain. These can relate to accountability for pain management, local

Table 3.4 The 10 most common perioperative nursing interventions.

Perioperative nursing interventions	Number (%)
Maintaining body temperature	344 (10)
Performing pain management	239 (7)
Preventing risks/perioperative injury	165 (7)
Monitoring fluid volume	160 (5)
Monitoring	147 (4)
Preventing risk for impaired skin integrity	146 (4)
Supporting patient's perioperative coping	135 (4)
Administering medicines	114 (3)
Implementing aseptic technique	104 (3)
Providing information about anaesthesia/procedure	103 (3)
Total	1700 (49)

Junttilla *et al.* (2005).

culture, trust or hospital policies regarding drug administration and resources available. Beyond the hospital, national policies can influence the availability of analgesics by restricting the prescribing or influencing service provision. There are also global barriers which affect pain management, such as influencing the importation of opioids. These policies have received considerable attention in recent years as it is increasingly recognised that these restrictions reduce the quality of life for many people including those in European countries (Blengini *et al.* 2003).

Accountability

Over 30 years ago, *The Politics of Pain Management* by Fagerhaugh & Strauss (1977) was published. The text detailed a research study involving observation and interviews with staff and patients in a hospital, with a consideration of how the organisation in which pain control took place influenced the patients' experience. They concluded that the discrepancy between actual pain relief and the potential was due to work demands in the clinical area, lack of accountability surrounding the management of pain and the complexity of the patient/staff relationship. In the perioperative area, who is accountable for pain management – the anaesthetist, surgeon, acute pain team, registrar, the nurse caring for the patient or indeed the patient? It is often difficult to determine exactly who is accountable as the person may change during the course of the patient's journey. Clear lines of accountability and communication are important aspects of pain management. Personally, I take the stance that the nurse is accountable for he or she is with the patient around the clock and is potentially in the most prominent position to influence the care for that person. Whilst recognising that they may not always be in a position to prescribe (although this is changing), they can influence and often have flexibility to decide on analgesic administration and non-pharmacological strategies to ameliorate pain.

The organisation in which we work can be powerful in tempering the 'norms' of practice. This moves beyond an individual's response to a person in pain but reflects a social collective where certain groups of patients may be disadvantaged in terms of the quality of their pain management. For example it has been found that ethnic group may influence analgesic practice (Todd *et al.* 2000) and older people in surgical settings may also not always fair as well as their younger counterparts (Prose 2007). There is also limited data to support the view that women are more likely to be undertreated for their pain than are men (Hoffmann & Tarzian 2001, McNeill *et al.* 2004).

Local policies

Despite the best will (and knowledge), sometimes local policies can inhibit effective pain management. These policies are frequently part of the rules and regulations and are rarely challenged. One example of a common hospital policy is where two nurses are required to check a controlled drug. Many hospitals continue to use this policy and indeed many nurses feel that this makes the administration of these drugs safer. In reality, errors are well documented even when two people check the drug, as part of the problem lies in the range of other factors that might contribute, such as poorly written prescriptions (Anderson & Webster 2001). The requirement for two nurses to check a controlled drug is not a legal one (Royal Pharmaceutical Society of Great Britain 2005). Another routine ritual is the blanket rule that morphine cannot be carried on a drug trolley, yet the oral preparation of 10 mg/5 mL does not fall into the same legal requirements for storage as those of other opioids. This preparation can be carried on a drug trolley for immediate administration, rather than taking the prescription and saying 'we'll come back later'. This often results in a delay, which means someone enduring further pain for perhaps another 30–40 min.

Reflect on your local policies and assess whether they hinder you in delivering analgesics. It might be helpful to time how long it takes to prepare and administer the analgesics over the period of a week by keeping a note on a piece of paper. All you need to do is note the start time (identifying patient in pain) and end time (giving analgesics). This information can be helpful when requesting a review of policy.

Local resources

Resources available to us such as access to high-quality analgesics, an epidural service and the availability of patient-controlled analgesia, all form part of our local resources. It has been reported, not surprisingly, that barriers such as workload and lack of staff impede pain management (Schafheutle *et al.* 2001). The advent of acute pain teams in hospitals has done a great deal to improve local acute pain management and would be considered a prime resource. The continuing fiscal demands in the National Health Services (NHS) have revealed the vulnerability of some of these teams and their activities have sometimes been curtailed or devolved to other professionals in an attempt to save money. Inadequate resources become a barrier to the effective delivery of pain management and monitoring the quality of patients' experiences of pain through audit activity can change the perspective. Too often, staff feel disempowered or anxious that patients' negative experiences may reflect badly upon them and are inhibited to reveal the extent of a problem. Ensuring that pain assessment (and documentation) and management are integrated in local audit activity is crucial if pain management is to be improved and appropriate resources given to support it.

The US developed a strategy to help change the management of pain by documenting the assessment of pain as the 'fifth vital sign' in an attempt to change heighten awareness and change behaviour (Berdine 2002). The Joint Commission on Accreditation of Health Care Organisations (2001) published a set of standards for accreditation in American hospitals. These standards provide a framework for good-quality pain management and can highlight areas where resources may be inadequate. For example the provision of a dedicated pain management team and a formal quality programme are cited as a standard. It is helpful to use published standards such as these in measuring performance and identifying areas for improvement. The importance of linking audit to improvement activities in pain management has been explored and there are published examples how this has been done (Carr 2002, Gordon & Dahl 2004, Stomberg *et al.* 2003). Critically look at local documents and note where pain assessment and information relating to interventions are recorded. Is pain assessment and documentation a routine part of care – does it appear as the fifth vital sign? These sorts of questions start to address barriers and identify areas for quality improvement work.

Harnessing published guidelines, on the management of pain, and linking these with your own audit activity is a powerful combination. In the UK, it begins to shift the culture of acceptance to challenge and enquiry. It focuses on learning about what is actually happening in practice and you will soon see lots of opportunities for small changes which have the potential to improve care.

National perspectives – new legislation on prescribing

One of the major barriers repeatedly reported in the literature, over several decades, has been associated with nurses who care for people experiencing pain and responsible for the safe administration of their analgesics but who are unable to prescribe or review them for the patient. Experienced nurses talk of their role in educating junior doctors and their prescribing of analgesics. The modernisation of the NHS and a review of nursing roles have helped to push forward legislation to widen prescribing beyond the medical practitioner. These changes in legislation and their influences on local policy are welcome as it will help remove barriers which impede effective and timely administration of analgesics. There are three key developments worth mentioning in relation to pain, supplementary prescribing, independent nurse prescribing and PGDs.

Supplementary prescribers are nurses, pharmacists, chiropodists/podiatrists, physiotherapists and radiographers who have undergone specialist training. They are permitted to prescribe any NHS medicine, provided it is in partnership with an independent prescriber who establishes the initial diagnosis and starts the treatment. The supplementary prescriber then monitors the patient and prescribes further supplies of medication when necessary. Initially aimed at chronic disease management in primary care, there has been a call for consideration in acute settings if the benefits are to be realised (Fitzpatrick 2004).

In May 2006, qualified nurse independent prescribers (previously known as extended formulary nurse prescribers) were permitted to prescribe any licensed medicine for any medical condition within their competence, including some controlled drugs. As noted earlier in this chapter, there is a possibility that the recent consultation on prescribing will result in an opening of the gate to widen prescribing access for nurses (and dentists) to include opioids across several patient groups, including postoperative and trauma. A recent national advert for an advanced perioperative practitioner required the applicant to work as an independent prescriber and give oral and parental medicines. The pace of change is fast and a range of health care professionals are eligible to take forward these changes in prescribing. Pain management is a central activity for clinicians working in the perioperative setting and ripe for development in this context.

Global barriers and policies

The increasing globalisation of health care is pertinent to the management of pain in the perioperative period as many countries strive to deliver high-quality care within tight fiscal policies. Rapid advancements in technology promise a range of improvements, such as reduced operating times and shorter inpatient stay. Acute pain guidelines published in Australia and New Zealand (Australian and New Zealand College of Anaesthetists, Faculty of Pain Medicine 2005) have utility and resonance with health care organisations thousands of miles away. Yet many countries continue to face barriers to delivering effective pain relief – not just of inadequate technology and facilities but in the inability to relieve pain through the fundamental use of opioids. Figure 3.1 shows a selection of countries and the mg per capita use of morphine.

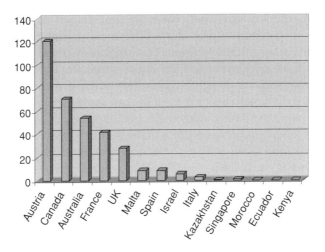

Figure 3.1 Selected countries' mg per capita from the International Narcotics Control Board (2005).

A recent paper highlighted the numerous barriers India faced when importing opioids for the management of pain (Rajagopal & Joranson 2007). These included requirements for several licences to procure one consignment of morphine, inadequate health profession knowledge and interruptions to morphine supplies. The Pain and Policy Studies Group, at the University of Wisconsin, has been instrumental in working with governments around the world to streamline regulations and policies which conspire to inhibit pain relief. Whilst much of their focus is within palliative care, there is recognition that such policies also limit the availability of opioids following surgery and many people undergo major surgical intervention without adequate postoperative pain relief. In the International Narcotics Control Boards Annual Report for 2004 (International Narcotics Control Board 2004, p. 24), they stated that the global use of narcotics for medical purposes was inadequate and identified three main reasons: unnecessarily strict rules and regulations, inappropriate attitudes by health care professionals and a lack of economic means and resources to treat pain.

It is salutary to reflect on the difficulties faced by many countries in their endeavours to provide opioids to people in pain. Many of the barriers which exist in the UK have not been provided by national regulations but are due to local interpretation and bureaucracy – thus self-imposed. It is only by critically reflecting on local policies and procedures and identifying those which impede or prevent timely administration of analgesics that this can be improved.

Conclusion

This chapter has brought together a range of patient, professional and organisational barriers which can impede the effective management of pain in the perioperative area. Anxiety is a major concern as it can have a detrimental effect on the experience of pain and is often amenable to pharmacological and non-pharmacological intervention. The experience of pain has long been accepted as an inevitable part of surgical intervention, but new understanding reveals a dynamic and complex nervous system which can change in response to unrelieved pain which can leave permanent damage. Professionals often endeavour to deliver good pain management, but inappropriate attitudes, beliefs and poor communication between those in the perioperative field can mitigate effective care. Beyond the vicinity of the perioperative arena is the organisation in which this care is carried out. Local regulations and policies can conspire to delay or impede the delivery of good-quality pain management. Practitioners may feel frustrated and powerless to do anything but accept the status quo. Improving pain management is more than good knowledge and clinical skills. It requires practitioners to continually ask critical questions, communicate openly with other professionals and recognise the wider organisational context in which care takes place.

References

Anderson, D.J. & Webster, C.S. (2001) A systems approach to the reduction of medication errors on the hospital ward. *Journal of Advanced Nursing*, **35** (1), 34–41.

Australian and New Zealand College of Anaesthetists, Faculty of Pain Medicine (2005) *Acute Pain Management: Scientific Evidence*, 2nd edn. Australian and New Zealand College of Anaesthetists, Melbourne. http://www.anzca.edu.au/publications/acutepain.htm. Accessed 30 July 2007.

Banks, A. (2007) Innovations in postoperative pain management: continuous infusion of local anesthetics. *Association of Perioperative Registered Nurses Journal (AORN)*, **85** (5), 904–914.

Barr, H., Koppel, I., Reeves, S., Hammick, M. & Freeth, D. (2005) *Effective Interprofessional Education: Argument, Assumption and Evidence.* Blackwell, Oxford.

Berdine, H.J. (2002) The fifth vital sign: cornerstone of a new pain management strategy. *Disease Management and Health Outcomes*, **10** (3), 155–165.

Blengini, C., Joranson, D.E. & Ryan, K.M. (2003) Italy reforms national policy for cancer pain relief and opioids. *European Journal of Cancer Care*, **12** (1), 28–34.

Boyd, A., Eastwood, V., Kalynych, N. & McDonough, J. (2006) Clinician perceived barriers to the use of regional anaesthesia and analgesia. *Acute Pain*, **8** (1), 23–27.

Breau, L.M., McGrath, P., Stevens, B., et al. (2006) Judgments of pain in the neonatal intensive care setting: a survey of direct care staffs' perceptions of pain in infants at risk for neurological impairment. *Clinical Journal of Pain*, **22** (2), 122–129.

Carr, E., Brockbank, K., Allen, S. & Strike, P. (2006) Prevalence and patterns of anxiety in patients undergoing gynaecological surgery. *Journal of Clinical Nursing*, **15** (3), 341–352.

Carr, E.C.J. (2002) Refusing analgesics: using continuous improvement to improve pain management on a surgical ward. *Journal of Clinical Nursing*, **11** (6), 743–752.

Carr, E.C.J. & Thomas, V.J. (1997) Anticipating and experiencing post-operative pain: the patients' perspective. *Journal of Clinical Nursing*, **6** (3), 191–201.

Chiu, L.H., Trinca, J., Lim, L.M. & Tuazon, J.A. (2003) A study to evaluate the pain knowledge of two sub-populations of final year nursing students: Australia and Philippines. *Journal of Advanced Nursing*, **41** (1), 99–108.

Coulling, S. (2005) Nurses' and doctors' knowledge of pain after surgery. *Nursing Standard*, **19** (34), 41–49.

Department of Health (2007) *Pain Relief Made Easier: Publication of Consultations on Improving Patients' Access to Medicines.* Department of Health, London.

Dihle, A., Bjolseth, G. & Helseth, S. (2006) The gap between saying and doing in postoperative pain management. *Journal of Clinical Nursing*, **15** (4), 469–479.

Ekstein, P., Szold, A., Sagie, B., Werbin, N., Klausner, J.M. & Weinbroum, A.A. (2006) Laparoscopic surgery may be associated with severe pain and high analgesia requirements in the immediate postoperative period. *Annals of Surgery*, **243** (1), 41–46.

Fagerhaugh, S.Y. & Strauss, A. (1977) *Politics of Pain Management: Staff–Patient Interaction.* Addison-Wesley Publishing Company, Menlo Park, CA.

Ferrell, B., Virani, R., Grant, M., Vallerand, A. & McCaffery, M. Analysis of pain content in nursing textbook. *Journal of Pain and Symptom Management*, **19**, 216–228.

Haythornthwaite, J.A., Menefee, L.A., Heinberg, L.J. & Clark, M.R. (1998) Pain coping strategies predict perceived control over pain. *Pain*, **77** (1), 33–39.

Hoffmann, D.E. & Tarzian, A.J. (2001) The girl who cried pain: a bias against women in the treatment of pain. *Journal of Law, Medicine and Ethics*, **29** (1) 13–27.

Ikonomidou, E., Rehnström, A. & Naesh, O. (2004) Effect of music on vital signs and postoperative pain. *American Operating Registered Nurse Journal*, **80** (2), 269–274, 277–278.

Joint Commission on Accreditation of Health Care Organisations (2001) *Pain Management Standards.* http://www.jointcommission.org. Accessed 30 July 2007.

Junttilla, K., Salantera, S. & Hupli, M. (2005) Developing terminology for documenting perioperative nursing interventions. *International Journal of Medical Informatics*, **74** (6), 461–471.

Fitzpatrick, R. (2004) It is time we shared good practice in supplementary prescribing? *Hospital Pharmacist* **11**, 442.

Gordon, D.B. & Dahl, J.L. (2004) Quality improvement challenges in pain management. *Pain*, **107** (1–2), 1–4.

Gottschalk, A. & Smith, D.S. (2001) New concepts in acute pain therapy: preemptive analgesia. *American Family Physician*, **63** (10), 1979–1984.

International Narcotics Control Board (2004) *Annual Report.* http://www.incb.org/incb/annual_report_2004.html. Accessed 6 August 2007.

International Narcotics Control Board (2005) *Annual Report.* http://www.incb.org/pdf/e/ar/2005/incb_report_2005_full.pdf. Accessed 6 August 2007.

Laffey, J.G., Coleman, M. & Boylan, J.F. (2000) Patients' knowledge of perioperative care. *Irish Journal of Medical Science*, **169** (2), 113–118.

Lebovitz, A.H., Florence, I., Bathina, R., Hunko, V., Fox, M. & Bramble, C. (1997) Pain knowledge and attitudes of health care providers: practice characteristic differences. *Clinical Journal of Pain*, **13** (3), 237–243.

Marks, R.M. & Sachar, E.J. (1973) Undertreatment of medical inpatients with narcotic analgesics. *Annals of Internal Medicine*, **78** (2), 173–181.

Martin, D. (1996) Pre-operative visits to reduce patient anxiety: a study. *Nursing Standard*, **10** (23), 33–38.

McCaffery, M. & Ferrell, B. (1997) Nurses' knowledge of pain assessment and management: how much progress have we made? *Journal of Pain and Symptom Management*, **14** (3), 175–188.

McNeill, J., Sherwood, G.D. & Starck, P.L. (2004) The hidden error of mismanaged pain: a systems approach. *Journal of Pain and Symptom Management*, **28** (1), 47–58.

Moiniche, S., Kehlet, H. & Dahl, J.B. (2002) A qualitative and quantitative systematic review of preemptive analgesia for postoperative pain relief. *Anesthesiology*, **96** (3), 725–741.

Puntillo, K.A., White, C., Morris, A., *et al.* (2001) Patients' perceptions and responses to procedural pain: results from Thunder II Project. *American Journal of Critical Care*, **10** (4), 238–251.

Prowse, M. (2007) Postoperative pain in older people: a review of the literature. *Journal of Clinical Nursing*, **16** (1), 84–97.

Puntillo, K., Stannard, D., Miaskowski, C., Kehrle, K. & Gleeson, S. (2002) Use of a pain assessment and intervention notation (P.A.I.N.) tool in critical care nursing practice: nurses' evaluations. *Heart & Lung*, **31** (4), 303–314.

Rajagopal, M.R. & Joranson, D.E. (2007) India: opioid availability: an update. *Journal of Pain Symptom and Management*, **33** (5), 615–622.

Royal Pharmaceutical Society of Great Britain (2005) *The Safe and Secure Handling of Medicines: A Team Approach*. Royal Pharmaceutical Society of Great Britain, London. Revised Duthie Report of 1988. http://www.rpsgb.org.uk/informationresources/downloadsocietypublications/. Accessed 30 July 2007.

Schafheutle, E.I., Cantrill, J.A. & Noyce, P.R. (2001) Why is pain management suboptimal on surgical wards? *Journal of Advanced Nursing*, **33** (6), 728–737.

Scudds, R. & Solomon, P. (1995) Pain and its management: a new pain curriculum for occupational therapists and physical therapists. *Physiotherapy in Canada*, **47** (2), 77–78.

Seers, K. (1987) *Pain, Anxiety and Recovery in Patients Undergoing Surgery*. PhD Thesis. University of London, London.

Shi, S.F., Munjas, B.A., Wan, T.T., Cowling, W.R., Grap, M.J. & Wang, B.B. (2003) The effects of preparatory sensory information on ICU patients. *Journal of Medical Systems*, **27** (2), 191–204.

Sloman, R., Rosen, G., Rom, M. & Shir, Y. (2005) Nurses' assessment of pain in surgical patients. *Journal of Advanced Nursing*, **52** (2), 125–132.

Stomberg, M.W., Wickström, K., Joelsson, H., Sjöström, B. & Haljamäe, H. (2003) Postoperative pain management on surgical wards – do quality assurance strategies result in long-term effects on staff member attitudes and clinical outcomes? *Pain Management in Nursing*, **4** (1), 11–22.

Strong, J., Tooth, L. & Unruh, A. (1999) Knowledge about pain among newly graduated occupational therapists: relevance for curriculum development. *Canadian Journal of Occupational Therapy*, **66** (5), 221–228.

Svensson, I., Sjöström, B. & Haljamäe, H. (2000) Assessment of pain experiences after elective surgery. *Journal of Pain and Symptom Management*, **20** (3), 193–201.

Titler, M.G., Herr, K., Schilling, M.L., *et al.* (2003) Acute pain treatment for older adults hospitalized with hip fracture: current nursing practices and perceived barriers. *Applied Nursing Research*, **16** (4), 211–227.

Todd, K.H., Deaton, C., D'Adamo, A.P. & Goe, L. (2000) Ethnicity and analgesic practice [Comment]. *Annals of Emergency Medicine*, **35** (1), 11–16.

Twycross, A. (2002) Educating nurses about pain management: the way forward. *Journal of Clinical Nursing*, **11** (6), 705–714.

Van Niekerk, L.M. & Martin, F. (2003) The impact of the nurse–physician relationship on barriers encountered by nurses during pain management. *Pain Management Nursing*, **4** (1), 3–10.

Vaughn, F., Wichowski, H. & Bosworth, G. (2007) Does preoperative anxiety level predict postoperative pain? *Association of Perioperative Registered Nurses Journal (AORN)*, **85** (3), 589–594, 597–604.

Visser, E. (2006) Chronic post-surgical pain: epidemiology and clinical implications for acute pain management. *Acute Pain*, **8** (2), 73–81.

Walker, K.J., Smith, A.F. & Pittaway, A.J. (2003) Premedication for anxiety in adult day surgery. *Cochrane Database of Systematic Reviews*, Issue 1, Art No CD002192. DOI: 10.1002/14651858.CD002192.

Wickström, K., Nordberg, G. & Gaston Johansson, F. (2005) Predictors and barriers to adequate treatment of postoperative pain after radical prostatectomy. *Acute Pain*, **7** (4), 167–176.

Wu, C., Berenholtz, S., Pronovost, P. & Fleisher, L. (2002) Systematic review and analysis of postdischarge symptoms after outpatient surgery. *Anesthesiology*, **96** (4), 994–1003.

Xie, W., Strong, J., Meij, J., Zhang, J.M. & Yu, L. (2006) Neuropathic pain: early spontaneous afferent activity is the trigger. *Pain*, **116** (3), 243–256.

Zwarenstein, M., Reeves, S., Barr, H., Hammick, M., Koppel, I. & Atkins, J. (2001) Interprofessional education: effects on professional practice and health care outcomes (Cochrane review). In: *The Cochrane Library 4*. Update Software, Oxford.

4 Psychosocial Perspectives of Acute Pain

Rachel Hagger-Holt

Key Messages

- In order to gain a good understanding of patients' experiences of pain, it is important to consider a range of psychosocial factors.
- Models and theories from psychology can provide frameworks to conceptualise pain.
- Patients' previous experiences – both of pain and generally – can affect their experiences of pain.
- Ways in which health care staff describe, respond to and understand patients' pain can affect patients' experiences of pain.
- Including a clinical or health psychologist within a pain team can assist staff in managing patients' pain.

Anita and Brian both are going to have an operation. Anita has been told in advance that this is a particularly risky operation because of the possibility of extensive tissue damage. She has been told that if she feels severe pain afterwards, then this indicates that the operation went wrong and left her with widespread physical injury.

Brian is due to have the same operation. He has been told that this operation cuts some nerve endings as a normal part of the procedure. There will be some pain as a result, so he is advised to ask for pain medication as necessary to control the expected feeling resulting from that.

How do you think Anita and Brian would experience pain in the postoperative period? What differences might there be, and how might any differences affect the intensity of their experiences? How might they influence their behaviour in seeking pain medication? Would it make a difference if they'd been given the information by a trusted friend who'd had the same operation or by the nurse registering them on admission? How might we make sense of these differences?

Introduction

Whilst clearly a medical aim in itself, there are many research findings that highlight the physical, emotional and social benefits of minimising patients' pain in the perioperative period. An increase in postoperative pain has been found to decrease a patient's quality of life in the immediate postoperative period (Level IV: Wu *et al.* 2003). Good control of postoperative pain is associated with reduced morbidity (Level I: Wu & Fleisher 2000), as well as a decreased likelihood of developing chronic pain (Level I: Perkins & Kehlet 2000) and improved rehabilitation (Level II: Gottschalk *et al.* 1998).

Pain can be subcategorised into two types: acute and chronic. Acute pain has at its source soft-tissue damage, infection and/or inflammation. It has traditionally been managed using medical interventions. Chronic pain is pain that persists longer than the temporal course of natural healing that is associated with a particular type of injury or disease process (Shipton & Tait 2005). There is a long history of including psychosocial factors within models of chronic pain and within chronic pain management (e.g. Anderson *et al.* 1977). This is likely to have occurred because of the low success rates in medical management of chronic pain.

The importance of psychosocial interventions in acute pain is slowly being realised (Symonds 1998). This is likely to be as a result of research suggesting that psychosocial variables are relevant when considering acute pain. There is a growing body of outcome research suggesting that adjusting psychosocial variables affects people's experiences of acute pain. As in chronic pain, the mind appears to play a role in processing and interpreting physical sensations, which contributes to a person's experience of acute pain. It is important to note, however, that brain-imaging studies have found that the brain network for chronic pain is at least partially distinct from that seen in acute pain perception (Apkarian *et al.* 2005). Currently, there are well-established psychosocial interventions for chronic pain. The imaging studies suggest that these should not be assumed to be relevant to acute pain, and instead the development of specific psychosocial interventions for acute pain needs to continue.

The International Association for the Study of Pain (Merskey & Bogduk 1994) defines pain as 'an unpleasant sensory and emotional experience associated with actual or potential tissue damage, or described in terms of such damage'. They note that if someone regards their experience as pain, and if they report it in the same ways as pain caused by tissue damage, it should be accepted as pain. This is the definition that will be used during this chapter, recognising that a patient's experience of acute pain does not have a simple relationship with tissue damage.

This chapter explores the ways in which medical approaches have been extended in the biopsychosocial model, which includes psychological and social perspectives of pain. These perspectives offer new understandings that can inform pain management to most effectively reduce the pain experiences in the perioperative period.

The medical model: a need for extension

The dominant approach to illness in the Western world is the medical model: an approach that treats the human body as a complex mechanism (e.g. Goffman 1961). Within this model is the assumption that problems result from part of a person's body physically failing to work as it should. Therefore, diagnosing the malfunction is key to determining a solution. The range of solutions considered spans physical interventions including surgery and medication.

From the perspective of the medical model, several questions need to be answered in order to effectively treat someone's pain. For example:

(i) Is a patient experiencing pain?
(ii) What is the physical damage that is causing that pain?
(iii) What medical treatment can best either address that damage or block its effects being felt?

This section outlines some of the research evidence that points towards limitations of these questions.

In patients with chronic pain, those who believe that pain signifies ongoing tissue damage report more suffering than those who believe that tissue damage will stay the same or improve (Level IV: Turk & Monarch 2003). This may be the experience of Anita. Similarly, those who believe that pain requires more medical intervention and that physical activity may cause more damage are unlikely to adhere to a physical exercise programme. In cancer patients, those who attribute their pain to a worsening of their disease have been found to experience more pain than patients with benign interpretations, independently of disease progression (Level IV: Spiegel & Bloom 1983).

Considering specifically the surgical environment, adolescents who expect to have high levels of postoperative pain have been found to report more pain and to use more opioid patient-controlled analgesia (PCA) medication than adolescents facing the same procedure who expect to have low levels of pain (Level IV: Logan & Rose 2005).

This evidence suggests that the assumptions of the medical model require closer examination.

The first question – is a patient experiencing pain? – assumes that there is a way to ascertain, from the outside, the nature and intensity of someone's internal experience. This is a problematic assumption, as highlighted in considering the complexities of measuring a patient's pain. Can we conclude this from observing the patient's behaviour (e.g. whether they are grimacing, crying or reporting pain)? Evidence would suggest not. When it comes to pain behaviours, marked differences have been found across cultures (Davidhizar & Giger 2004). This is unsurprising, given that culture shapes beliefs, norms and practices in a wide range of situations. Therefore, in some cultures, grimacing and reporting pain is viewed as appropriate, and in others it is not. Alongside consideration of the culture of the patient, Davidhizar & Giger (2004) found the culture of the health care provider to influence their understanding of a patient's pain behaviour. Differences in the ways in which pain is expressed by patients, and in the way that those expressions are interpreted by health care professionals, suggest that there are no reliable behavioural indicators that can measure a patient's pain experience.

The second question – what is the physical damage causing the pain? – assumes a direct link between physical injury and the experience of being in pain. However, research suggests that, if this connection exists, it has several mediating factors, including the circumstances of the pain, the person's previous experiences and personal factors. Early studies of soldiers wounded in World War II demonstrated that the pain they experienced was markedly less than that experienced by a civilian with a similar injury (Level III: Beecher 1956, 1959). Previous experiences have been shown to affect a person's experience of pain (Level IV: Skevington 1995). For example it has been found that women become more tolerant of pain after they have experienced childbirth (Level IV: Hapidou & De Catanzaro 1992). Personal factors including age and pre-existing signs of anxiety and depression have also been found to increase a patient's experience of pain (Level IV: Caumo *et al.* 2002, Level IV: Kain *et al.* 2000).

The third question – what medical treatment can best remove the pain? – addresses the techniques used to reduce the intensity of a patient's pain experience. As Symonds (1998) noted, management of acute pain has mainly involved medical management (e.g. rest or medication), without generally considering the psychological impact. However, Cassell (Level IV: 1982) reported one patient whose pain could easily be controlled with codeine when he attributed it to sciatica but required significantly greater amounts of opioid to achieve the same relief when he attributed it to metastatic cancer. This suggests that the management of pain, like the pain experience, is not directly related to the physical changes that medical treatment can influence and that psychological factors play a role here too.

In addition to the expectations and beliefs that patients hold about their pain experience, it is important to address the expectations and beliefs of health care professionals. Studies in Scandinavia have found that both nurses and physicians have a tendency to underestimate patients' pain (Sjöström 1997, Level III: Zalon 1993). This result has been replicated in studies carried out in many different countries (Calvillo & Flaskerud 1993, Level III: Seers 1987). In addition, it has been found that nurses offer pain medication to women more often than to men, and are more likely to refuse men's requests for analgesia than women's in the postoperative period (Level III: Bennett 2000). In a literature review in the US, people from minority ethnic groups were found to be undertreated for pain compared with people from the non-Hispanic white population (Level III: Green *et al.* 2003). Therefore, it is important to consider the perspective of health care professionals, as well as that of patients.

So it appears that, in order to obtain a more complete understanding of a patient's pain experience, a more complex model is required. A range of additional factors – from the persons' age to their understanding of the pain – appear to have an impact on the intensity, nature and distress of the pain experience; on the way in which the pain experience is communicated; and on the extent to which physical treatments are effective in relieving pain and the distress of pain.

Biopsychosocial model of pain

The biopsychosocial model was originally introduced by Engel in 1977, as a challenge to the biomedical model (Engel 1977). It has been seen from the evidence outlined in the previous section that there is more to the experience of pain than the medical and that consideration of these additional factors can offer something more to the understanding and treatment of pain. The biopsychosocial model proposes that biological, psychological and social factors all play a significant role.

Biological refers to viruses, bacteria, lesions, genes etc.

Psychological refers to behaviours, emotions, beliefs, coping strategies and motivation. Psychology is interested in mental processes and behaviour.

Social refers to society, family, ethnic background, culture and class. Sociology is interested in society and in human social interactions.

Thus, the biopsychosocial model includes roles for mind, body and society in understanding pain. Turk & Burwinkle (2006) provided a biopsychosocial model for pain, which is shown in Figure 4.1.

Nociception is generated by physical pathology or physical changes; however, within this model it is not experienced as pain until meaning has been

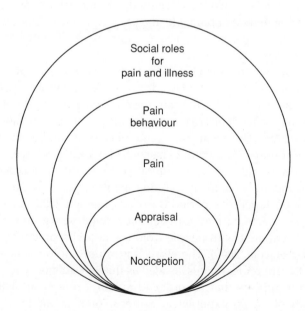

Figure 4.1   Biopsychosocial model of pain (Turk & Burwinkle 2006).

attributed to it. Thoughts and feelings that a patient experiences before, during and after an episode of pain stand between the nociceptive input and their experience of that pain.

The model also details that the meaning (appraisal) given to the sensation affects the patient's behaviour. For example how might Anita and Brian respond to being given PCA? How might they respond to the advice of a physiotherapist who, visiting shortly after the operation, advises them to get out of bed and move about as normally as possible?

Social roles for pain are wider than just those witnessed or expected on the ward, and will also depend on the person's previous experiences of both being in pain and observing others in pain.

This model suggests that psychosocial aspects of pain management are present in both the preoperative and the postoperative periods, as the beliefs and expectations that influence the pain experience and the patient's management of their pain can be formed or modified at both of these time points.

A biopsychosocial approach is starting to be recognised in guidance on pain management. There is no National Service Framework (NSF) for perioperative pain. However, the NSF for children, young people and maternity services (Department of Health 2003) specifies that treatment of pain from planned procedures, trauma or illness should include psychological therapies. In the US, the American Society of Anesthesiologists Task Force on Acute Pain Management (2004) advised that perioperative pain management should include psychological interventions.

Gate control theory of pain

The gate control theory (Melzack & Wall 1965) is another theory which tries to account for the complex research evidence of people's experiences of pain and, in particular, that cognitive and emotional factors affect people's experiences of pain. The theory is illustrated in Figure 4.2 and can be considered as the biological level of explanation for the biopsychosocial model.

The 'gate' refers to an area of the dorsal horn of the spinal cord, which is proposed to be able to facilitate or inhibit transmission of nerve impulses, i.e. to 'open' or to 'close'. Melzack & Wall suggested that signals descending from the brain are able to act on the gate. Thus, the patient's psychological state including their attention to the pain source, emotions, anxiety, coping skills etc. act on the gate and determine whether it will open to the nerve impulses coming from the area of damage or closed to those impulses. Some evidence has been found to support the existence of a gate (e.g. Hughes *et al.* 1975, Reynolds 1969).

Within this model, the pain experience is conceptualised to be a result of continuous interaction of multiple systems. There is therefore hypothesised to be considerable potential for shaping the pain experience. It is important to note that both the biological and the psychological, both medication and non-physical mediating factors, are proposed to play an important role in the management of pain.

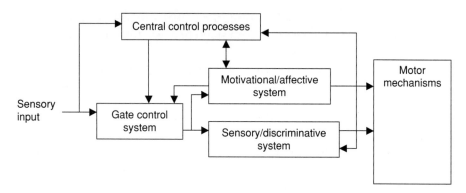

Figure 4.2 Gate control theory of pain (Melzack & Wall 1965). (© R. Melzack, 1965.)

This has been found to be the case, for example, in the following three examples of non-physical interventions. Chan *et al.* (Level II: 2006) investigated the effect of music on patients undergoing a painful procedure. Compared to a control group that did not hear music, the patients played music showed a statistically significant reduction in pain and in physiological reactions to pain (including heart rate and respiratory rate). A study by Pellino *et al.* (Level II: 2005) gave some patients a kit of non-pharmacological strategies for pain and anxiety, e.g. diverting attention from the pain. Patients who had been given the kit used less opioid on the 2 days immediately following the operation than those not given the kit. In a study with children undergoing surgery, canine visitation therapy – i.e. a dog visiting the ward – was found to significantly reduce perceived pain (Level IV: Sobo *et al.* 2006).

An advantage of this model is the relative ease with which it can be explained to patients, who based on their previous experiences may already have a good idea of what closes the gate for them. They may then be encouraged to use this knowledge to manage their pain in the perioperative period.

Psychological theories

In contrast to the medical model, which has physical matter as its subject, psychological approaches are concerned with things that cannot be seen and are instead part of individual and collective experience. The ideas and concepts that are used can be understood as theories of human experience.

A theory, according to the US Department of Health and Human Sciences (2005), is 'a systematic way of understanding events or situations. It is a set of concepts, definitions and propositions that explain or predict these events or situations by illustrating the relationships between variables. Like empty coffee cups, theories have shapes and boundaries, but nothing inside. They become useful when filled with practical topics, goals and problems' (p. 4).

Using this definition, two theories from psychology will now be introduced, which provide ways to understand some of the research findings about pain. The theories are ones generally used within psychology, which have been applied particularly to thinking about pain. Each theory focuses on different aspects of pain, explains different parts of the research findings and points towards possible interventions. Questions will be included that arise for practice.

Behavioural theory

Behavioural theory developed out of models of how animals learn. Two principles form a core of the theory, both of which can be applied to consideration of human pain.

The first principle is classical conditioning. Classical conditioning is the principle that the mind learns to link together things that are presented close together in time. Certain stimuli lead to certain responses as part of innate human wiring; for example unexpected loud noises generate a fearful response, the hearer's body is roused, their heart rate increases, and they may feel anxious, startled and hypervigilant for a while. This was used in a well-known study by Watson & Rayner (1920), who conditioned a child to become scared of a rat. Initially, the child was happy with the rat. However, he was innately anxious of loud noises. For a while, whenever the rat appeared, they played a loud 'bang'. Over time, the child showed anxiety to the rat – even when they stopped playing the noise. This can be understood as the mind making an association between the rat and an anxiety-provoking event, so that the child's anxious response came to be elicited by the rat. (The classical conditioning of Pavlov's dogs, who came to salivate in response to a bell, after hearing the bell at feeding time, is another well-known example of classical conditioning; Pavlov 1927.)

By classical conditioning, some environments may become associated with pain. This has been used historically in aversion therapy, where, for example, alcohol use is paired with an electric shock and thus conditioning that alcohol (or being in a pub) becomes paired with the anxiety that a painful electric shock produces. Such techniques are now not used, due to ethical concerns. However, patients who have previously experienced pain in a hospital environment, with health care professionals, may have a pain response to being in that environment, even without any physical pain being caused on this occasion.

The second key principle of behavioural theory is operant conditioning. This is the principle that if a behaviour results in a reward, then the behaviour is more likely to happen again. If there is no reward, then the behaviour is less likely to happen again. For example, if someone smiles cheerily and looks pleased when their neighbour says 'hello' over the fence, then the neighbour is more likely to say 'hello' the next time the situation arises. If they are ignored, the neighbour is less likely to give a greeting in the future.

One consequence of operant conditioning can be a result of the inherently aversive nature of pain, so that people stop or reduce anything that they have experienced as resulting in pain. For example, if certain movements have previously given the patient pain, then operant conditioning would suggest that the patient would be less likely to risk those movements in the future, in order to avoid further pain (Fordyce *et al.* 1982). For such a patient to 'relearn' that the movements no longer cause pain may require considerable encouragement and practice.

Turk & Monarch (2003) suggested that operant conditioning could also be used to understand possible consequences of the use of *pro re nata* (PRN) medication. They proposed that this could result in patients experiencing more pain, because they must pay attention to increased pain in order to receive medication. If the medication then reduces the pain experience, the patient is rewarded for paying careful attention to the pain. Using the terms of operant conditioning, the behaviour (recognising an increase in pain) results in a reward (being able to reduce the pain), making the behaviour more likely to happen in the future. This additional attention given to pain could lead to patients reporting higher levels of pain. Turk & Monarch suggest that an alternative, avoiding this reinforcement pattern, would be to use routine time-contingent medication, as this isn't dependent on the patient attending to their level of pain.

Questions for practice from behavioural theory include:

- Does this patient have previous experiences of being in pain in this environment? Can this be made easier for them? (For example would they have fewer reminders if their bed was in a different part of the ward?)
- How is it best to balance meeting patients' needs for pain medication and approaches that require them to be hypervigilant to their pain? (For example are there alternatives to PRN analgesia, such as by the clock analgesia doses or PCA that may be important to consider?)
- Are staff providing rewards for this patient being in pain? (For example encouraging them to take an extended time off work)
- Are staff ceasing to reward the patient when their pain fades? (For example are their needs overlooked in favour of other patients, at this time?)

Cognitive theory

Cognitive theory is based largely on the work of Aaron Beck (1976). This theory proposes that early experiences lead to the development of ways of understanding how the world works (called 'core beliefs'), from which we develop rules for life (called 'assumptions') to guide our journey through the world. The core beliefs are triggered in relevant situations and then produce a stream of automatic thoughts about the person, their situation and the future. These automatic thoughts result in emotional changes, behavioural changes and somatic changes. The processes are outlined in Figure 4.3.

For example someone may have a core belief that they are vulnerable. They may develop an assumption to guide their journey that if they never show they are suffering, then this will protect them against their vulnerability. When in pain, it may not be possible for this patient to completely hide their suffering.

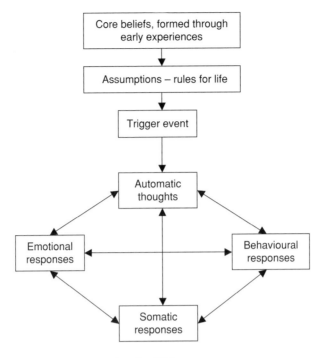

Figure 4.3 Cognitive theory (Beck 1976).

This may lead to a stream of automatic thoughts through their head that they have failed, they are not safe and they won't be able to survive this. These thoughts are likely to be accompanied by negative emotions of fear and anxiety; behaviours such as trying to keep 'a stiff upper lip', not asking for pain relief, and avoiding visitors; and somatic changes such as difficulty sleeping and eating.

Someone else may have a core belief that they are vulnerable, but they may develop an assumption that they must call on other people to protect them at all times, because they cannot manage their vulnerability themselves. When in pain, this patient may feel compelled to communicate their suffering and seek help from others, because they do not believe that they have the ability to survive their distress. These thoughts are also likely to be accompanied by negative emotions of fear and anxiety; however, this patient may constantly seek reassurance that their treatment is going to plan and ask continually for pain relief.

Turk *et al.* (1983) concluded that what distinguishes low- from high-pain-tolerant patients is their cognitive processing. It appears that ability to cope with and tolerate pain is determined by the meaning that had been given to that pain, rather than the level of pain itself. Cognitive theory would suggest that the patient's underlying beliefs, assumptions and thoughts need to be explored and, where necessary, challenged so that they can function in new, more helpful ways.

Critically, cognitive theory proposes that it is not the situation, but the person's understanding of the situation, that will determine what they think, feel and do. Thus, if people's understandings can be altered, then their thoughts and other related reactions will also be altered. A patient's pre-existing beliefs about pain, about their ability to tolerate pain and about what it means to them to be in pain are all open to investigation and adaptation.

It is important to note that patients' beliefs, assumptions and thoughts are created by their past experiences, and have been the best ways that they have found to make sense of their world. Exploring and challenging these beliefs involves inviting patients to consider for themselves how their beliefs affect them (for better and for worse) and what it might be like to take on different beliefs. It is not often helpful to tell people that they are thinking 'wrongly' and 'should' think differently.

Questions for practice from cognitive theory include:

- How might this patient be encouraged to explore their understanding of their pain? How might erroneous beliefs be helpfully challenged (e.g. a patient who believes, 'My pain means the operation has been a failure')?
- How might this patient be encouraged to explore the negative consequences of their beliefs about pain in a non-judgemental way (e.g. a patient who believes, 'My pain means that I am useless because I should be able to cope with everything')?
- How might health care professionals be encouraged to think about their own core beliefs and assumptions about pain and about patients' abilities to tolerate pain? How might this influence the ways in which staff work with patients in pain?

Recently, models combining cognitive and behavioural approaches have gained great favour within the health service. This may in part be due to the large amount of research produced that has focused on these approaches and on showing that treatments based on them are effective. It may also be because principles of these approaches can be incorporated into universal interventions such as preoperative information, as well as being used when specific patients show difficulties. Within chronic pain, cognitive–behavioural approaches are probably the most commonly accepted psychological intervention (Morley *et al.* 1999). There is growing evidence for cognitive–behavioural interventions for acute pain (e.g. Jay *et al.* 1995).

Application to a specific area

Preoperative preparation

There is a large literature on the benefits of preparing people for surgery and other medical procedures (Pitts & Phillips 1998). This preparation is informed by the biopsychosocial model outlined above, and includes information aimed

Box 4.1 Preoperative patient preparation.

Preoperative preparation can consist of:

(1) Sensation information (what sensations can be expected, such as nature and duration of pain)
(2) Behavioural instructions about which behaviours will promote recovery
(3) Cognitive coping training, which may involve an exploration of the thoughts and worries that a patients has and ways to manage them

---

at moderating patients' beliefs and expectations, a powerful cognitive factor in patients' experiences of pain.

The aspects of preparation in Box 4.1 can be considered in the light of the research and models given earlier in this chapter, and rest on the important observations that the way that a patient is prepared will impact on their experience of pain. This needs to be considered when preparing patient information booklets and when providing information verbally. For example Sjöling *et al.* (Level III: 2003) found that postoperative pain decreased more rapidly for patients who were given more specific information prior to surgery.

A study by Platow *et al.* (Level II: 2007) concluded that verbal reassurance can protect against pain – but only when it's from someone we identify with.

In a meta-analysis, Johnston & Vogele (Level I: 1993) found that all three of these preparation types had a significant impact on reducing patients' pain and their distress about their pain. Another study attempted to compare the different types of preparation and found that patients given cognitive interventions took fewer oral analgesics and received fewer injections for pain while in hospital and experienced fewer days of pain following discharge than those given sensation information (Level II: Ridgeway & Mathews 1982).

However, research has also shown that different patients react differently to preoperative preparation, some seeming to benefit in terms of pain reduction more than others. For example patients who don't want to know about the operation do better if they are not given information.

One way of understanding this is in terms of 'locus of control' – that is, who patients believe is in control of their situation. A patient who feels that they are in control is said to have an internal locus of control. A patient who believes that someone else is in control is said to have an external locus of control. A related, but distinct, concept is that of self-efficacy. Patients with a high sense of self-efficacy believe that actions they take will be effective, whereas patients with a low sense of self-efficacy believe that actions they take are unlikely to bring about goals they want to achieve. A study by Shelley & Pakenham (Level IV: 2007) found that within a group of patients with a high external locus of control, psychological preparation for surgery resulted in lower postoperative pain for the people who had high self-efficacy compared to those with low self-efficacy. However, within the group of patients with low external locus of control, psychological preparation for surgery decreased postsurgical pain for the subgroup with lower self-efficacy compared to those with high self-efficacy.

This suggests that a variety of beliefs are at play in a complex relationship between the patient, the preparation they receive for surgery and their pain. People with particular problems in managing pain might benefit from therapy from a clinical or health psychologist to explore their beliefs and assumptions related to their experience of pain.

Postoperative treatment

Research suggests that it is very difficult for a patient and health care professional to share an understanding of the pain that the patient experiences. Davidhizar & Giger (2004) suggested six strategies to assist in ensuring that assessment and management of pain is culturally appropriate. These are listed in Box 4.2.

Considering different methods of analgesia administration may assist a patient in managing their pain. For example published evidence reveals that patients consider the major benefit of PCA to be avoiding the difficulties of disclosing pain and securing pain relief within the nurse/patient relationship (Level IV: Taylor *et al.* 1996).

Alongside the consideration of medication, it has been found that acute pain can be relieved when patients focus on things other than the source of pain (Level I: Suls & Fletcher 1985). Health care professionals may find various ways to divert a patient's attention – from providing access to television, newspapers and other resources on the ward; gently encouraging visitors to discuss things other than the pain the patient feels; or ensuring the patient has other distractions such as a view of outside or the nursing station.

Exploring ideas from the gate control theory with patients may encourage them to think of what helps when they are in pain (e.g. they may report that telling themselves that the pain is only temporary helps when they have a headache, that watching TV distracts them from period pain or that talking with

Box 4.2 Strategies to ensure culturally appropriate pain assessment and management.

(1) Utilise assessment tools to assist in measuring pain
(2) Appreciate variations in affective response to pain
(3) Be sensitive to variations in communication styles
(4) Recognise that communication of pain may not be acceptable within a culture
(5) Appreciate that the meaning of pain varies between cultures
(6) Develop personal awareness of values and beliefs which may affect responses to pain.

Adapted from Davidhizar & Giger (2004).

friends made them forget the pain of a previous broken leg). This can be used to encourage patients to use their existing strategies to manage postoperative pain.

Summary

A medical approach to pain management is limited because it does not take into account mediating factors which impact on the pain experience. The biopsychosocial model extends the medical model and includes psychological and sociological aspects of the pain experience. Gate control theory offers a biological understanding of these non-physical mediating factors.

The psychological aspects of pain can be understood using psychological theories. Behavioural and cognitive theories have been found to be helpful in understanding the meaning, behaviours and distress of pain. These models can also offer new ideas about the management of pain, including preoperative preparation and postoperative management. However, not every patient will benefit from a standard, non-specific intervention, and input from a psychologist may be helpful in tailoring treatment to a specific patient.

Acknowledgements

With thanks to Robyn Vesey and Sarah Hagger-Holt for their comments on and input to this chapter.

References

American Society of Anesthesiologists Task Force on Acute Pain Management (2004) Practice guidelines for acute pain management in the perioperative setting: an updated report by the American Society of Anesthesiologists Task Force on Acute Pain Management. *Anesthesiology*, **100** (6), 1573–1581.

Anderson, T.P., Cole, T.M., Gullickson, G., *et al.* (1977) Behaviour modification of chronic pain: a treatment programme by a multidisciplinary team. *Clinical Orthopaedics and Related Research*, November–December (129), 96–100.

Apkarian, V., Bushnell, M.C., Treede, R.D. & Zubieta, J.K. (2005) Human brain mechanisms of pain perception and regulation in health and disease. *European Journal of Pain*, **9** (4), 463–484.

Beecher, H.K. (1956) Relationship of significance of wound to pain experienced. *Journal of the American Medical Association*, **161** (17), 1609–1613.

Beecher, H.K. (1959) *Measurement of Subjective Responses: Quantitative Effects of Drugs.* Oxford University Press, New York.

Beck, A.T. (1976) *Cognitive Therapy and the Emotional Disorders.* International Universities Press, New York.

Bennett, P. (2000) *Introduction to Clinical Health Psychology.* Open University Press, Buckingham.

Calvillo, E. & Flaskerud, J. (1993) Evaluation of pain response by Mexican American and Anglo-American women and their nurses. *Journal of Advanced Nursing*, **18** (3), 451–459.

Cassell, E.J. (1982) The nature of suffering and the goals of medicine. *New England Journal of Medicine*, **306** (11), 639–645.

Caumo, W., Schmidt, A.P., Schnieder, C.N., *et al.* (2002) Preoperative predictors of moderate to intense acute postoperative pain in patients undergoing abdominal surgery. *Acta Anaesthesiologica Scandinavica*, **46** (10), 1265–1271.

Chan, M.F., Wong, O.C., Chan, H.L., *et al.* (2006) Effects of music on patients undergoing C-clamp procedure after percutaneous coronary interventions. *Journal of Advanced Nursing*, **53** (6), 669–679.

Davidhizar, R. & Giger, J.N. (2004) A review of the literature on care of clients in pain who are culturally diverse. *International Nursing Review*, **51** (1), 47–55.

Department of Heath (2003) *Getting the Right Start: National Service Framework for Children, Young People and Maternity Services. Part 1: Standard for Hospital Services.* Department of Heath, London.

Engel, G.L. (1977) The need for a new medical model: a challenge for biomedicine. *Science*, **196** (4286), 129–136.

Fordyce, W.E., Shelton, J.L. & Dundore, D.E. (1982) The modification of avoidance learning and pain behaviours. *Journal of Behavioural Medicine*, **5** (4), 405–414.

Goffman, E. (1961) *Asylums: Essays on the Social Situation of Mental Patients and Other Inmates.* Doubleday, New York.

Gottschalk, A., Smith, D.S., Jobes, D.R., *et al.* (1998) Pre-emptive epidural analgesia and recovery from radical prostatectomy. *Journal of the American Medical Association*, **279** (14), 1076–1082.

Green, C.R., Anderson, K.O., Baker, T.A., *et al.* (2003) The unequal burden of pain: confronting racial and ethnic disparities in pain. *Pain Medicine*, **4** (3), 277–294.

Hapidou, E.G. & De Catanzaro, D. (1992) Responsiveness to laboratory pain in women as a function of age and childbirth pain experience. *Pain*, **48** (2), 177–181.

Hughes, J., Smith, T.W., Kosterlitz, H.W., *et al.* (1975). Identification of two related pentapeptides from the brain with potent opiate agonist activity. *Nature*, **258** (5536), 577–581.

Jay, S., Elliott, C.H., Fitzgibbons, I., *et al.* (1995) A comparative study of cognitive behaviour therapy versus general anaesthesia for painful medical procedures in children. *Pain*, **62** (1), 3–9.

Johnston, M. & Vogele, C. (1993) Benefits of psychological preparation for surgery: a meta-analysis. *Annals of Behavioural Medicine*, **15** (4), 245–256.

Kain, Z.N., Sevarino, F., Alexander, G.M., *et al.* (2000) Preoperative anxiety and postoperative pain in women undergoing hysterectomy. A repeated-measures design. *Journal of Psychosomatic Research*, **49** (6), 417–422.

Logan, D.E. & Rose, J.B. (2005) Is postoperative pain a self-fulfilling prophesy? Expectancy effects on postoperative pain and patient-controlled analgesia use among adolescent surgical patients. *Journal of Pediatric Psychology*, **30** (2), 187–196.

Melzack, R. & Wall, P.D. (1965) Pain mechanisms: a new theory. *Science*, **150** (699), 971–979.

Merskey, H. & Bogduk, N. (1994) *Classification of Chronic Pain: Descriptions of Chronic Pain Syndromes and Definitions of Pain Terms*, 2nd edn. IASP Press, Seattle.

Morley, S., Eccleston, C. & Williams, A. (1999) Systematic review and meta-analysis of randomised controlled trials of cognitive–behaviour therapy and behaviour therapy for chronic pain in adults, excluding headache. *Pain*, **80** (1–2), 1–13.

Pavlov, I. (1927) *Conditioned Reflexes*. Oxford University Press, Oxford.

Pellino, T.A., Gordon, D.B., Engelke, Z.K., *et al.* (2005) Use of nonpharmacologic interventions for pain and anxiety after total hip and total knee arthroplasty. *Orthopaedic Nursing*, **24** (3), 182–190.

Perkins, F.M. & Kehlet, H. (2000) Chronic pain as an outcome of surgery: a review of predictive factors. *Anesthesiology*, **93** (4), 1123–1133.

Pitts, M. & Phillips, K. (1998) *The Psychology of Health: An Introduction*, 2nd edn. Routledge, London.

Platow, M.J., Voudouris, N.J., Coulson, M., *et al.* (2007) In-group reassurance in a pain setting produces lower levels of physiological arousal: direct support for self-categorisation analysis of social influence. *European Journal of Social Psychology*, **37** (4), 649–660.

Reynolds, D.V. (1969) Surgery in the rat during electrical analgesia induced by focal brain stimulation. *Science*, **164** (878), 444–445.

Ridgeway, V. & Mathews, A. (1982) Psychological preparation for surgery: a comparison of methods. *British Journal of Clinical Psychology*, **21** (Part 4), 271–280.

Seers, K. (1987) *Pain, Anxiety and Recovery in Patients Undergoing Surgery*. PhD Thesis. University of London, London.

Shelley, M. & Pakenham, K. (2007) The effects of preoperative preparation on postoperative outcomes: the moderating role of control appraisals. *Health Psychology*, **26** (2), 183–191.

Shipton, E.A. & Tait, B. (2005) Flagging the pain: preventing the burden of chronic pain by identifying and treating risk factors in acute pain. *European Journal of Anaesthesiology*, **22** (6), 405–412.

Sjöling, M., Nordahl, G., Olofsson, N. & Asplund, K. (2003) The impact of preoperative information on state anxiety, postoperative pain and satisfaction with pain management. *Patient Education and Counseling*, **51** (2), 169–176.

Sjöström, B. (1997) Assessment of postoperative pain: impact of clinical experience and professional role. *Acta Anaesthesiologica Scandinavica*, **41** (3), 339–344.

Skevington, S.M. (1995) *The Psychology of Pain*. Wiley, Chichester.

Sobo, E.J., Eng, B. & Kassity-Krich, N. (2006) Canine visitation (pet) therapy. *Journal of Holistic Nursing*, **24** (1), 51–57.

Spiegel, D. & Bloom, J.R. (1983) Pain in metastatic breast cancer. *Cancer*, **15:52** (2), 341–345. Cited in Turk, D.C. & Monarch, E.S. (2003) Chronic pain. In: *Handbook of Clinical Health Psychology* (eds S. Llewelyn & P. Kennedy). Wiley, Sussex.

Suls, J. & Fletcher, B. (1985) The relative efficacy of avoidant and non-avoidant coping strategies: a meta-analysis. *Health Psychology*, **4** (3), 249–288.

Symonds, T. (1998) Pain: psychological aspects. In: *The Psychology of Health: An Introduction*, 2nd edn (eds M. Pitts & K. Phillips). Routledge, London.

Taylor, N., Hall, G.M. & Salmon, P. (1996) Is patient-controlled analgesia controlled by the patient? *Social Science and Medicine*, **43** (7), 1137–1143.

Turk, D.C. & Burwinkle, T.M. (2006) Coping with chronic pain. In: *The Handbook of Adult Clinical Psychology* (eds A. Carr & M. McNulty). Routledge, London.

Turk, D.C., Meichenbaum, D. & Genest, M. (1983) *Pain and Behavioural Medicine: A Cognitive–Behavioral Perspective*. Guilford Press, New York.

Turk, D.C. & Monarch, E.S. (2003) Chronic pain. In: *Handbook of Clinical Health Psychology* (eds S. Llewelyn & P. Kennedy). Wiley, Sussex.

US Department of Health & Human Sciences (2005) *Theory at a Glance: A Guide for Health Promotion Practice*, 2nd edn. National Cancer Institute & USA National Institutes of Health. www.cancer.gov. Accessed 25 August 2007.

Watson, J.B. & Rayner, R. (1920) Conditioned emotional reactions. *Journal of Experimental Psychology*, **3**, 1–14.

Wu, C.L. & Fleisher, L.A. (2000) Outcomes research in regional anaesthesia and analgesia. *Anesthesia and Analgesia*, **91** (5), 1232–1242.

Wu, C.L., Naqibuddin, M., Rowlingson, A.J., *et al.* (2003) The effect of pain on health-related quality of life in the immediate postoperative period. *Anaesthesia and Analgesia*, **97** (4), 1078–1085.

Zalon, M.L. (1993) Nurses' assessment of postoperative patients' pain. *Pain*, **54** (3), 329–334.

5 The Role of Personal Coping Strategies in the Management of Perioperative Pain

Dee Burrows and Elaine Taylor

Key Messages

- People develop a repertoire of personal pain-coping strategies in day-to-day life.
- Giving patients permission to use personal strategies perioperatively can enhance perceptions of control and value the person as a partner in care.
- If nurses actively support patients to use their strategies, postoperative outcomes related to pain and its management improve.
- Combining pharmacological and non-pharmacological techniques is appropriate for managing the multidimensional phenomenon of perioperative pain.

Introduction

Perioperative pain management tends to be orientated towards a 'medical management' approach in which the practitioner is in control. It is right and proper that practitioners are in control of the medical matters surrounding perioperative care because a lay patient may not have had any previous experience or understanding. However, all human beings (who survive to adulthood) have experience of pain and its management.

Human beings learn constantly. One of the areas we learn about is what to do when we are in pain. For example we learn from our parents to rub a banged knee, give and receive reassurance, take simple analgesics or maybe apply ice or heat. These strategies help us to deal with the pain and return to activity. When people come into hospital they tend to hand over control to practitioners and personal experiences get lost in the medicalised approach to care.

The goal of perioperative pain management is to ensure sufficient pain control to reduce patients' physical and emotional distress, enhance mobility and promote recovery. Although analgesics are regarded as the mainstay of post-operative pain management, several authors commented as early as 1988 on the limitations of analgesics in treating a multidimensional event, such as pain (McCaffery 1999, Melzack & Wall 1996, Sofaer 1998, Walker & Campbell 1988). They recommend that decisions about pain management should be based on Melzack & Wall's (1996) gate control theory and a multimodal approach. This would include using non-pharmacological strategies that prompt both peripheral and central action on the gate. It is possible that in doing so analgesic effect may be enhanced and holistic pain management improved.

Taught non-pharmacological strategies have been tested and used in a number of clinical settings and we look at some of these studies later in this chapter. The possibility that patients may have a range of coping strategies that they have used in their past to cope with pain has tended not to be acknowledged in acute areas. Conversely, practitioners working in chronic pain management have been used to working with individuals to promote their positive coping strategies to enhance perceptions of control and reduce pain intensity (Arnstein *et al.* 1999, Jenson *et al.* 1991).

If patients are given the opportunity to communicate their own coping strategies on admission to hospital and permission and active support are given to use them in the clinical setting, the impact on postoperative recovery may be significant.

This chapter presents the evidence for and practical guidance on the use of incorporating patient's own non-pharmacological strategies in perioperative pain management.

What do we mean by 'coping strategies'?

Oxford Pocket School Dictionary (2005) defines coping as:

> an ability to deal successfully with situations, such as stress or pain.

Coping strategies are developed in order to manage internal stressors, such as pain, and external factors, such as the environment someone is in. For example Alison, who is recovering from abdominal surgery, has to cope with her surgical pain and reliance on staff to provide painkillers. Alison may use problem- or emotion-focused coping.

Problem-focused coping involves trying to alter the situation and thereby eliminate the stress factor. Emotion-focused coping involves reinterpreting the situation so that it is not perceived as a threat. Thus, individuals need to evaluate the situation and ask themselves what they can do about it (Folkman *et al.* 1986). Coping is a dynamic process that changes over time as individuals are faced with new and different situations. Each new situation adds to their range of positive and negative coping strategies (Lazarus & Folkman 1984).

It seems reasonable to speculate that adults admitted to hospital have, through their everyday pain experiences, developed a range of pain-coping strategies. Faced with an operation, these strategies may be inadequate and be abandoned or they may be adapted and used together with analgesics to relieve postoperative pain.

An influencing factor is that of self-efficacy. Bandura (1977, 1997) defines self-efficacy as the belief that an individual has in their ability to connect to a particular action, so that a desired outcome is achieved. These beliefs are said to significantly influence the start of and continuation of specific behaviours. For example if Alison believes that relaxation will reduce muscle tension and pain and then uses this strategy, she is likely to be more successful at controlling her pain than if she did not believe in the power of relaxation to reduce pain.

Our initial survey aimed to identify the pain-relieving strategies used by 200 adult outpatients attending surgical and orthopaedic clinics for their first appointment. Consenting patients were given a questionnaire to complete and 10% also participated in an audiotaped structured interview.

The questionnaire asked:

- Are there any things you do (thoughts and actions) when you are in pain to help relieve your pain or discomfort?
- Are there any things your family and friends do for you when you are in pain to help relieve your pain or discomfort?
- What sort of things you think the nurses and doctors might do to help relieve your pain?

Interviewees were asked to provide an example of a time when they had ex-perienced physical pain and describe the strategies employed, what prompted them to choose that particular technique, the way in which the strategy helped and how successful it was in relieving pain. They were then asked to repeat the process when recalling experiences of everyday aches and pains. Finally, they were asked for their opinions about using their personal coping strategies in perioperative pain management.

The survey highlighted that most individuals acquire a range of personal coping strategies for dealing with pain. Strategies are learnt during childhood and developed through exposure to pain and the advice of family, friends and health care practitioners as the individual moves into adulthood. What is learnt during one pain episode is retested by the person in the next. Gradually, individuals identify those strategies that they think will either help relieve their pain or at least promote a sense of self-control.

The range of strategies employed is frequently wide and linked to the in-tensity of pain. In other words, it appears that the more intense the pain, the greater the number of strategies used. There was also evidence that intensity influenced the particular strategies adopted. For example relatively mild or short-lasting pain is typically ignored or managed through positive thinking and strategies such as distraction. As the intensity or duration of pain begins to increase, people use focused strategies, such as warm baths and going for a walk. The next step up tends to be mild analgesics, talking about the pain, physical contact with someone and seeking reassurance. Finally, resting alone,

Box 5.1   Self-generated pain-coping strategies (Burrows 2000).

Behavioural	35%	Positioning	4%
Analgesics	25%	Seeking treatment	2%
Resting alone	13%	Cognitive and expressive reassurance	1%
Cognitive control	10%	Other	5%
Mobilising	5%		

positioning, seeking treatment and medically prescribed analgesics are used for more serious pain. We concluded that as pain demands more of our attention, we use more personal pain-coping strategies.

In total, the 200 outpatients recorded 368 different self-generated strategies, which we collapsed into nine themes and ranked as shown in Box 5.1.

A tenth theme entitled 'general help' was identified as being used by family and friends to support the person with pain.

Many of those who participated in the survey were adamant that they wanted to use their preferred strategies in hospital, to be treated as individuals and to be fully involved in their pain management. However, they also expressed concern that they would lose control to health care practitioners. Conversely, others said that they would prefer practitioners to adopt a nurturing role. These individuals wanted to use their strategies in hospital but either expected not to be allowed to do so or stated that they would do so only if the doctors and nurses did not mind.

The historical context of personal pain-coping strategies

Historically, health care practitioners have tended to teach pain-coping strategies rather than consider that patients may have their own personal strategies that could be supported in the clinical setting. Rosenstiel & Keefe (1983) developed the Pain-Coping Strategy Questionnaire (PCSQ) to identify patients' preferred strategies. This tool was subsequently used in a number of studies and found to be reliable and valid for practice (e.g. Beckham *et al.* 1991, Keefe *et al.* 1992). It is now used by many pain services to identify which of the following patients are inclined to use: diverting attention, reinterpreting pain sensations, catastrophising (where a small disappointment becomes a disaster), ignoring pain sensations, praying and hoping, and coping self-statements and increased behavioural activities.

A study by Keefe *et al.* (1997) used the PCSQ to identify that the most frequently used strategies by a group of patients with osteoarthritis of the knee were coping self-statements, increasing behavioural activities and ignoring pain sensations. The researchers concluded that health care practitioners should focus on identifying patients' pain-coping strategies, intervening to reduce negative strategies and actively supporting positive ones.

However, Schanberg *et al.* (1997) in a study involving adolescents and young adults with juvenile arthritis concluded that practitioners should teach coping strategies rather than identify patients' own, as taught strategies would ensure positive rather than negatively focused coping. The assumption here of course is that people's own strategies may not be positive and that the health care practitioner 'knows best'. More recently, LaMontagne *et al.* (2003) also concluded that directing adolescents to learning coping strategies is more effective.

From taught to self-generated strategies in acute care

Moving from the chronic pain setting to acute care, the nursing literature appears to accept that there are benefits of teaching non-pharmacological strategies to patients undergoing surgery. The classical texts, such as those by McCaffery & Pasero (1999) and Sofaer (1998), contain chapters encouraging their use, without providing much evidence of benefit. Indeed, a meta-analysis by Sindhu in 1996 found little evidence to support the effectiveness of taught techniques, including biofeedback, relaxation, music, imagery, coping strategies and self-care education. However, she also noted that many of the earlier studies included few quality randomised controlled trials (RCTs).

More recently, a number of relatively large RCTs have found more significant effect of taught strategies. For instance, Roykulcharoen & Good's (2004) RCT with 102 adults following abdominal surgery examined the effects of a systematic method of relaxing the body on the sensory and affective components of postoperative pain, anxiety and opioid intake after initial ambulation. Substantial reductions in sensation and distress of pain were found when postoperative patients used systematic relaxation. Participants also commented that they felt more in control, perhaps highlighting the link with self-efficacy.

Good *et al.* (2005) tested three non-pharmacological nursing interventions – relaxation, chosen music and their combination – with 167 patients undergoing intestinal surgery. In her RCT, pain sensation and distress were significantly reduced by 16–40%.

In 100 patients undergoing open-heart surgery, Kehettry-Vibhu *et al.* (2006) evaluated the feasibility, safety and impact of guided imagery, massage and music. This RCT's findings showed that pain and tension scores decreased significantly during early recovery.

As well as teaching coping strategies nurses are also known to employ imagery, talking, repositioning, distraction, warm baths and ice (Burrows 1997), to provide emotional support and comforting touch (Carr & Thomas 1997) and to 'engage with the patient's pain' by providing information and sharing control (Nagy 1999).

An interesting, though old, study by Chaves & Brown (1987) with dental surgery patients discovered that 28 of 63 used a variety of personal coping strategies in addition to those being taught. They concluded that:

there are indications that administered cognitive strategies may interact in complex ways with spontaneous self-generated strategies, that are already within the patient's repertoire. (p. 276)

The importance of Chaves & Brown's (1987) work is that it provides evidence for the use of personal pain-relieving strategies in acute pain episodes. It is possible that studies on taught strategies have been compromised by a lack of awareness regarding the existence of self-generated strategies. For instance, if Alison was enrolled on a trial on taught relaxation, she might use her own relaxation strategy in addition to, or in place of, the taught technique. Indeed, Pick *et al.* (1990) found that postoperative patients recorded a variety of self-generated pain-coping strategies and that pain intensity and distress were reduced in those using positive techniques.

An early study by one of the authors provided some evidence for the possible benefits of identifying and using patients' strategies in perioperative settings. However, nurses' knowledge of, and therefore ability to support, interventions other than analgesics was found to be limited. Thus, it was not possible to fully incorporate patients' self-generated strategies into the plan of care (Burrows 1997).

Following this study, the authors were encouraged to explore the use of personal self-generated pain-coping strategies further. The first stage of the study was the survey in outpatients, already described. The second stage was an RCT involving 80 inpatients undergoing orthopaedic and general surgery.

Engaging patients in their own pain management

The aim of the study was to test the hypothesis:

> Overt identification and systematic incorporation of patients' self-generated strategies into the plan of care, reduces postoperative pain intensity and distress, analgesic consumption, anxiety and length of stay, and enhances patient satisfaction with their postoperative pain management.

We also sought to empower nurses to deliver effective pain management and promote evidence-based practice. To achieve this we wanted to actively involve nursing staff in the process. We chose to use action research as a method of achieving our aims. Our survey formed the first cycle of the study, followed by a second cycle, which considered the following:

- What are the effects on postoperative pain of patients using their own pain-relieving strategies? (The RCT.)
- How can these strategies be integrated and supported by nurses in postoperative pain management? (A strategies booklet was devised and carried by each nurse throughout the time of the study, evaluated and revised. We also kept field notes and involved staff in focus groups and in completing questionnaires.)

Table 5.1 A summary of instruments used by Burrows in their study.

Instrument	Time of completion
Preoperative patient questionnaire (included Short-Form Spielberger State-Trait Anxiety Inventory (STAI), pain intensity and distress ratings)	Following written consent, prior to randomisation
Pain strategies questionnaire (to identify the self-generated pain-coping strategies of subjects in the intervention group)	Following randomisation, prior to surgery
Self-report pain intensity scales (0 = no pain, 10 = unbearable pain)	12.00–14.00, day 1 – day of discharge
Self-report distress scales (0 = not at all distressing, 10 = extremely distressing)	12.00–14.00, day 1 – day of discharge
Analgesic and antiemetic consumption record	Daily, from day 0 post-surgery to discharge
Pain strategies questionnaire (included STAI, length of stay and perceived control scale 0 = not at all in control, 10 = completely in control)	The day prior to, or the morning of, discharge
Postoperative strategies questionnaire (to identify self-generated pain-coping strategies used by patients in both groups during their hospital stay)	The day prior to, or the morning of, discharge

As the focus of this book is on perioperative nursing, we would like to share the process and findings of the RCT.

All adult patients scheduled for booked surgery on the study ward, able and willing to give written, informed consent were approached. Following consent and the collection of baseline data, participants were randomly allocated to an intervention or control group. Table 5.1 summarises the data collection instruments used during the RCT.

The Pain Strategies Questionnaire (PSQ) shown in Figure 5.1 contains a list of strategies devised from the survey data. The questionnaire was administered to the experimental group preoperatively and to both groups prior to discharge. Respondents were asked to identify the pain-relieving techniques that they had used in the past (or postoperatively); then indicate how helpful they found each strategy in relieving pain (please note this column has been removed for the clinical version of the PSQ); and on the preoperative questionnaire only, experimental subjects were asked to identify any strategy they wished to use in hospital following surgery.

PAIN STRATEGIES QUESTIONNAIRE

Many people use strategies at home to help relieve pain. If you continue to use them in hospital it can help to reduce the amount of pain you experience. Please fill in this questionnaire and hand it to your nurse who will advise you how to adapt your strategies to the hospital setting.

- Please place a ✓ in column A against all of the strategies that you use when in pain.
- In column B, place a ✓ against any of the strategies that you would like to use in hospital.

Strategy	Column A Strategies You Use When in Pain	Column B Strategies You Would Like to Use in Hospital
Painkillers (state which if known)		
Distraction e.g. reading, watching TV		
Relaxation		
Breathing exercises		
Imagery (using your senses to imagine a place or experience)		
Music		
Massage		
Warmth		
Cold		
Resting alone e.g. peace & quiet, lying down, trying to sleep Please state which:		
Grin & bear, mind over matter, positive thinking		
Mobilising e.g. walking, moving about, exercise Please state which:		
Positioning e.g. changing position, supporting painful area Please state which:		
Treatment e.g. seeking medical attention, advice or information Please state which:		
Reassurance e.g. talking about the pain, physical contact with someone, confidence in someone else Please state which:		
General help with activities		
Other Please state what:		
None/not sure		

Thank you for completing this questionnaire

Figure 5.1 Pain Strategies Questionnaire. (©Dee Burrows (2000), reproduced with permission from Dr D. Burrows.)

Both patients and staff commented on the benefits of completing the PSQ and using it to guide pain management interventions. Patients felt valued that their strategies were considered; staff felt they gained useful in-depth information about the patients' strategies quickly. Working together, patients in the experimental group along with the nurses used the PSQ to determine which strategies the patient would use postoperatively and the support that they needed to do so. For example it was usual ward practice to walk patients to the 'balcony' postoperatively. Practice changed during the RCT so that those who wished to use television as a distraction were walked to the day room where a television is available. These and other ideas were included in the strategies booklet.

Nurses were advised how to manage patients in the control group should the issue of self-generated strategy use arise.

Findings

There was little difference in the number of personal pain-coping strategies used by the two groups postoperatively. Out of the 80 subjects, 505 self-generated strategies were used postoperatively: 265 by the experimental group participants and 240 by control group participants. Two hundred eighty-six practitioner-generated strategies were recorded (including analgesic administration). Again there was little difference between the two groups. The key difference was that the experimental group regarded their strategies as effective and used them continuously with overt support from staff, whereas control subjects quickly abandoned their strategies.

The RCT showed that identifying and supporting patient's self-generated strategies perioperatively significantly reduces pain intensity and pain distress (see Table 5.2). Furthermore, anxiety from admission to discharge was significantly reduced in the experimental group ($p = 0.006$).

Pharmacological management was also influenced as experimental subjects received fewer opioids ($p = 0.024$). They were also more likely to step down from patient-controlled analgesia (PCA)/epidural to non-steroidal anti-inflammatory drugs (NSAIDs) ($p = 0.009$), while control subjects tended to

Table 5.2 Pain intensity and pain distress, results from the RCT.

	Pain intensity		Pain distress	
	Control	Experimental	Control	Experimental
Range of pain intensity scores on 0–10 scale	0.0–8.5	0.0–7.0	0.0–9.5	0.0–5.5
Mean	3.95	2.74	3.08	1.91
Statistical significance	$p = 0.005$		$p = 0.005$	

transfer to intramuscular (IM) or oral opioids ($p = 0.009$). Experimental subjects received 68 fewer doses of IM and oral opioids than the control group ($p = 0.024$). This impacted positively on the pharmacy budget and reduced the amount of time nurses spent administering controlled drugs.

There were no statistically significant differences between length of stay and patient satisfaction.

The role of personal coping strategies

Both experimental and control subjects used pain-relieving strategies postoperatively. Although there were some differences observed in the type of strategies used, the total number employed by each group was similar. Explanations for the statistically significant differences in postoperative pain intensity and distress therefore needed to be carefully considered.

Experimental subjects had the opportunity to overtly identify their personal pain-relieving strategies on admission and enter into discussions with nursing staff regarding the necessary resources and mechanisms required to support them postoperatively. This patient-centred approach valued the actions of patients in the experimental group, enhanced understanding of the choices available and enabled them to be actively involved in decision making. By approaching the patient as an equal partner, nurses sought to empower patients to draw upon their own personal previous pain-coping experiences. As a consequence, experimental subjects came to understand that they had 'permission' to use their strategies in hospital. This simple action appeared sufficient to enable them to actively engage in their strategies postoperatively.

In the immediate postoperative period, when all subjects were using PCAs or epidurals, there were no statistical differences between the two groups. As the anaesthetic wore off, and the use of morphine reduced, experimental subjects became actively engaged in their pain management, employing self-generated strategies and seeking appropriate practitioner assistance. This is consistent with the literature, which suggests that as patients become less acutely ill, they are more able to participative in their care (Caress 1997, Elliott & Turrell 1996). One of the main differences between the two groups was that patients in the experimental group found their strategies considerably more helpful than those in the control group. This offers a further explanation for the differences observed in pain intensity and distress.

Self-efficacy theory would suggest that people who believe in the effectiveness of their actions will achieve their goals, whereas those who do not will not. Patients who were given permission and offered support were more able to utilise their strategies effectively and thereby reduce their pain. Conversely, patients in the control group were unaware of whether they could use their strategies in hospital and, if they did so, of the ensuing value for postoperative pain management. Interestingly, this suggests that patients in both groups were influenced by external powerful others – in this case the ward nurses (see

Chapter 4 for discussion on locus of control). It is likely that whatever one's usual locus of control, when faced with admission to a busy surgical ward or recovering from an operation, one's sense of personal control will be reduced. This may be able to be changed simply by giving permission to patients to use their strategies. The study by Shelley & Pakenham (2007) referred to in Chapter 4 highlights that people with a high external locus of control are more likely to take on board psychological preparation to reduce postoperative distress if they have high self-efficacy.

Subjects in the experimental group were told that they could continue to use their pain-relieving strategies in the hospital setting and were shown where and how to access any resources they required. Suggestions were also made as to how strategies could be adapted from home to hospital. For instance, hot-water bottles are not allowed on the ward; however, heat pads could be provided through the physiotherapists. Equipment on which to listen to music could be used with headphones. The ability of patients to initiate and maintain strategies in a hospital setting is thus facilitated through the provision of information and resources.

In 2004, the American Society of Anesthesiologists Task Force on Acute Pain Management highlighted the importance of including non-pharmacological approaches in postoperative pain management. This recognised the increasing number of applied studies on non-pharmacological strategies in acute care settings. For instance, in addition to those already mentioned, Prensner *et al.* (2001) have found that burns patients have a significant positive response to music therapy, while Pellino *et al.* (2005) used a kit of non-pharmacological strategies to support orthopaedic patients' pain management postoperatively.

At a more abstract level, we believe that overtly identifying and supporting individual's strategies values the patient as an expert in their pain management. In this sense, patients are regarded as possessing social power which has arisen as a result of increasing knowledge, skills and experience (Buchmann 1997) in the employment of pain-coping strategies. If patients are to be able to exercise their social power, nurses need to act as 'significant others' who hold the patient and their actions in genuine high regard.

Turk & Okifuji (2003) point out that individuals are active processors of information and that their thoughts will influence and be influenced by their emotions and environmental factors. The consequences will serve to direct social behaviour. Furthermore, these actions will have an active impact on the gate, modifying pain processing (McMahon & Koltzenburg 2005). Indeed, this point is highlighted in Chapter 4, where the author suggests that people use their tried-and-tested pain-coping strategies to close the gate. She also discusses the classical work by Beck (1976) who proposed that our core beliefs, developed through early experience, guide our later social action.

As previously mentioned, The American Society of Anesthesiologists Task Force on Acute Pain Management (2004) advocates a multidimensional approach to acute pain management, which of course also includes analgesics. In our study we showed a significant reduction in the need for opioids in the experimental group compared to the control group. Pellino *et al.* (2005) looked at opioid use with a similar group of patients undergoing orthopaedic surgery and using non-pharmacological strategies and found a reduction in opioid use on day 2. We surmised from our findings that patients in the experimental group stepped down quicker from PCA and epidurals on day 3. We concluded that using personal pain-coping strategies reduces opioid consumption postoperatively.

To engage patients in using their personal coping strategies in a busy surgical setting, you may want to ask yourself the following:

- What strategies do I use when I am in pain and what do my colleagues use?
- Do we believe that personal coping strategies make a difference to postoperative pain?
- How can we identify patients' strategies on admission?
- How can we support those strategies postoperatively?
- How can we encourage patients to feel empowered to use their strategies?

Summary

People develop a repertoire of self-generated personal pain-relieving strategies in day-to-day life, which they are able to transfer to more serious acute pain contexts. Combining pharmacological and non-pharmacological techniques appears appropriate for managing the multidimensional phenomenon of perioperative pain. If nurses encourage and support patients to use their strategies in perioperative settings, postoperative outcomes related to pain and its management should improve. Giving patients permission to use their strategies can enhance perceptions of control and will value the person as a partner in care.

References

American Society of Anesthesiologists Task Force on Acute Pain Management (2004) Practice guidelines for acute pain management in the perioperative setting: an updated report by the American Society of Anesthesiologists Task Force on Acute Pain Management. *Anesthesiology*, **100** (6), 1573–1581.

Arnstein, P., Caudill, M., Mandle, C.L., Norris, A. & Beasley, R. (1999) Self efficacy as a mediator of the relationship between pain intensity, disability and depression in chronic pain patients. *Pain*, **80**, 483–491.

Bandura, A. (1977) Self-efficacy theory: toward a unifying theory of behavioural change. *Psychological Review*, **84** (2), 191–215.

Bandura, A. (1997) *Self Efficacy: The Exercise of Control.* W.H. Freeman, New York.

Beck, A.T. (1976) *Cognitive Therapy and the Emotional Disorders.* International Universities Press, New York.

Beckham, J.C., Keefe, F.J., Caldwell, D.S. & Roodman, A.A. (1991) Pain coping strategies in rheumatoid arthritis: relationships to pain, disability, depression, and daily hassles. *Behavioural Therapy*, **22**, 113–124.

Buchmann, W.F. (1997) Adherence: a matter of self-efficacy and power. *Journal of Advanced Nursing*, **26** (1), 132–137.

Burrows, D. (1997) Action on pain. In: *Nurse Teachers as Researchers: A Reflective Approach* (ed. S. Thomson). Edward Arnold, London, pp. 86–117.

Burrows, D. (2000) *Engaging Patients in Their Own Pain Management*. Unpublished PhD Thesis, Brunel University.

Caress, A.L. (1997) Patient roles in decision-making. *Nursing Times*, **93** (31), 45–48.

Carr, E.C.J. & Thomas, V.J. (1997) Anticipating and experiencing post-operative pain: the patients' perspective. *Journal of Clinical Nursing*, **6** (3), 191–201.

Chaves, J.F. & Brown, J.M. (1987) Spontaneous cognitive strategies for the control of clinical pain and stress. *Journal of Behavioral Medicine*, **10** (3), 263–276.

Elliott, M. & Turrell, A. (1996) Understanding the conflicts of patient empowerment. *Nursing Standard*, **10** (45), 43–47.

Folkman, S., Iazarus, R.S., Dunkel-Schetter, C., DeLongis, A. & Gruen, R.J. (1986) Dynamics of a stressful encounter: cognitive appraisal, coping and encounter outcomes. *Journal of Personality and Social Psychology*, **50** (5), 992–1003.

Good, M., Anderson, G., Cranston, A.S., Cong, X. & Stanton-Hicks, M. (2005) Relaxation and music reduce pain following intestinal surgery. *Research in Nursing and Health*, **28** (3), 240–251.

Jenson, M.P., Turner, J.A., Romano, J.M. & Karoly, P. (1991) Coping with chronic pain: a critical review of the literature. *Pain*, **47**, 431–438.

Keefe, F.J., Kashikar-Zuck, S., Robinson, E., *et al.* (1997) Pain coping strategies that predict patients' and spouses' ratings of patients' self-efficacy. *Pain*, **73** (2), 191–199.

Keefe, F.J., Salley, A.N. & Lefebvre, J.C. (1992) Coping with pain: conceptual concerns and future directions. *Pain*, **51** (2), 131–134.

Kehetry-Vibhu, R., Files, C.L., Henly, S.J., *et al.* (2006) Complementary alternative medical therapies for heart surgery patients: feasibility, safety, and impact. *The Annals of Thoracic Surgery*, **81** (1), 201–205.

LaMontagne, L., Hepworth, J.T., Salisbury, M.H. & Cohen, F. (2003) Effects of coping instruction in reducing young adolescents' pain after major spinal surgery. *Orthopaedic Nursing*, **22** (6), 398–403.

Lazarus, R.S. & Folkman, S. (1984) *Stress, Appraisal and Coping*. Springer, New York.

Nagy, S. (1999) Strategies used by burns nurses to cope with the infliction of pain on patients. *Journal of Advanced Nursing*, **29** (6), 1427–1433.

McCaffery, M. (1999) *Pain: Clinical Manual*, 2nd edn. Mosby, St Louis.

McCaffery, M. & Pasero, C. (1999) *Pain: Clinical Manual*, 2nd edn. C.V. Mosby, St. Louis.

McMahon, S. & Koltzenburg, M. (2005) *Wall and Melzack's Textbook of Pain*, 5th edn. Churchill Livingstone, Edinburgh.

Melzack, R. & Wall, P.D. (1996) *The Challenge of Pain*, 3rd edn. Penguin, London.

Oxford Pocket School Dictionary (2005) Oxford University Press, Oxford.

Pellino, T.A., Gordon, D.B., Engelke, Z.K., *et al.* (2005) Use of non-pharmacologic interventions for pain and anxiety after total hip and total knee arthroplasty. *Orthopaedic Nursing/National Association of Orthopaedic Nurses*, **24** (3), 182–190.

Pick, B., Pearce, S. & Legg, C. (1990) Cognitive responses and the control of postoperative pain. *British Journal of Clinical Psychology*, **29**, 409–415.

Prensner, J.D., Yoeler, C.J., Smith, L.F., *et al.* (2001) Music therapy for assistance with pain and anxiety management in burn treatment. *Journal of Burn Care and Rehabilitation*, **22** (1), 83–88.

Rosenstiel, A.K. & Keefe, F.J. (1983) The use of coping strategies in chronic low back pain patients: relationship to patient characteristics and current adjustment. *Pain*, **17** (1), 33–44.

Roykulcharoen, V. & Good, M. (2004) Systematic relaxation to relieve postoperative pain. *Journal of Advanced Nursing*, **48** (2), 140–148.

Schanberg, L.E., Lefebvre, J.C., Keefe, F.J., *et al.* (1997) Pain coping and the experience in children with juvenile chronic arthritis. *Pain*, **73** (2), 181–189.

Shelley, M. & Pakenham, K. (2007) The effects of preoperative preparation on postoperative outcomes: the moderating role of control appraisals. *Health Psychology*, **26** (2), 183–191.

Sindhu, F. (1996) Are non-pharmacological nursing interventions for the management of pain effective? A meta-analysis. *Journal of Advanced Nursing*, **24** (6), 1152–1159.

Sofaer, B. (1998*) Pain: Principles, Practice and Patients,* 3rd edn. Stanley Thornes, Cheltenham.

Turk, D.C. & Okifuji, A. (2003) A cognitive-behavioural approach to pain management. In: *Handbook of Pain Management; a Clinical Companion to Wall and Melzack's Textbook of Pain* (eds R. Melzack & P.D. Wall). Churchill Livingstone, Edinburgh, pp. 533–541.

Walker, J. & Campbell, S. (1988) Pain assessment and the nursing process. *Senior Nurse*, **88** (5), 28–31.

Useful websites

American Pain Society: *www.ampainsoc.org*.
American Society of Anesthesiologists: *www.asahq.org/*.
Bandolier: *www.jr2.ox.ac.uk/bandolier*.
British Pain Society: *www.britishpainsociety.org*.
The British Psychological Society: *www.bps.org.uk/*.

6 How Analgesics Work

Kirsty Scott

Key Messages

- Analgesia aims to relieve pain by altering or inhibiting the body's response to pain.
- The World Health Organization analgesic ladder remains a cornerstone of acute pain management.
- Every patient's experience of pain is different as is their response to analgesia.
- Paracetamol, non-steroidal anti-inflammatory drugs and adjuvant agents can reduce pain intensity and provide an opioid-sparing effect.
- The addition of a low-dose opioid to a low-dose local anaesthetic infusion for neuraxial analgesia produces a synergistic effect.

Introduction

The aim of analgesia is to achieve relief from or to prevent an unpleasant sensation – pain. Analgesia may be provided using pharmacological or non-pharmacological means (or a combination of both), depending on the type and nature of the pain, its duration and its responses to previous treatments. This chapter concentrates on the main pharmacological interventions that can be made to achieve relief of pain and how they work.

In order to achieve pain relief, the body's response to pain must be altered or inhibited. It is essential to understand the physiology of pain (described in Chapter 1) before trying to understand how medicines provide analgesia.

There are three main possibilities for intervention because of the nature of pain:

(1) Pain is a receptor-mediated response. To bind or inhibit the receptors involved would block the process.
(2) Transmission of pain is along nerve fibres. Transmission of neurotransmitters could be blocked.
(3) Pain is a sensation with neurological involvement. Alter the perception of pain within the brain.

Table 6.1 Examples of opioid and non-opioid analgesics.

Opioids	Non-opioids
Morphine analogues, e.g. morphine, codeine	Paracetamol
Synthetic derivatives Phenylpiperidines, e.g. fentanyl Semisynthetic thebaine derivatives, e.g. buprenorphine	Non-steroidal anti-inflammatory drugs, e.g. diclofenac, ibuprofen, ketorolac
Tramadol	Cyclooxygenase-2 inhibitors (COX-2), e.g. etoricoxib, parecoxib
Oxycodone	

Analgesics are generally classified into two main groups, opioid and non-opioid analgesics. These groups then contain different classes of drugs. The modes of action within classes will be similar; however, the different classes have very different actions and may be used in combination to optimise pain relief (see Table 6.1).

In addition to the two main groups of analgesics, local anaesthetic agents can be used for pain relief, via a peripheral (Chapter 8) or central route (Chapter 9). Agents termed adjuvant analgesics may also be used. There are also medicines used for analgesia under special circumstances that are unlicensed for analgesia, but reported as being effective, e.g. clonidine. These drugs are being used 'off label' and should only be used by experienced practitioners. The basic principles of acute pain management are outlined in the introduction together with a review of the use of the World Health Organization (WHO) analgesic ladder in acute pain.

Non-opioid analgesics

Anti-inflammatory agents

The anti-inflammatory agents belonging to non-steroidal anti-inflammatory drugs (NSAIDs) and cyclooxygenase-2 (COX-2) inhibitors are closely related in their pharmacological actions.

When a painful stimulus is applied, nociceptors (pain receptors) respond by releasing sensitising chemicals such as prostaglandins and substance P amongst others to stimulate an effective response to the insult. This stimulus causes an opening of channels in the receptor membrane, which allows a process called depolarisation to occur. Depolarisation is the change in electrical charge across a membrane and in this instance the change is due to the movement of sodium (Na^+) ions through Na^+ channels in the nociceptor membrane.

By causing this electrical change and influx of Na^+ ions to the associated nerve fibres, there is a resultant rush of activity along the fibres at speeds of up to 100 m/sec. These fibres are fast A fibres and are responsible for the initial sensation of pain, which occurs rapidly in response to an insult. This pain is a sharp sensation and usually causes withdrawal from the stimulus (see Chapter 1 for further detail related to the physiology of pain).

NSAIDs mode of action

NSAIDs primarily work by inhibiting arachidonate COX that is necessary in the synthesis of prostaglandins and thromboxanes from arachidonic acid.

As a result of this inhibition, NSAIDs have three major beneficial effects: antipyretic, analgesic and anti-inflammatory, although the extent to which they exert each effect varies between each drug.

By interfering with prostaglandin synthesis and hence dampening the sensitisation of nociceptors and opening of Na^+ channels, NSAIDs cause analgesia by blocking the rapid response to a painful stimulus.

Although prostaglandins are one of a number of substances released to trigger inflammation and pain responses to an injury, they do also have a protective role within the human body. The synthesis of the protective prostaglandins is via an enzyme called cyclooxygenase-1 (COX-1), whereas the synthesis of the prostaglandins released in response pain and inflammation is via an enzyme called cyclooxygenase-2 (COX-2).

After an initial insult and rapid sharp pain associated with it, there is often tissue damage of some degree, whether it is due to accidental damage or due to surgery. The pain experienced is duller and is accompanied by heat, redness and swelling, all of which are characteristic of the term inflammation.

This inflammatory response is caused by the release of the chemical substances at the original site, which cause a leaking of the white blood cells from blood vessels in the area and results in pressure on the nerve cells and a painful sensation in the injured area. At this point in the process the chemicals released by the noxious stimulus have been transported by slow C fibres to the brain and spinal cord and there is central nervous system (CNS) involvement.

Once again the inhibition of prostaglandin synthesis by NSAIDs will dampen the pain experienced by an individual.

NSAIDs inhibit both COX-1 and COX-2 (see Figure 6.1) and it is the inhibition of COX-1 and the resulting inhibition of protective prostaglandins that contributes to the high incidence of gastrointestinal (GI) side effects and ulceration with long-term usage. NSAIDs also need to be avoided or used with the utmost caution in patients with renal impairment and cardiac failure. This is due to a tendency to cause fluid retention, which is detrimental to both of these patient groups.

Commonly used NSAIDs in acute pain relief and the surgical setting are ibuprofen, diclofenac, parecoxib and ketorolac. Aspirin is rarely used in the hospital setting for analgesia now, although it is still commonly used at home. The potency of NSAIDs varies and is illustrated by the Oxford Analgesic League Table (Chapter 7). The general rule is that the more potent, i.e. the lower the number needed to treat (NNT), the greater the risk of GI side effects from an NSAID.

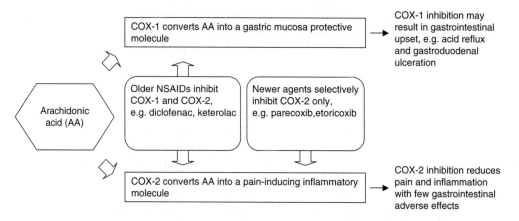

Figure 6.1   Arachidonic acid and the actions of COX-1 and COX-2.

In recent years, new, more selective anti-inflammatory agents have been developed and have created a 'second generation' of NSAIDs. These agents are usually referred to as COX-2 inhibitors due to the selectivity they possess for blocking COX-2 over COX-1 and the decrease in GI side effects. They are not, however, without side effects and cautions and are contraindicated in patients with ischaemic heart disease (Level I: Chen & Ashcroft 2007). Their role is predominantly in the postoperative setting when used for acute pain and the available forms are intravenous (IV) (e.g. parecoxib) and oral (e.g. celecoxib and etoricoxib).

Paracetamol

Paracetamol is a non-opioid analgesic. It not only has analgesic properties but also has antipyretic properties; however, its anti-inflammatory properties are very weak. It is a simple analgesic used at home as well as widely throughout hospitals. It is now available as an IV formulation as well as orally and rectally and plays a very important role in postoperative analgesia. Due to the simple nature of paracetamol it is often underutilised by patients but, taken regularly with or without combination of opioids, it is a very useful analgesic (Level I: Barden *et al.* 2004) and has been shown to reduce postoperative opioid requirement by 20–30% (Level I: Remy *et al.* 2005, Level I: Rømsing *et al.* 2002).

When given orally, it is easily absorbed with peak plasma concentrations being obtained approximately 30–60 min after administration. The half-life is usually 2–4 hr; however, this can increase if toxic doses have been taken.

If patients are unable to swallow or nil by mouth during the perioperative period, then it may also be administered rectally or intravenously. Until recently the only non-oral option was the rectal route. Absorption via this route is relatively good with peak plasma concentrations being reached after 2–3 hr, again with a half-life of 2–4 hr.

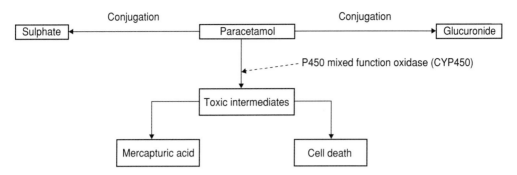

Figure 6.2 The metabolism of paracetamol.

In some cases the rectal route is not appropriate and the newer IV preparation is required. This reaches peak plasma concentrations after 15 min (at the end of the infusion) and has a half-life of 2.7 hr.

Metabolism is predominantly via the liver and uses two of the major hepatic metabolism pathways. Both involve conjugation, one of glucuronic acid and the other of sulphuric acid (see Figure 6.2). The other method of metabolism involves formation of a reactive intermediate by cytochrome P450 that then undergoes reduction followed by conjugation and is eliminated in the urine. Because the pathway using glucuronic acid conjugation is easily saturable, these toxic metabolites can easily accumulate during overdosage with paracetamol causing long-term irreversible liver damage.

The precise mechanism of paracetamol is yet to be clearly understood; however, it is thought that it works on COX in a similar manner to NSAIDs and has an effect on prostaglandins within the brain. It does not however have the GI side-effect profile of NSAIDs.

There is suggestion of the presence of a third enzyme (COX-3) and maybe paracetamol plays a role in inhibition of this pathway rather than the same as the NSAIDs or COX-2 inhibitors.

Opioid analgesics

Opioids are a large class of analgesics and can be split into two main groups – weak and strong (see Table 6.2).

In addition, there are partial opioids, e.g. tramadol, that work by more than one mechanism and partial opioid agonists, e.g. buprenorphine.

The choice of opioid depends on the type and severity of pain to be treated, the route of administration and the onset and duration of action required. Table 6.3 outlines the properties of the different routes of the more common opioids seen in practice.

Opioids work via a receptor-based mechanism of action. There are several opioid receptors. They all possess different properties and the beneficial

Table 6.2 Strong and weak opioids.

Strong opioids	Weak opioids
Morphine	Codeine
Diamorphine	Dihydrocodeine
Pethidine	Dextropropoxyphene
Fentanyl	
Alfentanil	
Oxycodone	
Hydromorphone	

pharmacological effects of the drugs depend on the receptors involved. Some opioid receptors do not have any analgesic properties and only contribute to the side effects of the drugs. The properties of the different receptors known to exist are shown in Table 6.4.

Opioid receptors (particularly mu) are mainly located in synapses in the dorsal horn of the spinal cord and this is where opioids exert their analgesic effect. There are also some receptors located in the brainstem and in other CNS locations which contribute to the side effects regularly experienced by patients, e.g. nausea and vomiting, and euphoria.

Opioid mode of action

When the initial painful stimulus is made as well as prostaglandins being released, a neurotransmitter called substance P that is specific to pain fibres is also released. It is involved in the transmission of pain along the neurons,

Table 6.3 Opioid analgesia comparison.

Opioid	Route	Onset of action	Duration of action
Morphine	Intravenous	5–7 min	2 hr
	Short-acting oral	10–20 min	2–4 hr
	Modified release oral	90 min	8–12 hr
Oxycodone	Intravenous	<5 min	6–8 hr
	Oral	10–20 min	4–12 hr
Buprenorphine	Sublingual	30 min	4 hr
	Transdermal patch	12–24 hr	96 hr
Fentanyl	Transdermal patch	12–24 hr	72 hr
	Buccal lozenge	5–10 min	2 hr (max)
Codeine	Oral	30–60 min	4–6 hr

Table 6.4 Effects produced at different opioid receptors.

Property	Mu(μ) MOP1	Kappa (κ) KOP1	Delta (δ) DOP1	Sigma (σ)
Analgesia	✓	✓	✓	✗
Respiratory depression	✓	✓	✓	✓
Euphoria	✓	✗	✗	✗
Dependence	✓	✗	✓	✗
Gut motility	✓	✗	✗	✗
Sedation	✗	✓	✗	✗
Dysphoria	✗	✗	✗	✓
Hallucinations	✗	✗	✗	✓
Delusions	✗	✗	✗	✓

sending impulses to different senses within the body. It affects pain perception, emotional response to the pain and localises where the pain can be felt.

If the opioid receptors at the synapses are occupied by another substance, e.g. a drug molecule, then it is impossible for substance P to be transmitted and the pain impulse is halted.

Figure 6.3 shows opioid receptors being bound by naturally occurring opioids within the body (endorphins) that will block a pain impulse. When opioid analgesics bind to the opioid receptors, they form a complex similar to a lock and key and block the receptor sites in a similar manner and augment the naturally occurring analgesia. This halts pain transmission since substance P can no longer send impulses across the synaptic junction and along the pain fibres.

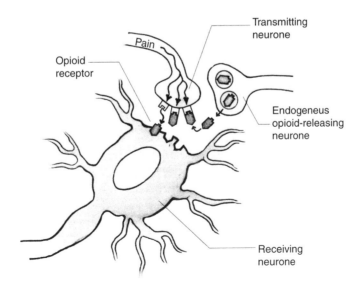

Figure 6.3 Mechanism of pain transmission and interference.

The different properties of the opioid analgesics are due to the varying affinities for the different opioid receptors. The greater the affinity for the receptor, the longer the duration of action, irrespective of plasma half-life.

Morphine

Morphine is a pure opioid agonist. It has a high affinity for μ receptors with weak agonist properties on δ and κ receptors. It is generally the gold-standard opioid by which all others are judged and there is no ceiling effect on its dosage. Unfortunately as with any opioid, dependence and tolerance due to receptor downregulation (decrease in opioid receptors) can occur and this will affect its efficacy and the dosage required to maintain a long-term analgesic effect. Morphine is metabolised in the liver to morphine-3-glucuronide (M3G), morphine-6-glucuronide (M6G), normorphine and codeine all of which are renally excreted. M6G is an active metabolite that is a more potent analgesic than morphine. It crosses the blood–brain barrier and thus can cause CNS side effects even after discontinuation. In patients with renal dysfunction, metabolites may accumulate, causing increased therapeutic and adverse events. Dose reduction and opioid choice in renal impairment are described in Chapter 12.

Fentanyl

Fentanyl is another pure agonist and is more potent than morphine. It has a more rapid onset of action; however, it has a short duration of action and generally needs to be given by infusion. Fentanyl does not appear to have any active metabolites and is therefore suitable for patients with renal dysfunction, although dose reduction should be considered. For breakthrough or procedural pain, fentanyl may be administered as a transmucosal lozenge. For chronic pain it can also be administered transdermally as a matrix or reservoir patch. These routes are described in Chapter 11.

Oxycodone

Oxycodone is a relatively new opioid which has an important role in analgesia in patients unable to tolerate morphine. The oral bioavailability of oxycodone is two to three times greater than that for morphine. Oxycodone has two metabolic pathways – N-demethylation (accounting for 45%) and O-demethylation (accounting for 10%) of a dose. Oxycodone is metabolised principally to noroxycodone and oxymorphone in the first pathway. Oxymorphone has some analgesic activity but is present in the plasma in low concentrations and is not considered to contribute to oxycodone's pharmacological effect. The second pathway uses CYP450 2D6 enzymes that may be genetically influenced, as some patients have multiple copies of the gene (with rapid metabolism) and some none at all (slow or absent metabolism). The active drug and its metabolites are excreted in both urine and faeces. The plasma concentrations of oxycodone are only minimally affected by age, being 15% greater in elderly as compared to young subjects.

Buprenorphine

Buprenorphine is a partial agonist with a very high affinity for opioid receptors and hence a long duration of action. It has a ceiling analgesic effect and if given in greater than optimum doses, it may actually reduce the analgesic effect and increase side effects.

If it has been administered to a patient who wishes to change to a pure agonist, e.g. morphine, it can pose a problem because it can take a large dose of morphine to successfully compete with the buprenorphine already bound to the receptors and despite high doses of opioids the patient may not be receiving adequate analgesia.

Antagonists, e.g. naloxone, have no analgesic properties; however, they will compete with agonists for receptors and have a useful role in reversing opioid effects in overdose. Buprenorphine is only partially reversed by naloxone since it is only a partial agonist.

Codeine

Codeine is a week opioid and is also metabolised via the CYPD26 pathway to codeine-6-glucuronide (C6G) predominantly, morphine (10%), normorphine (2%) as well as M6G, M3G and small amounts of other metabolites. Renal clearance of the metabolites is decreased in patients with renal dysfunction.

Along with other weak opioids it is less potent and often the side effects compared with the degree of analgesia obtained will prevent the dose from reaching the maximum.

Tramadol

Tramadol is termed as a partial opioid. This is because although it binds to opioid receptors in the same way as other opioids and produces an analgesic effect, it also augments spinal pathways as a non-opioid, resulting in enhanced serotinergic and adrenergic mechanisms. This is of benefit in patients who have not responded to non-opioids but do not require a strong opioid. It has a relatively rapid onset of action but does still have the typical opioid side effects.

Local anaesthetics

When a painful stimulus is received, as mentioned earlier, an action potential across the nociceptor membrane is created by naturally occurring sensitising agents causing the opening of sodium channels and a movement of Na^+ ions in turn causing depolarisation and rapid pain impulse. Local anaesthetic agents act on the sodium channels, inhibiting them all along nerve fibres. Since depolarisation cannot occur, the nerve impulse is blocked and hence the pain impulse is blocked. It is not a receptor-based action like the other agents previously discussed.

There are varying routes of administration of local anaesthetics. The route used will affect the distribution to some extent to all body tissues, with high concentrations found in highly perfused organs, e.g. liver, lungs, heart and brain.

The rate of systemic absorption will depend on the dose, concentration, route of administration and the vascularity of the administration site. Systemic absorption produces effects on both the cardiovascular and central nervous systems. At normal therapeutic doses, cardiac changes and peripheral vascular resistance are minimal but at toxic doses cardiac conduction and excitability may be decreased. This sometimes results in atrioventricular block, ventricular arrhythmias and cardiac arrest. In addition, cardiac output can be decreased as a result of weakened myocardial contractility and peripheral vasodilatation leading to hypotension.

Lidocaine

Lidocaine (lignocaine) causes stabilisation of the neuronal membrane by inhibiting the movement of Na^+ ions required for the initiation and conduction of impulses and as a result gives rise to a local effect. The onset of action is rapid as is its metabolism by the liver. Metabolites and unchanged drug are excreted by the kidneys. The pharmacological actions of the metabolites are weaker but similar to those of the parent drug.

In patients with liver dysfunction, the half-life of lidocaine may be prolonged more than twofold. Therefore, it must be used with extreme care, if at all, in any patient with a condition that affects liver function. This is because of the rapid rate at which it is metabolised under normal circumstances. Renal dysfunction does not affect lidocaine kinetics, but it may increase the accumulation of renally excreted metabolites.

Bupivacaine hydrochloride

Bupivacaine hydrochloride is a racemic mixture of an amide-type local anaesthetic. The onset of action is relatively fast. After an injection for caudal, epidural or peripheral nerve block, peak blood levels of bupivacaine can be reached within 30 min of administration. Analgesia is also long-lasting, since although it may remain effective for as little as 3 hr, analgesia can last for as long as 6 hr. The duration of block is longer with bupivacaine hydrochloride than with any of the other common local anaesthetics, and in some patients analgesia may persist after the return of sensation, which reduces the requirement for strong opioid analgesia.

As with lidocaine, bupivacaine hydrochloride undergoes extensive metabolism by the liver and patients with hepatic disease, especially those with severe hepatic disease, will be more likely to experience toxicity with bupivacaine hydrochloride. Only 6% of bupivacaine is excreted unchanged in the urine.

In addition to various pharmacokinetic parameters of bupivacaine being significantly altered by hepatic or renal disease, the route of drug administration, age of the patient and the addition of adrenaline (epinephrine) can also affect the pharmacokinetics. A dilute concentration of adrenaline (epinephrine) usually reduces the rate of absorption and peak plasma concentration of bupivacaine due to local vasoconstriction. This delay permits the use of moderately larger total doses and sometimes prolongs the duration of action by as much as 50%.

The most feared side effect is as a result of inadvertent intravascular local anaesthetic toxicity inducing a prolonged cardiac arrest. The National Patient Safety Agency (2007) has issued an alert to minimise the risk.

Bupivacaine is available in ampoules for infiltration and peripheral nerve blockade and commercially prepared ready-to-administer epidural infusions with or without fentanyl.

Levobupivacaine

Levobupivacaine is the S-enantiomer only of bupivacaine rather than a racemic mixture. It is a long-acting local anaesthetic and analgesic. Like bupivacaine it blocks nerve conduction in sensory and motor nerves by interacting with voltage-sensitive sodium channels on the cell membrane. Potassium and calcium channels are also blocked.

It has an improved side-effect profile and a longer duration of action compared with bupivacaine.

It is equipotent to bupivacaine. There are no relevant data in patients with hepatic or renal impairment. Levobupivacaine is extensively metabolised and unchanged levobupivacaine is not excreted in urine. Studies indicate that the metabolism of levobupivacaine and bupivacaine are similar in that they both are CYP3A4 and CYP1A2 pathways. Levobupivacaine is available in ready-to-use licensed commercially prepared infusions and in an unlicensed ('special') but stable preparation in combination with fentanyl.

Ropivacaine

Ropivacaine is a long-acting amide-type local anaesthetic with both anaesthetic and analgesic effects. Both onset and duration of action depend on the dose and site of administration. In contrast to bupivacaine, the addition of adrenaline (epinephrine) does not improve the effect or duration of action. Higher doses provide surgical anaesthesia, whilst lower doses produce a sensory block.

The mechanism of action is via a reversible reduction of the membrane permeability of the nerve fibres to sodium ions. As a result, the rate of depolarisation decreases and the excitable threshold increases, resulting in a local blockade of nerve impulses.

Ropivacaine is available as the pure S-(−)-enantiomer and is highly lipid soluble, enabling effective distribution throughout the tissue. Like lidocaine, the metabolites have a local anaesthetic effect but of considerably lower potency and shorter duration than that of ropivacaine.

One advantage of ropivacaine is the potentially reduced risk of cardiotoxicity, although this is a reduced risk rather than complete avoidance. Like bupivacaine, inadvertent intravascular injection has resulted in cardiac arrest, which required prolonged resuscitation. The treatment of cardiotoxicity is outlined in Chapter 8. Like the other agents it also has to be used with extreme care in liver impairment due to its metabolism by the liver.

Ropivacaine is available in ampoules and in a prediluted presentation for epidural infusion.

Combining a local anaesthetic with an opioid

Local anaesthetics are often used in combination with opioids when given epidurally because they each have a different pharmacological effect and they act in a synergistic manner. This synergistic effect enables effective analgesia at lower doses of each agent and thus fewer side effects. The use of local anaesthetic and opioid mixtures for central blockade is described in Chapter 9.

Other agents

NMDA receptor antagonists

NMDA (*N*-methyl-D-aspartate) receptor antagonists, e.g. ketamine, act as an antagonist at the NMDA receptor. NMDA receptors are located both peripherally and in the spinal cord and are known to produce an opioid-sparing effect. They may also be useful in severe pain that is not opioid responsive. The action of NMDA receptor antagonists and the evidence for their use is outlined in Chapter 7.

α_2-Adrenergic agonists

Medicines that act as α_2-adrenergic agonists inhibit pain transmission. This class of medicines includes clonidine and dexmedetomidine. Clonidine is more widely used as it provides an opioid-sparing effect when administered intravenously and can reduce the intensity of withdrawal in opioid-dependent patients. The addition of clonidine to solutions for peripheral and central can increase the duration of action of the solution. The evidence for the use of clonidine in acute pain is described in Chapter 7 alongside its mode of action and side-effect profile.

Summary

The choice of analgesic and route of administration is dependent on the patient and the type of pain that they are experiencing. This chapter has focused primarily on the agents used for acute pain in the perioperative period. However, it must be remembered that a patient admitted for surgery is quite likely to have other underlying medical complaints (maybe the reason for surgery) that may result in them experiencing chronic pain.

The WHO analgesic ladder remains a building block for perioperative pain management, although it was introduced to standardise and improve cancer pain management. The use of regular paracetamol-based analgesia is fundamental to effective acute pain management. NSAIDs and paracetamol exert an opioid-sparing effect and when used in combination with a mild opioid can relieve mild-to-moderate pain. If pain persists or increases, patients should receive an appropriate dose of a strong opioid by an appropriate route. If patients are able to swallow and tolerate oral medicines, they should receive analgesia via that route.

The use of low-dose combinations of opioids and local anaesthetics for neuraxial analgesia produces a synergistic effect that reduces the overall required dose of each and the incidence of side effects. Other agents are available that can provide an opioid-sparing effect and improve pain intensity.

References

Barden, J., Edwards, J., Moore, A. & McQuay, H. (2004) Single dose oral paracetamol (acetaminophen) for postoperative pain. *Cochrane Database of Systematic Reviews*, Issue 1, Art No CD004602.

Chen, L.C. & Ashcroft, D.M. (2007) Risk of myocardial infarction associated with selective COX-2 inhibitors: meta-analysis of randomised controlled trials. *Pharmacoepidemiology and Drug Safety*, **16** (7), 762–772.

National Patient Safety Agency (2007) *PSA 21 Safer Practice with Epidural Injections and Infusions*. http://www.npsa.nhs.uk/patientsafety/alerts-and-directives/alerts/epidural-injections-and-infusions/. Accessed 19 December 2007.

Remy, C., Marret, M. & Bonnet, F. (2005) Effects of acetaminophen on morphine side-effects and consumption after major surgery: meta-analysis of randomized controlled trials. *British Journal of Anaesthesia*, **94** (4), 505–513.

Rømsing, J., Møiniche, S. & Dahl, J.B. (2002) Rectal and parenteral paracetamol, and paracetamol in combination with NSAIDs, for postoperative analgesia. *British Journal of Anaesthesia*, **88** (2), 215–226.

Useful websites

American Society of Regional Analgesia and Pain Medicine: *www.asra.com.*

Bandolier – 'Evidence-based thinking about health care': *www.jr2.ox.ac.uk/bandolier/.*

International Association for the Study of Pain: *www.iasp-pain.org.*

National Patient Safety Agency: *http://www.npsa.nhs.uk/patientsafety/alerts-and-directives/alerts/epidural-injections-and-infusions/.*

Special Product Characteristics for medicines: *www.medicines.org.uk.*

The Royal Pharmaceutical Society of Great Britain: *www.rpsgb.org.uk.*

7 The Evidence for Acute Perioperative Pain Management

Jane Quinlan

Key Messages

- All evidence is not equal. Systematic reviews of well-designed studies give us the most accurate information as to the effectiveness of analgesia.
- Evidence cannot be viewed in isolation. It should be considered together with the clinical context and individual patient circumstances.
- Multimodal analgesia, using a combination of drugs acting on different parts of the pain pathway, provides the best form of pain relief with an associated reduction in side effects.
- Non-opioid analgesics such as ketamine, gabapentin, clonidine and magnesium may prove useful in postoperative pain, but further studies are needed to clarify the optimal doses and the patient groups most likely to benefit.
- Our goal should not be simply to provide a pain-free convalescence, but to use the best analgesia possible with minimal side effects to enable a swift return to full function.

Introduction

The use of good scientific evidence to provide best-quality analgesia for our patients is fraught with difficulties. We are not just dealing with tissue damage stimulating a pain receptor (nociception) and producing a predictable outcome (pain perception). Instead, we have to consider the emotional effect of pain: the patient's personality, coping ability, previous pain experiences, mood, culture, beliefs and understanding. En route between the nociceptor and the cortical and thalamic interpretation, we have a multitude of chemical messengers in the nervous system and neurones, which may have already undergone changes related to previous pain.

Evidence-based medicine provides us with a recipe book for the best treatments available for a given type of pain. These recipes present us with probabilities, not certainties, and so constitute a guide to treatments most likely to work, all other things being equal. But of course, all other things are not equal.

Patients bring with them expectations, fears, beliefs and misconceptions about both pain and its treatment. Some views may be based on previous experiences of pain, some relate to the tolerability of side effects, while other views may be strongly held but without foundation: a reluctance to take strong opioids for fear of addiction, for example.

Patients also have individual clinical circumstances with, possibly, atypical features of the pain, other comorbidities and differing contexts for the pain. Postoperatively, two patients with abdominal pain will have different pain experiences if one has just had a caesarean section and a healthy baby delivered, while the other has undergone a hysterectomy for malignancy.

To use evidence effectively, therefore, and to provide the best treatment for our patients, we need to consider four elements (Straus *et al.* 2005):

1. Best research evidence
2. Clinical expertise
3. Patient values: expectations, concerns and preferences
4. Patient circumstances

Next, we need to consider how to judge the quality and accuracy of the evidence available to us, for which it may be useful to clarify a few terms.

Randomisation

The computer-generated equivalent of tossing a coin for each patient to determine whether they will receive the treatment under investigation (heads) or receive the placebo or control drug (tails). This gives each participant an equal chance of being assigned to any of the groups and thus reduces the likelihood of selection bias.

Bias

In a clinical trial, bias is a flaw in the study design, method of collecting or the interpretation of information. Biases can lead to incorrect conclusions about what the study or trial showed.

Double-blind

A scientific technique used to eliminate bias in a study, where neither the investigators nor the subjects know which drug or treatment the subject is receiving.

Meta-analysis

A statistical technique that summarises the results of several studies, giving a greater weighting to higher quality studies. Data obtained from combined studies must be comparable in order to be evaluated by this method.

Systematic review

A summary of the medical literature that uses explicit methods to perform a thorough literature search and critical appraisal of individual studies. It uses appropriate statistical techniques (meta-analysis) to combine these valid studies. The combining of data from several different research studies provides a better overview of a topic than that available in any single investigation.

Confidence intervals

Confidence intervals are a measure of the accuracy of an estimated effect. They define a range of values within which the population mean is likely to lie. Usually 95% confidence limits are quoted, where there is a 95% probability that the true population mean will lie somewhere between the upper and lower confidence limits. The width of the confidence interval gives us some idea about the uncertainty of the unknown parameter. A very wide interval indicates a large spread of results in the study population, while a narrow interval shows that the results fall within a small range and are therefore likely to be more accurate.

Levels of evidence

In 1784, James Moore, the Glasgow-born London-based surgeon, provided the first record of opium use after surgery: 'Opium is highly expedient to abate the smarting of the wound after the operation is over ...' (Moore 1784). Clinicians and researchers have been assessing the effectiveness of postoperative analgesia ever since.

We need to use studies to find out the answer to a clinical question. Is drug X an effective analgesic and, if so, what is the optimal dose? The clinical trials addressing that question must be sufficiently well thought out and executed to be able to give us an accurate answer. If a trial is poorly planned with too few patients, is biased or doesn't answer the right question, then a conclusion may be drawn that is just wrong.

Studies that are not randomised or poorly randomised can exaggerate the treatment effect by up to 40%, risking a false positive result, i.e. showing a benefit to the treatment that doesn't really exist. Studies where there is not full blinding, so that the data collectors know whether the study patient is receiving the trial drug or a placebo, risk overestimating the treatment benefit by up to 17% (Schulz *et al.* 1995).

Box 7.1 Levels of evidence.

Levels of evidence (according to the NHMRC[a] designation 1999)

I Evidence obtained from a systematic review of all relevant randomised controlled trials

II Evidence obtained from at least one properly designed randomised controlled trial

III-1 Evidence obtained from well-designed pseudorandomised controlled trials (alternate allocation or some other method)

III-2 Evidence obtained from comparative studies with concurrent controls and allocation not randomised (cohort studies), case-controlled studies or interrupted time series with a control group

III-3 Evidence obtained from comparative studies with historical control, two or more single-arm studies or interrupted time series without a parallel control group

IV Evidence obtained from case series, either post-test or pre-test and post-test

[a]National Health and Medical Research Council, Canberra.
National Health and Medical Research Council (1999). © Commonwealth of Australia reproduced by permission.

Trials with large numbers of patients reduce the risk of getting a skewed population. With the development of systematic reviews of clinical trials, we can pool evidence of postoperative interventions to establish which work effectively. By reviewing all valid, good quality, randomised controlled clinical trials of an intervention we can produce the best evidence available and therefore get closest to the truth (McQuay & Moore 1998).

In 2005, the Australian and New Zealand College of Anaesthetists and Faculty of Pain Medicine produced 'Acute Pain Management: Scientific Evidence'. This impressive piece of work presents recommendations on treatments for acute pain (including postoperative pain) based on the robustness of the evidence available (Box 7.1). Levels of evidence are used to judge the reliability of conclusions, with a lower number (I) being the most likely to be closest to the real answer.

Pain measurement in research

Clinically, pain is usually measured with *pain intensity scales* either as verbal descriptors (none, mild, moderate or severe), which may then be assigned numbers (0–3 respectively), with a numerical rating scale (0–10) or with visual analogue scales where the patient marks a scale (0–100 mm) from no pain to the worst pain imaginable.

Box 7.2 Pain relief scale.

Categorical verbal-rating pain relief scale
0 = none
1 = slight
2 = moderate
3 = good
4 = complete

In research, *pain relief scales* (Box 7.2) are often more convenient, as all patients start from zero – no pain relief – before the intervention. With effective analgesia, they should reach a score of 4 – complete pain relief.

Using the pain relief scores plotted against time, the total pain relief (TOTPAR) achieved by an analgesic can be measured by calculating the area under the curve. Conventionally, pain relief scores have been measured, and their totals calculated, over 4–6 hr, as this is the duration of effect of most oral analgesics. To reach maximum TOTPAR (maxTOTPAR) then, a patient would need to get complete pain relief (score 4) immediately and sustain it for the next 6 hr (Moore *et al.* 1996). TOTPAR can then be used to compare the effectiveness of analgesics.

In Figure 7.1, drug A provides full pain relief (4 out of 4) within 1 h and sustains this for the full 6 h. The area under the curve is high, so the TOTPAR will be high. Drug B takes longer to reach its full effect and fails to provide

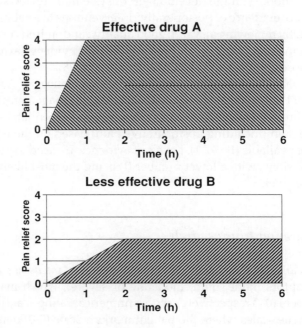

Figure 7.1 Total pain relief (TOTPAR).

complete pain relief at any point, so has a low TOTPAR and is a less effective analgesic.

Number needed to treat

The number needed to treat (NNT) is a clinically useful means of assessing the effectiveness of a treatment. It was developed to establish how many patients would need to be treated with a particular intervention to prevent one adverse event occurring, for example the prevention of stroke by treating patients with antihypertensive medication (Cook & Sackett 1995).

The number needed to harm (NNH) uses a similar concept, but reflects the incidence of side effects. This in itself provides interpretive difficulties: side effects range from minor to severe, so there is no definite end point. As a result, NNH is usually based on the number of patients withdrawn from a study owing to side effects sufficient to require cessation of the drug. For example a recent review of treatments for neuropathic pain (Finnerup *et al.* 2005) found that in trigeminal neuralgia, carbamazepine had an NNT of 1.7 (for every 1.7 patients treated, one will derive benefit) and a combined NNH of 21.7 (for every 22 patients treated, one will suffer problematic side effects).

Moore *et al.* (2003) used the concept of NNT to assess the effectiveness of anal-gesia and produced the Oxford League Table of Analgesic Efficacy (Table 7.1). The full table is available on the Bandolier website (http://www.jr2.ox.ac.uk/bandolier). The NNT here tells us the number of patients who receive an active drug for one patient to achieve 50% of the TOTPAR compared with placebo over a 4- to 6-hr period. An effective analgesic will have a low NNT, e.g. di-clofenac 100 mg *NNT 1.8*, while a high NNT, e.g. codeine 60 mg *NNT 16.7*, implies a poorer analgesic response.

The table provides a useful guide but is not definitive. Data are based on double-blind studies of only a single dose of the drug compared to placebo, so may not fully reflect clinical practice where simple analgesics are given reg-ularly. Also, data analysed were pooled from studies of a variety of surgical procedures and patient groups, so there may be differences between popula-tions. The nature of the pain and, therefore, the most effective analgesia follow-ing dental extraction, for example, may be very different from that following oesophageal or hip surgery. To avoid this problem of large heterogeneous pa-tient populations, some argue that procedure-specific evidence would be more useful (Gray *et al.* 2005).

The placebo effect

A placebo is a drug or intervention that has no treatment value, given as if it were a real treatment. Many trials in pain use a placebo to establish the efficacy of an analgesic, so that some patients in the trial will receive a possible effec-tive analgesic, while other patients will be given a placebo with no analgesic

Table 7.1   Oxford League Table of Analgesic Efficacy (2007).

Analgesic and dose (mg)	Number of patients in comparison	Percent with at least 50% pain relief	Number needed to treat	Lower confidence interval	Higher confidence interval
Etoricoxib 180/240	248	77	1.5	1.3	1.7
Etoricoxib 120	500	70	1.6	1.5	1.8
Diclofenac 100	545	69	1.8	1.6	2.1
Celecoxib 400	298	52	2.1	1.8	2.5
Paracetamol 1000+ Codeine 60	197	57	2.2	1.7	2.9
Rofecoxib 50	675	54	2.3	2.0	2.6
Aspirin 1200	279	61	2.4	1.9	3.2
Ibuprofen 400	5456	55	2.5	2.4	2.7
Oxycodone IR 10+ Paracetamol 650	315	66	2.6	2.0	3.5
Diclofenac 25	502	53	2.6	2.2	3.3
Ketorolac 10	790	50	2.6	2.3	3.1
Naproxen 400/440	197	51	2.7	2.1	4.0
Piroxicam 20	280	63	2.7	2.1	3.8
Lumiracoxib 400	370	48	2.7	2.2	3.5
Naproxen 500/550	784	52	2.7	2.3	3.3
Diclofenac 50	1296	57	2.7	2.4	3.1
Ibuprofen 200	3248	48	2.7	2.5	2.9
Pethidine 100 (intramuscular)	364	54	2.9	2.3	3.9
Tramadol 150	561	48	2.9	2.4	3.6
Morphine 10 (intramuscular)	946	50	2.9	2.6	3.6
Naproxen 200/220	202	45	3.4	2.4	5.8
Ketorolac 30 (intramuscular)	359	53	3.4	2.5	4.9

(*continued*)

Table 7.1 Oxford League Table of Analgesic Efficacy (2007). (*Cont.*)

Analgesic and dose (mg)	Number of patients in comparison	Percent with at least 50% pain relief	Number needed to treat	Lower confidence interval	Higher confidence interval
Paracetamol 500	561	61	3.5	2.2	13.3
Celecoxib 200	805	40	3.5	2.9	4.4
Ibuprofen 100	495	36	3.7	2.9	4.9
Paracetamol 1000	2759	46	3.8	3.4	4.4
Paracetamol 600/650 + codeine 60	1123	42	4.2	3.4	5.3
Paracetamol 650 + dextropropoxyphene (65-mg hydrochloride or 100-mg napsylate)	963	38	4.4	3.5	5.6
Aspirin 600/650	5061	38	4.4	4.0	4.9
Paracetamol 600/650	1886	38	4.6	3.9	5.5
Ibuprofen 50	316	32	4.7	3.3	8.0
Tramadol 100	882	30	4.8	3.8	6.1
Tramadol 75	563	32	5.3	3.9	8.2
Aspirin 650 + codeine 60	598	25	5.3	4.1	7.4
Paracetamol 300 + codeine 30	379	26	5.7	4.0	9.8
Tramadol 50	770	19	8.3	6.0	13.0
Codeine 60	1305	15	16.7	11.0	48.0
Placebo	>10000	18	N/A	N/A	N/A

IR, immediate release.

properties. This may raise concerns that it is ethically wrong to provide the placebo group with no analgesia. The counterargument is that, in order to establish whether a drug provides effective analgesia, the study must be robust enough to provide a definite, reproducible and comparable answer. For example if drug X is compared to drug Y (where drug X is the test drug and Y is a drug with known analgesic properties), we can then say that drug X is better, worse or the same as drug Y in providing pain relief. In a separate study, drugs A and B could be analysed and result in the same conclusions. But is X better than A? We cannot tell as the results are not comparable. If drugs X and A were both compared to placebo, however, we could then compare the two without the need for a separate trial. It would also enable us to compare doses of the same drug.

The placebo effect is a positive medical response to a placebo, simply because the patient expects it to work. The more a person believes they are going to benefit from a treatment, the more likely it is that they will experience a benefit.

In a study of placebo expectations post-thoracotomy, patients were divided into three groups and each received a continuous infusion of saline. One group was told that the infusion was a painkiller, while a second group were told that they were in a clinical trial and the infusion could be either a painkiller or a placebo. The third group was given no information about the infusion. The amount of opioid analgesia requested by the patients was then measured. The first group, with high expectations of analgesia, required 33.8% less opioid than the third 'no-expectation' group, while the second ('double-blind') group used 20.8% less opioid than the 'no-expectation' group (Level IV: Pollo *et al.* 2001).

It is difficult to predict who will be a 'placebo responder'. It used to be thought that about a third of patients will show a response to placebo, but it has now been established that there is no predictable fraction of responders. In a large review of patients suffering from postoperative pain, 18% described at least 50% pain relief with placebo (McQuay & Moore 2005). Interestingly, people who receive a placebo may also experience negative effects, for example nausea, diarrhoea and constipation. A negative placebo effect is called the nocebo effect.

Petrovic and colleagues have used neuroimaging techniques to show that placebo and opioid analgesia share common neuronal networks, with both producing an increase in activity in the rostral anterior cingulate cortex, part of the medial pain system responsible for the affective (emotional) component of pain (Petrovic *et al.* 2002). The placebo and opioid connection is also reflected in the fact that the placebo effect can be reversed by naloxone, an opioid antagonist (Benedetti 1996, Levine *et al.* 1978).

Evidence for effectiveness of specific drugs

Paracetamol (acetaminophen)

Paracetamol is an effective analgesic (Level I: Barden *et al.* 2004a) with few side effects, and has been shown to reduce postoperative opioid requirement by 20–30% when given regularly (Level I: Remy *et al.* 2005, Level I: Rømsing *et al.* 2002). Morphine use can be reduced yet further by the combination of regular paracetamol with regular non-steroidal anti-inflammatory drugs (NSAIDs) (Level I: Hyllestad *et al.* 2002, Level II: Montgomery *et al.* 1996). Its mode of action is still unclear, but is thought to act centrally, inhibiting brain prostaglandin synthetase. Paracetamol may be given orally, intravenously or rectally, although rectal absorption is poor, necessitating doses of 35–45 mg/kg to attain therapeutic blood levels (Stocker & Montgomery 2001). Intravenous doses of paracetamol provide faster, more effective analgesia than the equivalent oral dose (Level II: Jarde & Boccard 1997).

Non-steroidal anti-inflammatory drugs

NSAIDs inhibit cyclooxygenase and reduce the production of proinflammatory prostaglandins and leukotrienes. They are effective analgesics for postoperative pain (Level I: Barden *et al.* 2004b) and work well as part of a multimodal approach to pain in combination with regular paracetamol, thus decreasing opioid requirements (Level I: Hyllestad *et al.* 2002). Parenteral or rectal NSAIDs provide no advantages over oral administration: they are all equally efficacious, with a similar speed of onset and no reduction in side effects (Level I: Tramèr *et al.* 1998). Side effects related to NSAIDs limit their use in many patients, however.

Oral opioids

As demonstrated in the Oxford Analgesic Table, weak opioids alone are just that: weak. Codeine 60 mg has an NNT of 16.7 and tramadol 50 mg has an NNT of 8.3. However, when combined with paracetamol, the NNT improved to 2.2 for codeine+paracetamol and 2.6 for tramadol+paracetamol. That said, the analysis used to develop the table was based on single doses of drug, rather than on repeated doses given regularly.

Intramuscular opioids

A review by Dolin and colleagues in 2002 compared the incidence of moderate-to-severe and severe postoperative pain with three analgesic techniques: intramuscular (IM) morphine, patient-controlled analgesia (PCA) and epidural analgesia (Table 7.2).

The authors conclude that, despite published studies showing that IM morphine can be very effective when used with strict protocols (Harmer & Davies 1998), this does not happen in clinical practice, so support the general view that IM morphine is the least effective technique. Epidural analgesia appears to be the most effective technique. Epidurals can certainly provide excellent postoperative analgesia but are vulnerable to technical failure including unilateral or patchy block. In this review, the rate of epidural catheter dislodgement was 5.7%. The problem then is that the patient will be left in pain while alternative analgesia is set up – the 'analgesic gap'.

Table 7.2 A comparison of the incidence of moderate-to-severe postoperative pain between three techniques.

	Mean (%) of patients reporting pain	
	Moderate-to-severe pain (>3/10)	Severe pain (>7/10)
IM	67.2	29.1
PCA	35.8	10.4
Epidural	20.9	7.8

IM, intramuscular; PCA, patient-controlled analgesia.
Dolin *et al.* (2002).

Patient-controlled analgesia

PCA is covered fully in a separate chapter, but there are issues surrounding the interpretation of studies that merit comment.

Intravenous opioids delivered by PCA provide, arguably, the most flexible form of strong analgesia in the postoperative period. The bolus can be adjusted to cover dynamic pain, e.g. pain on movement, while, if necessary, a background infusion can be added for constant pain. Patients with opioid tolerance following treatment for chronic pain or patients with a history of illicit drug use require higher doses of opioid to achieve analgesia and this can easily be accommodated by further adjustment. Despite this, most studies assessing analgesic efficacy use a set prescription when PCA is compared to other methods of postoperative analgesia.

A recent study comparing various fixed-dose PCA prescriptions of morphine or hydromorphone found that 75% of the patients in the study described moderate-to-severe pain. The authors' conclusion was not that PCA provides poor analgesia, but that good postoperative analgesia is difficult to achieve with PCA unless treatment is individualised (Level IV: Larijani *et al.* 2005).

Similarly, the assessment of changes made to a PCA protocol often fails to appreciate the need to titrate the PCA to the individual patient. In one frequently quoted study, children undergoing appendicectomy were randomised to receive a morphine PCA alone postoperatively or a morphine PCA with a background infusion of 20 mcg/kg/hr. The authors found that the group that received a background infusion on the PCA had no benefit in analgesia, but experienced a higher incidence of side effects such as sedation and hypoxaemia (Level IV: Doyle *et al.* 1993a). The conclusion from many, based on this study, is that background infusions should never be used as they simply increase risk.

However, a second paper by Doyle *et al.* (Level IV: 1993b) repeated the first study but used a morphine PCA with a low-dose background infusion of morphine 4 mcg/kg/hr (B4) or 10 mcg/kg/hr (B10) and compared these to a no background group (B0). All three groups used similar amounts of morphine, had similar pain scores and had similar levels of sedation. They also found that group B4 suffered no increase in side effects, experienced less hypoxaemia and had better sleep patterns than those with no background infusion (B0).

PCA is not a 'one size fits all' or a 'set and forget' therapy (Macintyre 2001). Thought must be given to the nature of surgery, the patient circumstances and their previous opioid use to provide a sensible PCA prescription. This original prescription may then require further adjustment to achieve maximal benefit for the patient.

Epidural analgesia

Epidural analgesia is also fully discussed elsewhere, but again, there are observations to be made about the interpretation of studies that are worth mentioning.

The term 'epidural analgesia' encompasses a variety of drugs (opioids, local anaesthetics or a combination), delivery modes (continuous infusion, intermittent bolus or PCA), field of analgesia (thoracic or lumbar) and duration (one-off injection intraoperatively or postoperative continuation). This makes analysis difficult when clinical studies compare other forms of postoperative analgesia with 'epidural analgesia' as a generic concept.

Having said that, a recent meta-analysis by Wu *et al.* (Level I: 2005) compared epidural analgesia with intravenous opioid PCA for postoperative pain. They found that epidural analgesia provided superior postoperative analgesia compared with intravenous PCA, regardless of the epidural regimen. Epidurals containing local anaesthetic with or without opioid or opioid alone all performed better than intravenous PCA, as did continuous epidural infusion or patient-controlled epidural analgesia.

This then provides us with the opportunity to apply Straus' model for the use of evidence in the clinical scenario.

(i) Currently, the best research evidence available suggests that epidural analgesia may be preferable to intravenous PCA following major surgery.

(ii) Our clinical expertise (and common sense) leads us to use a thoracic, rather than a lumbar, epidural for upper abdominal surgery and a lumbar epidural, not thoracic, for lower limb procedures.

(iii) The patient's concerns may include severe nausea and vomiting while using an intravenous morphine PCA following previous surgery, so an opioid-alone epidural would not be suitable.

(iv) The patient circumstances may involve a requirement for early mobilisation postoperatively.

Therefore, an epidural infusion of low-dose local anaesthetic combined low-dose opioid would be preferable.

Ketamine

Ketamine is an antagonist at the NMDA (*N*-methyl-D-aspartate) receptor.

NMDA receptors, with glutamate as the neurotransmitter, are located both peripherally and in the spinal cord. NMDA receptor activation, produced by strong nociceptive (pain stimulus) input, will increase neuronal hyperexcitability and induce long-lasting changes in the spinal cord, such as central sensitisation, wind-up and pain memory (Dickenson 1995). As a result, rather than nociceptive pain fading once the stimulus causing the pain is removed, the pain will continue and show features more typical of neuropathic pain. These include allodynia, where light touch is felt as pain, or hyperalgesia, an exaggerated response to pain stimulation. By blocking NMDA receptors with ketamine, central sensitisation and wind-up should be reduced, thus reducing pain. Unfortunately, ketamine produces unpleasant side effects, such as nausea, hallucinations, confusion, unpleasant dreams and delirium, which can limit its dose and thus its effectiveness.

Ketamine alone does not provide as much analgesia as that produced by opioids, but can reduce postoperative opioid requirement when administered as a low-dose intravenous infusion or when given epidurally (Level I: Subramaniam *et al*. 2004). Ketamine has also proved useful in the treatment of opioid-insensitive neuropathic and cancer pain and has been used to good effect in the acute setting for patients with opioid tolerance and escalating opioid requirement (Level IV: Eilers *et al*. 2001)

Gabapentin

Gabapentin is an anticonvulsant that has a well-established role in the treatment of chronic pain and has now been reviewed for use in acute postoperative pain. It binds to voltage-gated calcium channels which inhibit calcium influx and thus inhibit the release of excitatory neurotransmitters in the pain pathways (Rowbotham 2006). When given preoperatively, gabapentin has been found to reduce opioid requirement in the postoperative period, with dizziness as its major side effect (Level I: Ho *et al*. 2006). It may also prove useful in reducing the development of chronic pain after surgery (Macrae 2001).

Clonidine

Norepinephrine (previously noradrenaline) and serotonin (5-HT) are involved in descending pain pathways which modulate the transmission of pain signals in the spinal cord. These descending pathways originate in the cortex, midbrain, pons and medulla and can amplify or inhibit incoming pain signals. Clonidine is an α_2-adrenoceptor agonist that produces analgesia via these descending pathways at both spinal and supraspinal levels (Ongjoco *et al*. 2000).

Clonidine administered intravenously for postoperative analgesia is effective in reducing opioid requirement, with a consequent reduction in opioid-related side effects (Level IV: De Kock *et al.* 1992, Level IV: Jeffs *et al.* 2002). It may also be administered orally, epidurally, in a peripheral nerve block and as an intrathecal injection (Eisenach *et al.* 1996). A study of patients undergoing colonic surgery randomised patients to receive an intrathecal injection of clonidine, bupivacaine or saline before induction of general anaesthesia. Those who received intrathecal clonidine or bupivacaine had lower pain scores during the immediate postoperative period than the saline group. Furthermore, the clonidine group went on to have less residual pain over the next 6 months and, more specifically, less hyperalgesia around the wound (Level IV: De Kock *et al.* 2005). For chronic-pain patients, clonidine may be administered as an epidural or intrathecal infusion. Side effects of clonidine via any route include sedation, hypotension and dry mouth, which can limit its usefulness. Research evidence is not yet robust enough to sanction its routine use.

Magnesium

Magnesium is an antagonist at the NMDA receptor and as such could be expected to provide analgesia. This has been confirmed in studies where intravenous magnesium, infused perioperatively, has been found to reduce postoperative morphine consumption (Level IV: Koinig *et al.* 1998, Tramèr *et al.* 1996). Magnesium is not an effective analgesic alone, however, which suggests that it potentiates morphine antinociception (Kroin *et al.* 2000). It is currently unclear how useful magnesium will prove to be in routine postoperative analgesia, owing to its side effects and the interaction of magnesium with other drugs (Dubé & Granry 2003).

Multimodal analgesia

It should be perfectly possible to provide adequate postoperative analgesia with opioids alone, but opioid side effects make this a rather unappealing prospect: nausea, vomiting, sedation, constipation and respiratory depression will not enhance recovery. By combining non-opioid and opioid analgesics postoperatively we can reduce the opioid requirement and thus, surely, the opioid side effects.

Unfortunately, despite providing a reduction in morphine use when paracetamol (Level I: Remy *et al.* 2005, Level I: Rømsing *et al.* 2002) and NSAIDs (Level I: Hyllestad *et al.* 2002) are given regularly postoperatively, most studies do not find a reduction in opioid-related complications. So we may then question the benefit of going to the trouble of reducing opioid consumption for no advantage (and exposing the patient to an increased risk of side effects from NSAIDs) or we may question the attribution of these side effects to opioids alone (Kehlet 2005). In most studies assessing opioid use, nausea and vomiting are documented as a primarily opioid-related effect, despite the knowledge that postoperative nausea and vomiting (PONV) is multifactorial, related to gender, previous history, type of surgery and, indeed, pain itself.

As opioid-related side effects are usually viewed as secondary end points (with morphine consumption and a reduction in pain scores as the primary end points), single studies alone do not have sufficient power to address the side-effect issue. By pooling the results of these studies, a meta-analysis improves the statistical power and can provide more robust conclusions.

Marret *et al.* (Level I: 2005) performed a meta-analysis of randomised controlled trials where NSAIDs were used with PCA morphine and looked specifically at the incidence of morphine-related side effects. They found that NSAIDs reduced nausea and vomiting by 30% and sedation by 29%. Indeed, using regression analysis, they demonstrated that for every milligram of morphine spared, nausea was reduced by 0.9% and vomiting by 0.3%. Other side effects such as pruritus, urinary retention and respiratory depression were not significantly decreased.

Respiratory depression is difficult to interpret using meta-analysis, owing to the difference in criteria used in the studies (respiratory rate <8 breaths per minute or <10 breaths per minute; oxygen saturation <84% for 2 min or <90% for 10 min; or the need for naloxone administration). There is also likely to be a difference in the incidence of respiratory complications according to the type of surgery, for example upper gastrointestinal versus orthopaedic surgery.

Interestingly, a study of the dose–response pharmacology of morphine showed that as morphine dose increased, the incidence of vomiting and sedation increased, but no such correlation was found for pruritus or urinary retention (Bailey *et al.* 1993).

Recovery from surgery

It is increasingly recognised that to improve and expedite recovery from surgery, a multidisciplinary approach is required. Kehlet and colleagues have pioneered fast-track programmes after colorectal and urological surgery, involving analgesia with a thoracic epidural infusion of combined local anaesthetic and opioid, and enforced early mobilisation and oral feeding on the first postoperative day (Brodner *et al.* 2001). He concludes that 'multimodal interventions lead to an improved recovery and reduction in postoperative morbidity' (Kehlet 1997).

Many studies have shown that good postoperative analgesia does not result in early mobilisation and reduction in hospital stay. Kehlet argues that this is an opportunity missed: early physiotherapy and mobilisation, enabled by effective pain relief, will facilitate early discharge from hospital; patients languishing in bed, albeit pain free, will not.

Summary

Pain is a complex, individual experience. Research into the effectiveness of drugs and analgesic interventions is essential to provide accurate information as to the best treatment available. This research must be high quality, unbiased, reproducible and sufficiently well designed to answer the question asked. Those producing systematic reviews of these studies must apply the same rigour to their statistical methodology and guide us closer to the truth. We, in turn, have a duty to use this evidence-based medicine and apply it appropriately in the clinical situation.

References

Australian and New Zealand College of Anaesthetists and Faculty of Pain Medicine (2005) *Acute Pain Management: Scientific Evidence*, 2nd edn. Australian and New Zealand College of Anaesthetists and Faculty of Pain Medicine. http://www.anzca.edu.au/resources/books-and-publications/acutepain.pdf. Accessed 21 October 2007.

Bailey, P.L., Rhondeau, S., Schafer, P.G., *et al.* (1993) Dose–response pharmacology of intrathecal morphine in human volunteers. *Anesthesiology*, **79** (1), 49–59.

Bandolier. www.jr2.ox.ac.uk/bandolier. Accessed 22 October 2007.

Barden, J., Edwards, J., Moore, A. & McQuay, H. (2004a) Single dose oral paracetamol (acetaminophen) for postoperative pain. *The Cochrane Database of Systematic Reviews*, Issue 1, Art No CD004602. DOI: 10.1002/14651858.CD004602.

Barden, J., Edwards, J., Moore, A. & McQuay, H. (2004b) Single dose oral diclofenac for postoperative pain. *The Cochrane Database of Systematic Reviews*, Issue 2, Art No CD004768. DOI: 10.1002/14651858.CD004768.

Benedetti, F. (1996) The opposite effects of the opiate antagonist naloxone and the cholecystokinin antagonist proglumide on placebo analgesia. *Pain*, **64** (3), 535–543.

Brodner, G., Van Aken, H., Hertle, L., *et al.* (2001) Multimodal perioperative management – combining thoracic epidural analgesia, forced mobilization, and oral nutrition – reduces hormonal and metabolic stress and improves convalescence after major urologic surgery. *Anesthesia and Analgesia*, **92** (6), 1594–1600.

Cook, R.J. & Sackett, D.L. (1995) The number needed to treat: a clinically useful measure of treatment effect. *British Medical Journal*, **310** (6986), 452–454.

De Kock, M., Lavand'homme, P. & Waterloos, H. (2005) The short-lasting analgesia and long-term antihyperalgesic effect of intrathecal clonidine in patients undergoing colonic surgery. *Anesthesia and Analgesia*, **101** (2), 566–572.

De Kock, M.F., Pichon, G. & Scholtes, J.-L. (1992) Intraoperative clonidine enhances postoperative morphine patient-controlled analgesia. *Canadian Journal of Anaesthesia*, **39** (6), 537–544.

Dickenson, A.H. (1995) Spinal cord pharmacology of pain. *British Journal of Anaesthesia*, **75** (2), 193–200.

Dolin, S.J., Cashman, J.N. & Bland, J.M. (2002) Effectiveness of acute postoperative pain management: evidence from published data. *British Journal of Anaesthesia*, **89** (3), 409–423.

Doyle, E., Harper, I. & Morton, N.S. (1993b) Patient-controlled analgesia with low dose background infusions after lower abdominal surgery in children. *British Journal of Anaesthesia*, **71** (6), 818–822.

Doyle, E., Robinson, D. & Morton, N.S. (1993a) Comparison of patient-controlled analgesia with and without a background infusion after lower abdominal surgery in children. *British Journal of Anaesthesia*, **71** (5), 670–673.

Dubé, L. & Granry, J.-C. (2003) The therapeutic use of magnesium in anesthesiology, intensive care and emergency medicine: a review. *Canadian Journal of Anesthesia*, **50** (7), 732–746.

Eilers, H., Philip, L., Bickler, P., McKay, W. & Schumacher, M. (2001) The reversal of fentanyl-induced tolerance by administration of 'small-dose' ketamine. *Anesthesia and Analgesia*, **93** (1), 213–214.

Eisenach, J.C., De Kock, M. & Klimscha, W. (1996) Alpha-2-adrenergic agonists for regional anesthesia: a clinical review of clonidine (1984–1995). *Anesthesiology*, **85** (3), 655–674.

Finnerup, N.B., Otto, M., McQuay, H.J., Jensen, T.S. & Sindrup, S.H. (2005) Algorithm for neuropathic pain treatment: an evidence based proposal. *Pain*, **118** (3), 289–305.

Gray, A., Kehlet, H., Bonnet, F. & Rawal, N. (2005) Predicting postoperative analgesia outcomes: NNT league tables or procedure-specific evidence? *British Journal of Anaesthesia*, **94** (6), 710–714.

Harmer, M. & Davies, K.A. (1998) The effect of education, assessment and a standardised prescription on postoperative pain management. *Anaesthesia*, **53** (5), 424–430.

Ho, K.-Y., Gan, T.J. & Habib, A.S. (2006) Gabapentin and postoperative pain – a systematic review of randomized controlled trials. *Pain*, **126** (1–3), 91–101.

Hyllestad, M., Jones, S., Pedersen, J.L. & Kehlet, H. (2002) Comparative effect of paracetamol, NSAIDs or their combination in postoperative pain management: a qualitative review. *British Journal of Anaesthesia*, **88** (2), 199–214.

Jarde, O. & Boccard, E. (1997) Parenteral versus oral route increases paracetamol efficacy. *Clinical Drug Investigation*, **14** (6), 474–481.

Jeffs, S.A., Hall, J.E. & Morris, S. (2002) Comparison of morphine alone with morphine plus clonidine for postoperative patient-controlled analgesia. *British Journal of Anaesthesia*, **89** (3), 424–427.

Kehlet, H. (1997) Multimodal approach to control postoperative pathophysiology and rehabilitation. *British Journal of Anaesthesia*, **78** (5), 606–617.

Kehlet, H. (2005) Postoperative opioid sparing to hasten recovery: what are the issues? *Anesthesiology*, **102** (6), 1083–1085.

Koinig, H., Waller, T., Marhofer, P., Andel, H., Hörauf, K. & Mayer, N. (1998) Magnesium sulphate reduces intra- and postoperative analgesic requirements. *Anesthesia and Analgesia*, **87** (1), 206–210.

Kroin, J.S., McCarthy, R.J., Von Roenn, N., Schwab, B., Tuman, K.J. & Ivankovich, A.D. (2000) Magnesium sulphate potentiates morphine antinociception at the spinal level. *Anesthesia and Analgesia*, **90** (4), 913–917.

Larijani, G.E., Sharaf, I., Warshal, D.P., Marr, A., Gratz, I. & Goldberg, M.E. (September 2005) Pain evaluation in patients receiving intravenous patient-controlled analgesia after surgery. *Pharmacotherapy*, **25** (9), 1168–1173.

Levine, J.D., Gordon, N.C. & Fields, H.L. (1978) The mechanism of placebo analgesia. *Lancet*, **2** (8091), 654–657.

Macintyre, P.E. (2001) Safety and efficacy of patient-controlled analgesia. *British Journal of Anaesthesia*, **87** (1), 36–46.

Macrae, W.A. (2001) Chronic pain after surgery. *British Journal of Anaesthesia*, **87** (1), 88–98.

Marret, E., Kurdi, O., Zuffery, P. & Bonnet, F. (2005) Effects of nonsteroidal anti-inflammatory drugs on patient-controlled analgesia morphine side effects. *Anesthesiology*, **102** (6), 1249–1260.

McQuay, H. & Moore, A. (1998) *An Evidence-Based Resource for Pain Relief.* Oxford University Press, Oxford.

McQuay, H. & Moore, R.A. (2005) Placebo. *Postgraduate Medical Journal*, **81** (953), 155–160.

Montgomery, J.E., Sutherland, C.J., Kestin, I.G. & Sneyd, J.R. (1996) Morphine consumption in patients receiving rectal paracetamol and diclofenac alone and in combination. *British Journal of Anaesthesia*, **77** (4), 445–447.

Moore, A., Edwards, J., Barden, J. & McQuay, H. (2003) *Bandolier's Little Book of Pain.* Oxford University Press, Oxford.

Moore, A., McQuay, H. & Gavaghan, D. (1996) Deriving dichotomous outcome measures from continuous data in randomised controlled trials of analgesics. *Pain*, **66** (2–3), 229–237.

Moore, J. (1784) *A Method of Preventing or Diminishing Pain in Several Operations of Surgery.* J. Caddell, London. Cited in Hamilton, G.R. & Baskett, T.F. (2000) In the arms of Morpheus: the development of morphine for postoperative pain relief. *Canadian Journal of Anaesthesia*, **47**, 367–374.

National Health and Medical Research Council (1999) *A Guide to the Development, Implementation and Evaluation of Clinical Practice Guidelines.* National Health and Medical Research Council, Canberra.

Ongjoco, R.R.S., Richardson, C.D., Rudner, X.L., Stafford-Smith, M. & Schwinn, D.A. (2000) α_2-adrenergic receptors in human dorsal root ganglia. *Anesthesiology*, **92** (4), 968–976.

Petrovic, P., Kalso, E., Petersson, K.M. & Ingvar, M. (2002) Placebo and opioid analgesia – imaging a shared neuronal network. *Science*, **295** (5560), 1737–1740.

Pollo, A., Amanzio, M., Arslanian, A., Casadio, C., Maggi, G. & Benedetti, F. (2001) Response expectancies in placebo analgesia and their clinical relevance. *Pain*, **93** (1), 77–84.

Remy, C., Marret, M. & Bonnet, F. (2005) Effects of acetaminophen on morphine side-effects and consumption after major surgery: meta-analysis of randomized controlled trials. *British Journal of Anaesthesia*, **94** (4), 505–513.

Rømsing, J., Møiniche, S. & Dahl, J.B. (2002) Rectal and parenteral paracetamol, and paracetamol in combination with NSAIDs, for postoperative analgesia. *British Journal of Anaesthesia*, **88** (2), 215–226.

Rowbotham, D.J. (2006) Gabapentin: a new drug for postoperative pain? *British Journal of Anaesthesia*, **96** (2), 152–155.

Schulz, K.F., Chalmers, I., Hayes, R.J. & Altman, D.G. (1995) Empirical evidence of bias. Dimensions of methodological quality associated with estimates of treatment effects in controlled trials. *Journal of the American Medical Association*, **273** (5), 408–412.

Stocker, M. & Montgomery, J.E. (2001) Serum paracetamol concentrations in adult volunteers following rectal administration. *British Journal of Anaesthesia*, **87** (4), 638–640.

Straus, S.E., Richardson, W.S., Glasziou, P. & Haynes, R.B. (2005) *Evidence-Based Medicine: How to Practice and Teach EBM*, 3rd edn. Elsevier, Edinburgh.

Subramaniam, K., Subramaniam, B. & Steinbrook, R.A. (2004) Ketamine as adjuvant analgesic to opioids: a quantitative and qualitative systematic review. *Anesthesia and Analgesia*, **99** (2), 482–495.

Tramèr, M.R., Schneider, J., Marti, R.-A. & Rifat, K. (1996) Role of magnesium sulphate in postoperative analgesia. *Anesthesiology*, **84** (2), 340–347.

Tramèr, M.R., Williams, J.E., Carroll, D., Wiffen, P.J., Moore, R.A. & McQuay, H.J. (1998) Comparing analgesic efficacy of non-steroidal anti-inflammatory drugs given by different routes in acute and chronic pain: a qualitative systematic review. *Acta Anaesthesiologica Scandinavica*, **42** (1), 71–79.

Wu, C.L., Cohen, S.R., Richman, J.M., *et al.* (2005) Efficacy of postoperative patient-controlled and continuous infusion epidural analgesia versus intravenous patient-controlled analgesia with opioids. *Anesthesiology*, **103** (5), 1079–1088.

Useful websites

Bandolier (Evidence-based thinking about health care): *//www.jr2.ox.ac.uk/bandolier/*.
The Cochrane Collaboration: *www.cochrane.org./*.

8 Regional Anaesthesia and Analgesia, Part 1: Peripheral Nerve Blockade

Barbora Parizkova and Shane George

Key Messages

- Regional anaesthesia requires the same standard of preparation and monitoring as general anaesthesia.
- Regional anaesthesia alone or with general anaesthesia can decrease complications associated with surgery.
- The effects may persist for several hours after surgery.
- Appropriate care of the anaesthetised area is required in the postoperative period.
- Regular observation and vigilance can prevent or detect serious complications earlier and reduce the extent of complications.

Introduction

Regional anaesthesia and analgesia comprise a range of techniques that provide isolated localised anaesthesia (ability to perform surgery) or analgesia (pain relief). These techniques may be used alone, with sedation, or as part of a general anaesthetic technique, and often the analgesia can be extended into the postoperative period.

It is perhaps surprising that regional anaesthesia does not have the long history of anaesthetic techniques that included the use of alcohol, morphia, hemp, mandrake etc. The arrival of the coca leaf from South America, the detailed description of anatomy and the development of the syringe and needle allowed Koller and Freud to start the experience in the mid-nineteenth century.

The specific benefits of avoiding or minimising the complications of general anaesthesia, including respiratory and neurological compromise, are attractive. This is relevant in subgroups of patients, such as the elderly, the obese or those with chronic respiratory disease. Moreover, the development of newer

127

pharmaceutical agents and better techniques to identify nerves (including specific needles and cannulae, nerve stimulators and ultrasound) has increased the safety and success rate of individual procedures. Regional anaesthesia may also have additional useful non-analgesic benefits, such as regional sympathetic blockade.

Nevertheless, as in every procedure there are recognised complications, which should be proactively searched for to limit the extent of damage. This chapter does not aim to detail the specifics of undertaking procedures (there are many excellent textbooks that would be more appropriate), but aims to inform the general considerations about managing various regional anaesthetic techniques in the perioperative period.

General considerations

All regional anaesthesia is based on the exposure of nerves to local anaesthetics, or other drugs, that have been introduced close to the relevant nerves usually with a needle. General contraindications to the use of any regional block are patient refusal, infection of the area and significant coagulation abnormalities (Level II: Horlocker *et al.* 2003).

The peripheral nerves have a uniform structure (see Fig. 8.1). The neurone is the basic functional unit responsible for the conduction of nerve impulses.

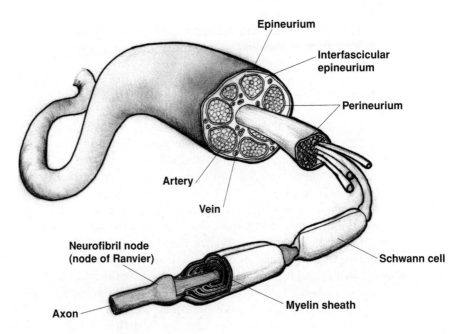

Figure 8.1 The peripheral nerve.

Neurons are the longest cells in the body. The cell body has a several branching processes, called dendrites, and a single axon. Dendrites receive information and axons conduct outgoing information. In peripheral nerves, axons are very long. The peripheral nerve is composed of three parts – somatosensory or afferent neurons, motor or efferent neurons and autonomic neurons. In the peripheral nerve, individual axons are enveloped in connective tissue, the endoneurium, which is a delicate layer around each nerve suspended within perineurium. Small groups of axons form a bundle called a nerve fascicle. The perineurium surrounds each fasciculus and splits with it at each branching point. The epineurium surrounds the entire nerve and holds it loosely to the connective tissue through which it runs. Nerves receive blood from the adjacent blood vessels running along their course.

The thinner the nerves, or those not protected by a myelin sheath, are the more easily penetrated (Fig. 8.2). Most nerves have a combination of fibres and the thinnest nerves are blocked preferentially and for longer. Sympathetic fibres are blocked with the lowest concentration of drug, followed by pain, touch and finally motor fibres.

Unlike general anaesthesia, there is a failure rate for regional anaesthetic techniques, and a plan for management of failure should be in place. Additionally, some complications, e.g. inadvertent intravenous injection of local anaesthetics or respiratory depression, may require urgent induction of general anaesthesia. Therefore, apart from the most minor procedures, patients should be prepared for regional anaesthesia as they would for general anaesthesia, including being nil-by-mouth and premedication as necessary. The standard of equipment and monitoring should similarly allow safe general anaesthesia if required. Infective complications can be quite devastating and full aseptic precautions, including a sterile field with surgical preparation and gloves and gown, are required for the major techniques.

Inadvertent intravenous injection or excessive dosage can result in high blood levels and is characterised by tingling of the lips and tongue, confusion, light-headedness, unconsciousness, convulsions and coma (Fig. 8.3).

Postoperatively, a number of complications may have a delayed presentation and therefore need continued vigilance (Table 8.1). For frequently done procedures, a separate assessment form may be the most appropriate tool. Additionally, unlike general anaesthesia, the effects of regional anaesthesia may persist for a few hours postoperatively and requires the anaesthetised region to be appropriately cared for. Some examples include anaesthetised limbs that are heavy and poorly controlled, which unless protected can cause injury. Similarly the loss of sensation means that these areas cannot protect themselves from temperature (hot tea or coffee) or pressure (prolonged immobility) and appropriate advice must be given to protect against damage.

For continuous infusions, regular observations are required to adjust the dose and rate of infusions so that the level of block is adequate, to treat side effects early and to be vigilant for more difficult but rare complications, such as abscesses and haematoma with compression syndromes of the relevant nerves.

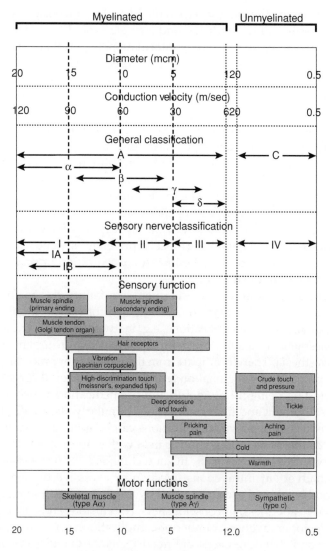

Figure 8.2 Classification and function of peripheral nerves. (From *Hadzic Text-book of Regional Anaesthesia*, McGraw-Hill.)

Figure 8.4 provides an algorithm for the early investigation and management of these rarer complications as this can lead to better eventual outcomes.

Commonly used agents

Local anaesthetic agents may be grouped as the short-acting ester and the moderate and long-acting amide drugs (see Chapter 6 for a more extensive

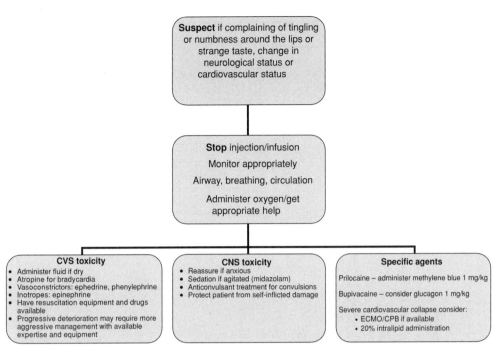

Figure 8.3 Complications of local anaesthetics used in regional anaesthesia.

discussion of their pharmacology). Examples of esters include procaine, chlorprocaine and tetracaine. Amides examples are bupivacaine, levobupivacaine, ropivacaine and lidocaine. Table 8.2 lists the commonly used local anaesthetics and maximum recommended doses. These agents typically act by penetrating the nerve structure and stabilising the nerves, so they fail to depolarise with the nerve impulse and therefore block the transmission of the nerve impulse.

Additional agents may be used with the local anaesthetics, including vasoconstrictors (epinephrine) or bicarbonate (used to prolong or improve the efficacy of the local anaesthetic and opioids) and clonidine (for their synergistic action).

Review of evidence in different populations

The evidence for the use of regional anaesthetic techniques can be compelling but, despite this, local preference or technical expertise and enthusiasm are the drivers of its use. The one area where its use is almost universal is in the *obstetric* population where the use of regional techniques is credited with significantly decreasing maternal mortality (Douglas 2004). Other advantages include reduction of gastric aspiration, avoidance of depressant anaesthetic drugs and allowing the mother to be awake during delivery. Regional techniques have

131

Table 8.1 General complications of regional anaesthesia.

Local	Nerve trauma/intraneural injection	Suspect with severe pain on injection	Avoid with short bevel/blunt needles
	Vascular	Ischaemia/haematoma	Some nerves are particularly susceptible to ischaemia, e.g. sciatic nerve
		Many nerves run in a neurovascular bundle, so damage to vascular structures can give rise to dissection of arteries and ischaemia, false aneurysms and shunt formation and haematoma	
	Neurotoxic injectate	Inappropriate solution used, e.g. preservative solutions	Longer term – arachnoiditis very rare
	Infection/abscesses		
Regional/remote	Related to technique/approach used		Some examples include: Pneumothorax with supraclavicular block
			Subdural/intrathecal migration of epidural catheters
			Pressure/temperature damage of anaesthetised areas
Drug related	Toxicity	Intravascular injection	Use safer newer agents – levobupivacaine and ropivacaine
		Overdose	
	Anaphylaxis		More commonly seen with the ester agents

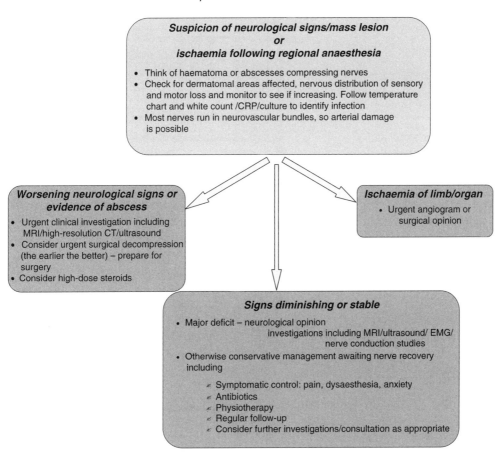

Figure 8.4 Suspicion of neurological signs following regional anaesthesia.

become an accepted form of pain relief during labour and vaginal or caesarean delivery.

Regional anaesthesia can be particularly challenging in *high-risk surgical* patients undergoing orthopaedic, thoracic, abdominal or vascular surgery but, on the other hand, can offer perioperative benefits with stress-response attenuation, a shorter hospital stay and intense postoperative analgesia (Level II: Stritesky *et al.* 2004). Diabetics and the elderly benefit from the selective anaesthesia provided by peripheral nerve blocks.

In *elderly* patients, the anaesthesia-related morbidity and mortality remain increased due to the higher incidence of coexisting age-related diseases. Regional anaesthesia may reduce the incidence of thromboembolic complications in this group, especially in orthopaedic and lower limb vascular surgery (Donadoni *et al.* 1989).

Patients with coexisting severe *pulmonary disease* undergoing regional anaesthesia have improved pulmonary outcomes in comparison with those

Table 8.2 Typical doses of local anaesthetic agents and maximum recommended doses.

Agent (%) 1% = 10 mg/mL	Spinal			Epidural			Peripheral nerve blockade		
	Volume (mL)	Onset (min)	Duration of action (min)	Volume (mL)	Onset (min)	Duration of action (min)	Volume (mL)	Onset (min)	Duration of action (min)
Lignocaine (5%)	1–2	3–5	30–90	15–30	10–15	80–120	30–50	10–20	120–240
Bupivacaine (0.5%)	3–4	5–8	75–150	15–20	18–30	160–220	30–50	10–20	360–720
Levobupivacaine (0.5%)	3–4	5–8	75–150	15–20	15–20	160–220	30–50	10–20	360–720
Ropivacaine (0.5%)				15–30	10–20	180–360	15–30	15–30	120–360

undergoing general anaesthesia (Van Zundert *et al.* 2006). For *obese* patients, regional anaesthesia can be the only option because of cardiopulmonary and airway complications during general anaesthesia (Noble & McCallum 2004).

Regional anaesthesia in *infants* and *children* remains uncommon. Infants exposed to significant pain in the neonatal period may experience behavioural changes with advancing age (Taddio *et al.* 1997). Analgesia can be easily improved by using epidural (caudal – the most commonly used, lumbar and thoracic) or spinal blocks. Spinal blocks are used in the preterm infant undergoing hernia repair (Gerber 2000). Earlier ambulation and rapid weaning from ventilators are the benefits.

Peripheral neural blockade

Any patient scheduled for surgery on an extremity should be considered a candidate for peripheral nerve block anaesthesia (Grant *et al.* 2001). Most patients can benefit from infiltrative local anaesthesia at least. One of the most important advances in regional anaesthesia was the introduction of the portable peripheral nerve stimulator in the late 1970s and early 1980s. Over the last decade, ultrasound has also developed into a promising method for nerve localisation.

Continuous peripheral nerve blocks provide many advantages in the perioperative period, including the ability for long-term (days to weeks) pain management to enhance comfort for sleep, rehabilitation, dressing changes and transport. These techniques provide the possibility to prolong anaesthesia while avoiding the risks of general anaesthesia. After surgery there is superior analgesia, reduced opioid consumption and decreased opioid-related side effects. There is evidence that patients receiving continuous pain relief have a smoother postoperative period, better respiratory function and less morbidity. A variety of different techniques are available and some of the more common ones are described below.

Upper limb regional analgesia

The nerves of the upper extremity (i.e. the arm and hand) originate in the neck (Fig. 8.5) where they exit from the spinal cord. These nerves form a complicated web of nerves known as the brachial plexus. The plexus is formed by the ventral rami of the fifth to eight cervical nerves and the greater part of the ventral ramus of the first thoracic nerve. This network of nerves gives rise to the three main nerves (median, radial and ulnar). These nerves (the brachial plexus) can be blocked at different levels to provide regional anaesthesia to the arm. The different approaches to the brachial plexus favour different branches within it and include interscalene (for shoulder surgery), infraclavicular (for catheter placement) and the older techniques of axillary and supraclavicular

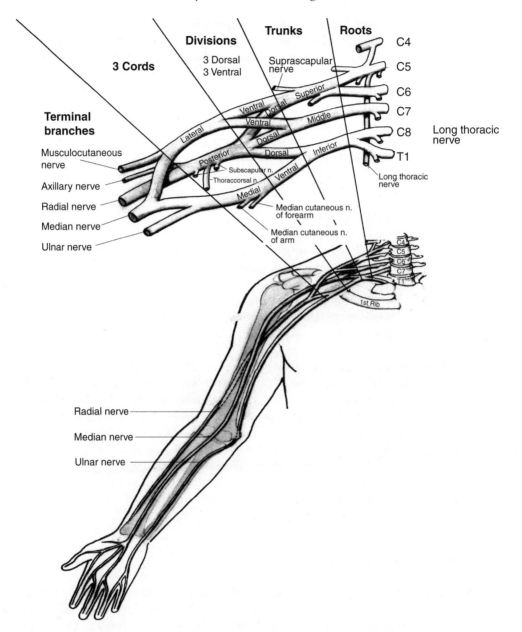

Figure 8.5   The nerves of the upper extremity.

block. More distal elbow and wrist blocks are also available for the specific nerves or to improve patchy brachial plexus blockade.

Brachial plexus blockade

Axillary block is probably the most widely taught and thus most frequently used approach to the brachial plexus. It has low risk of serious complications because the brachial plexus is relatively superficial in the axilla. This approach is typically chosen for anaesthesia of the distal upper limb (forearm, wrist or hand). In the axilla, the median and musculocutaneus nerves lie superior to the artery, whereas the ulnar and radial lie inferior to it. The most common technique is the triple-injection nerve stimulator approach with electrolocation of the median, musculocutaneus and radial nerves. The continuous axillary block is used for acute postoperative pain and management of chronic pain (Koscielnik-Nielsen 2007).

Infraclavicular blockade has similar indications like axillary block (hand, forearm, elbow and arteriovenous fistula surgery) but has a particular advantage over the axillary approach for continuous pain management (Clark 2007), as it is preferable for catheter placement.

The supraclavicular block is performed by inserting the needle just behind the collarbone, or clavicle, and is often used for surgery or managing pain related to the elbow. While easy to perform, its use has fallen out of favour because of the associated risk of pneumothorax.

The interscalene block is very similar to the supraclavicular block but differs in that the site of injection is closer to the base of the neck, behind the lateral edge of the sternocleidomastoid muscle in the interscalenic groove (Borgeat & Blumenthal 2007). It is most commonly used for postoperative pain management following surgery on the shoulder.

Lower limb regional analgesia

The lower limb is innervated by nerves which leave the lumbar area and the sacral area (Fig. 8.6). The lumbar nerves join to form the lumbar plexus which gives rise to nerves, including the femoral and obturator nerves, which innervate the front of the leg, while the sacral nerves join to form the sciatic nerve that innervates the back of the leg. Effective blockade for surgical procedures often needs more than one block, although analgesia may require only a single block.

Common techniques include

- Lumbar plexus block: anterior, posterior approach and continuous blockade
- Saphenous nerve block
- Sciatic nerve block: posterior and lateral approach

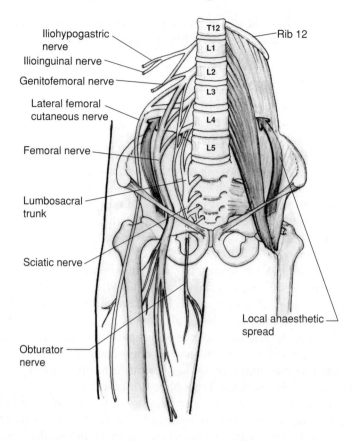

Figure 8.6   The lumbar and sacral plexus origin and lower limb innervations.

- Tibial and common peroneal nerve
- Popliteal fossa block
- Common peroneal nerve block at the neck of the fibula
- Ankle nerve blocks

Femoral nerve blockade

The femoral nerve block is easy to perform and is associated with a low risk of complications. Used for surgery on the anterior aspect of the thigh, it can also be employed to provide postoperative pain management after femur and knee surgery. In the emergency room this block can facilitate physical and radiologic examination of the fractured femur or hip. The femoral nerve is the largest nerve of the lumbar plexus. A useful mnemonic LOVAN (lymph nodes, vein, artery, nerve) describes the medial to lateral relationship of the femoral nerve to the vessels in the inguinal crease.

The needle insertion (connected to the nerve stimulator) is below the inguinal crease and immediately lateral (1 cm) to the pulse of the femoral artery. The needle is advanced through the fascia lata until quadriceps muscle contractions (patellar twitch) are obtained. The catheter is inserted 5–10 cm beyond and secured in place. A bolus of 20 mL of local anaesthetic is injected and followed by a continuous infusion.

For knee surgery, continuous femoral nerve block is as effective as continuous lumbar plexus block or continuous epidural analgesia (Chelly *et al.* 2001).

Lumbar plexus blockade

Continuous lumbar plexus blockade has been used for femoral shaft and neck fractures and knee procedures. The needle is introduced perpendicular through the skin in search of the transverse process of L5 and then oriented slightly cranially. At a depth of 3 cm, a quadriceps contraction was elicited, indicating the stimulation of the lumbar plexus. Continuous infusion is always initiated after an initial bolus of dilute local anaesthetic through the catheter. Large volumes of local anaesthetic are used to achieve anaesthesia of entire plexus.

Sciatic nerve blockade

Sciatic nerve block (SNB) is usually performed in conjunction with femoral nerve block or with a lumbar plexus block. This approach gives good perioperative and postoperative analgesia for hip, knee or foot surgery. In the classical posterior approach, the needle is inserted 4 cm distal to the midpoint between the greater trochanter and posterosuperior iliac spine. Newer approaches using nerve stimulators or ultrasound are also available. 'Single-shot' SNB usually can provide analgesia for up to 36 h, and continuous SNB is therefore indicated in special circumstances (amputation of a lower extremity).

Postoperative care

Limb blocks are not associated with major systemic effects. Postoperative care includes protection of the anaesthetised limb and introducing alternative analgesia as the blocks wear off.

For maintaining analgesia with continuous peripheral nerve blocks, dilute solutions of a long-acting local anaesthetic (usually 0.125% bupivacaine, 0.125% levobupivacaine or 0.2% ropivacaine) as continuous infusions can be utilised. Ropivacaine is preferable because of its relative sparing effect on the motor neurons and its lower cardiotoxicity (Table 8.2).

Different modes of administration can be used, including continuous background infusion, repeated boluses and a combination of both (in which the bolus administration is patient controlled). The use of boluses to produce analgesia relatively promptly offers the advantage of adjusting the level of analgesia to individual needs and allows the patient to manage his/her pain, which has a beneficial psychological effect. For a typical infusion regimen, see Table 8.3.

Table 8.3 Examples of local anaesthetic infusion regimens.

Catheter	Infusion rate (mL/hr)	Patient-controlled infusion
Interscalene	5–8	5 mL/hr with 2-mL bolus/20-min lockout
Super/infraclavicular	5–10	5–8 mL/hr with 2-mL bolus/20-min lockout
Axillary	5–10	5–8 mL/hr with 2-mL bolus/20-min lockout
Paravertebral	5–10	5 mL/hr with 2-mL bolus/20-min lockout
Lumbar plexus	8–15	8–10 mL/hr with 2-mL bolus/20-min lockout
Sciatic	5–10	5 mL/hr with 2-mL bolus/20-min lockout

Paravertebral blockade

Efficacy, indications, contraindications

Paravertebral nerve block (PVB) produces ipsilateral analgesia through injection of local anaesthetic alongside the vertebral column. It is advocated predominantly for unilateral surgery, e.g. thoracotomy, chest-wall trauma, breast surgery, cholecystectomy or renal surgery, although it can be used as a bilateral technique (Baumgarten & Greengraand 2006).

In chronic pain, it is used for the treatment of benign or malignant neuralgia and angina pectoris. Specific absolute contraindications for paravertebral block are empyema and a neoplastic mass occupying the paravertebral space.

Techniques

The paravertebral space is a wedge-shaped area sandwiched between the heads and necks of the ribs (Fig. 8.7). The nervous contents of each paravertebral space are the spinal (intercostal) nerve, its dorsal ramus, the rami communicantes and anteriorly the sympathetic chain. The spinal nerve as it emerges from the intervertebral foramen is devoid of a fascial sheath and is often broken up into small nerve rootlets, which are therefore easily penetrated by local anaesthetic.

The standard technique of space location is by loss of resistance to air or saline. The patient can be in the prone, lateral or sitting position. Two or three centimetres lateral to the spinous process a Tuohy needle (if a catheter is required) is advanced perpendicular to all skin planes. At approximately 2–5 cm in an adult, the transverse process should be contacted. On bony contact, the needle is re-angled superiorly and advanced 1.0 or 1.5 cm over the top of the process until loss of resistance to air or saline is appreciated. A 'click' may be appreciated as the superior costotransverse ligament is penetrated. The depth

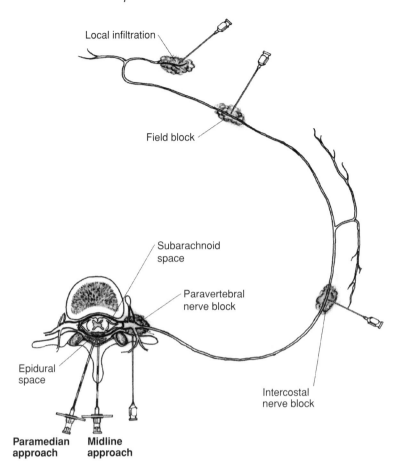

Figure 8.7   Central and peripheral techniques.

from the skin is variable but in the thoracic region the paravertebral space is usually 4–6 cm.

Catheter techniques may need greater force in feeding the catheter in comparison with epidural catheterisation.

PVB nursing care, observations and side effects

Routine postoperative observations (respiratory rate, blood pressure and heart rate) should be performed and possible side effects treated. Blood pressure should be checked every 15 min for the first hour and then 1/2 hourly for the next 2 h post-procedure.

Inadvertent epidural anaesthesia can occur because of misplacement or migration of the catheter. This results in loss of motor power to the lower torso. Any complication of epidural anaesthesia is therefore also possible with PVB techniques, although they are much less frequent.

141

Other techniques

It is not possible to cover every technique, but this chapter has explored those techniques that are most commonly extending into the postoperative period. A number of techniques such as ophthalmic blocks, dental blocks, intravenous regional anaesthesia (Bier's block) and digital ring blocks are performed relatively commonly but have not been discussed in detail and the reader is encouraged to read a comprehensive text to learn more of these techniques.

Summary

Peripheral nerve blockade can contribute significantly to a safe and more pleasant operative experience. Although a number of different techniques are in use, similar principles are required in managing them postoperatively.

References

Baumgarten, R.K. & Greengraand, R.A. (2006) Thoracic paravertebral block: is single-injection really safer? *Regional Anesthesia and Pain Medicine,* **31** (6), 584–585.

Borgeat, A. & Blumenthal, S. (2007) Interscalene brachial plexus block. In: *Textbook of Regional Anesthesia and Acute Pain Management* (ed. A. Hadzic). McGraw-Hill, New York, pp. 403–417.

Chelly, J.E., Gebhard, R., Coupe, K., *et al.* (2001) Local anesthetic delivered via a femoral catheter by patient-controlled analgesia pump for pain relief after an anterior cruciate ligament outpatient procedure. *American Journal of Anesthesiology,* **28,** 192–194.

Clark, L. (2007) Infraclavicular brachial plexus block. In: *Textbook of Regional Anesthesia and Acute Pain Management* (ed. A. Hadzic). McGraw-Hill, New York, pp. 427–440.

Donadoni, R., Baele, G., Devulder, J., *et al.* (1989) Coagulation and fibrinolytic parameters in patients undergoing total hip replacement: influence of anaesthesia technique. *Acta Anaesthesiologica Scandinavica,* **33** (7), 588–592.

Douglas, J. (2004) General anaesthesia for obstetrics: a deadly or winning combination. *Canadian Journal of Anaesthesia,* **51,** R5.

Gerber, A. (2000) Spinal and caudal anaesthesia in ex-premature babies. *Best Practise and Research Clinical Anaesthesiology,* **14** (4), 673–685.

Grant, S.A., Nielsen, K.C., Greengrass, R.A., *et al.* (2001) Continuous peripheral nerve lock for ambulatory surgery. *Regional Anesthesia and Pain Medicine,* **26** (3), 209–214.

Horlocker, T.T., Wedel, D.J., Benzon, H., *et al.* (2003) Regional anesthesia in the anti-coagulated patient: defining the risks (The Second ASRA Consensus Conference on Neuraxial Anesthesia and Anticoagulation). *Regional Anesthesia and Pain Medicine,* **28** (3), 172–197. http://www.asra.com/consensus-statements/2.html. Accessed 21 October 2007.

Koscielnik-Nielsen, Z. (2007) Axillary brachial plexus block In: *Textbook of Regional Anesthesia and Acute Pain Management* (ed. A. Hadzic). McGraw-Hill, New York, pp. 441–451.

National Patient Safety Agency (2007) *Patient Safety Alert 21. Safer Practice with Epidural Injections and Infusions.* National Patient Safety Agency, London. http://www.npsa.

nhs.uk/site/media/documents/2462_Epidural_alert_FINAL.pdf. Accessed 21 October 2007.

Noble, D. & McCallum, F. (2004) Anaesthesia for the obese patient. *Anaesthesia and Intensive Care Medicine*, **5** (3), 92–95.

Taddio, A., Katz, J., Ilierish, A.L. & Koren, G. (1997) Effect of neonatal circumcision on pain response during subsequent routine vaccination. *Lancet*, **349** (9052), 599–603.

Van Zundert, A., Stultiens, G., Jakimowicz, J., *et al.* (2006) Segmental spinal anaesthesia for cholecystectomy in a patient with severe lung disease. *British Journal of Anaesthesia*, **96** (4), 464–466.

Useful websites

American Society of Regional Anesthesia: *http://www.asra.com/*.
New York School of Regional Anesthesia: *http://www.nysora.com/*.
Regional Anesthesia and Pain Medicine (journal): *http://www.rapm.org/*.

9 Regional Anaesthesia and Analgesia, Part 2: Central Neural Blockade

Barbora Parizkova and Shane George

Key Messages

- Central neural blockade can cover a wide area.
- Significant effects on the cardiovascular system need to be managed appropriately.
- Standardised prescriptions and medicines can reduce the number of prescription errors associated with regional anaesthesia.
- Regular observation and vigilance can detect serious complications earlier and reduce extent of complications.
- Use of a catheter can allow continued postoperative analgesia but requires continued vigilance.

Neuraxial techniques – spinals and epidurals

Anatomy

Safe and effective exploitation of central neural blockade requires a thorough understanding of the anatomy of the vertebral column, ligaments, blood supply, the epidural space, spinal canal and peripheral nerves.

The vertebral column consists of seven cervical, twelve thoracic and five lumbar vertebrae (see Figure 9.1). The five sacral vertebrae form the sacrum and four coccygeal form the coccyx. The main functions of the vertebral column are to maintain erect posture and to protect the spinal cord. The vertebrae articulate at the intervertebral joints and are connected by a series of ligaments.

The spinal canal formed by vertebral foramina provides support and protection to the spinal cord and its nerve roots. From the spinal cord extend spinal nerves which contain motor, sensory and very often autonomic fibres (see Figure 9.2). Preganglionic fibres of the sympathetic nervous system leave the

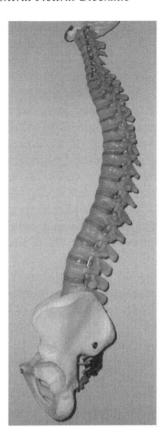

Figure 9.1 The vertebral column.

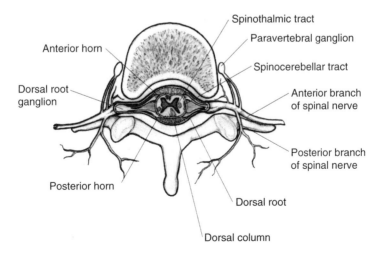

Figure 9.2 Transverse view of vertebral anatomy, including the origin of the spinal nerves.

spinal cord between T1 and L2. They emerge with spinal nerves and form the sympathetic chain which forms the stellate ganglion, splanchnic nerves and the coeliac plexus.

Three layers of membranes surround the spinal cord and its roots. Close to the surface of the spinal cord and roots of the spinal nerves is a thin layer – the pia mater. This is enclosed by a second layer – the arachnoid mater – and the resulting enclosed area is the subarachnoid space. This space is filled with cerebrospinal fluid (CSF) and blood vessels to and from the spinal cord pass through it. Superficial to the arachnoid is the thicker dura mater, and the enclosed area is the subdural space. The space superficial to the dura mater is the epidural space, which is bound posteriorly by the ligamentum flavum and laterally by the pedicles and the intervertebral foramina. It is filled with fat veins, lymphatics and nerve roots, but there is no free fluid. A decrease in epidural fat with age explains the age-related changes in epidural dose requirements (see Figure 9.3).

The safest point of entry into epidural space is below the lower border of the L1 vertebrae because of possible spinal cord injury. In adults, it means the lower border of the L1 vertebrae, and in children, at the lower border of the L3 vertebrae. The connection between the superior aspect of the iliac crests crosses either the spinous process of L4 or the L4–5 interspace.

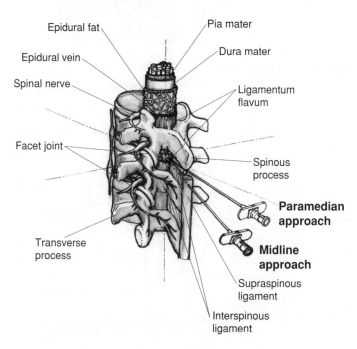

Figure 9.3 Anatomy for neuraxial techniques.

Specific contraindications to neuraxial anaesthesia

Absolute contraindications to neuraxial anaesthesia include patient refusal, infection at the site of injection, hypovolaemia, indeterminate neurologic disease (Vadalouca *et al.* 2002), severe coagulopathy and increased intracranial pressure. Relative contraindications include sepsis at a site distant from the puncture, the uncooperative patient and severe anatomic abnormalities of spine.

Anticoagulant and antiplatelet therapies are increasingly used for general medical conditions but this increases the risk of haematoma formation in regional techniques with subsequent nerve damage. The American Society of Regional Anesthesia and Pain Medicine (Horlocker *et al.* 2003) recommends the epidural block to be placed 4 hr after the last dose of subcutaneous heparin and 12 hr after the last dose of low-molecular-weight heparin (LMWH). Non-steroidal anti-inflammatory drugs (NSAIDs) including aspirin and internationalised ratio (INR) <1.5 are not considered to be contraindications to epidural placement. GIIa/IIb inhibitors should be withheld for at least 4 weeks after epidural placement and epidural placement should be avoided for 7 days after clopidogrel and 14 days after ticlopidin use. A further discussion on the risks associated with anticoagulation and thromboprophylaxis with neuraxial analgesia can be found in Chapter 14.

Side effects and complications of neuraxial blockade

Inadequate analgesia

Inadequate analgesia may be present for a number of reasons, including incomplete coverage of the surgical area, septated epidural spaces or migration of catheters. These are usually managed by repositioning, by increasing the concentration or rate of the epidural infusion, or by introducing other agents such as opioids or alpha agonists into the epidural space. Systemic agents – including NSAIDs, paracetamol and tramadol – can also ameliorate breakthrough pain.

Cardiovascular effects

The intense cardiac sympathetic blockade may result in bradycardia, which should respond to anticholinergics such as atropine. Similarly, hypotension is seen as a result of autonomic blockade and venous pooling. The aetiology of the hypotension should be determined and may be accompanied by nausea and vomiting. Administer intravenous (IV) fluids, elevate the patient's legs and closely monitor blood pressure (BP). Subsequently, a vasopressor such as ephedrine or phenylephrine may be required. Ephedrine may exert its effects for up to 1 hr after IV administration, while phenylephrine's effect may last for only 15 min. A falling BP associated with an increased pulse rate, decreasing urine output, loss of skin turgor and a dry mouth should indicate the need for volume replacement. Sympathetic blockade commonly causes vasodilatation below the level of block.

Pruritus

Pruritus (itching) occurs in up to in 8.5% of patients. It is thought to result from activation of opioid receptors in the spinal cord (Ballantyne *et al.* 1988) and is seen when opioids are used in the epidural or spinal space. It can be managed with antihistamines or failing this a small dose of parenteral naloxone.

Nausea and vomiting

The causes of postoperative nausea and vomiting (PONV) can be multifactorial (Kovac 2000) but are usually related to opioid use or significant hypotension. PONV usually responds to $5HT_3$ inhibitors such as ondansetron or dolasetron. Resistant nausea may respond to a bolus of low-dose parenteral steroids (e.g. dexamethasone) or a change or dose reduction of the neuraxial opioid.

Urinary retention

Urinary retention is more common in men with receiving opioids and inhibition of the parasympathetic nervous system of the bladder (Level III: Sand *et al.* 1998). These are among the last autonomic fibres to regain function. Significant retention usually occurs in the first 24–48 hr and often resolves spontaneously, but regular pelvic palpation or urinary catheterisation may be required.

Oversedation and respiratory depression

Respiratory depression can occur due to the absorption of opioids into the circulation or CSF (Hepner 2000). Regular assessment of the level of sedation, the character of respiration and O_2 saturation are essential and reduction of the epidural infusion rate or even naloxone as a continuous infusion may sometimes be required.

Postdural puncture headache

Postdural puncture headache, also known as spinal headache, indicates leak of CSF through the dura. Signs and symptoms of leakage, which may occur from 6 to 12 hr after the procedure up to the second postoperative day, include frontal or occipital head pain, tinnitus, double vision, nausea and photophobia. The headache is position dependent and worsens when the patient's head is elevated (Lybecker *et al.* 1995). The headache can be one of the most disabling complications after epidural blocks, but is more frequent with spinal anaesthesia as the mechanism requires dural puncture. The pain is usually located in the occipital region and may be associated with neck stiffness. Mild cases respond to regular simple analgesics, such as paracetamol or other NSAIDs, caffeine or gabapentin (Level I: Choi 2001). Hydration with regular oral or IV fluids should be maintained. More persistent headache may require an epidural blood patch, where 10–20 mL of the patient's blood is injected into the epidural space to stop the CSF leak ('epidural blood patch'). The clot serves as a haemostatic plug, closing the dural tear and preventing further CSF leakage. This technique is usually rapidly effective in 70–80% of cases (Level II: Oedit *et al.* 2005).

Epidural abscess and haematoma

Epidural abscesses and haematoma are much rarer complications but have devastating consequences if not managed appropriately. Epidural haematoma is as likely to occur on removal of the epidural catheter as on insertion and anticoagulants must be timed appropriately. Haematoma have developed where thrombolytic drugs have been used when an epidural is in situ. Abscess formation should be suspected in the presence of pyrexia, localised pain or increasing sensory and motor dysfunction. Early investigation with magnetic resonance imaging or other suitable investigation followed by early (<12 h) intervention leads to the best results. Further information on risk of abscess and haematoma formation can be found in Chapter 14.

Epidural blockade

Epidural blockade can be placed at any level of the spine and is often used for procedures involving the lower limbs, pelvis, perineum and lower abdomen. Its most common use is for maternal analgesia in labour. More uncommonly, high thoracic epidural anaesthesia is used in cardiac surgery (Level II: Scott *et al.* 2001). Michalek reported the use of cervical epidural anaesthesia at the C6–7 level for a total parathyroidectomy with parathyroid gland implantation into the forearm (Michalek *et al.* 2004).

Epidural blockade can provide anaesthesia and analgesia, but is also used in the diagnosis and treatment of chronic disease syndromes. Epidural analgesia can supplement general anaesthesia, decreasing the need for deep levels of general anaesthesia, therefore providing a more haemodynamically stable operative course. It provides effective postoperative pain management and more rapid recovery from surgery.

Epidural anaesthesia or analgesia also reduces the adverse physiological responses to surgery, such as autonomic hyperactivity, cardiovascular stress (Beattie *et al.* 2001), increased metabolic rate, pulmonary dysfunction (Level I: Ballantyne *et al.* 1998) and immune system dysfunction (Level II: Kawasaki *et al.* 2007), and is especially useful in patients with concomitant pulmonary disease.

Thoracic epidural anaesthesia has been shown to decrease the incidence of myocardial infarction and postoperative pulmonary complications (Level II:

Stritesky *et al.* 2004) and to promote the return of gastrointestinal (GI) motility without compromising fresh suture lines in the GI tract (Holte & Kehlet 2001).

Well-conducted randomised trials (Level I: Rodgers *et al.* 2000) have demonstrated the perioperative use of epidural anaesthesia and analgesia may reduce overall mortality and morbidity by approximately 30% compared with general anaesthesia using systemic opioids. Neuraxial blockade reduced the odds of deep-vein thrombosis by 44%, pulmonary embolism by 55%, pneumonia by 39% and respiratory depression by 59%.

Epidural techniques

Appropriate patient positioning aids successful placement of the epidural needle and catheter. For the obese patient, the midline sitting approach is easier than lateral decubitus position. Oxygen by mask should be administered prior to sedation (10–50 mcg/kg of midazolam with remifentanil 0.3–0.5 mcg/kg or fentanyl). Electrocardiography, BP and pulse oximetry monitoring are the minimum requirements.

Prepared sterile, disposable, epidural trays, with a styletted Tuohy needle (a curved tip needle to reduce accidental dural puncture) (Figure 9.4), are available. The spine is prepared and draped in a sterile fashion. Different techniques

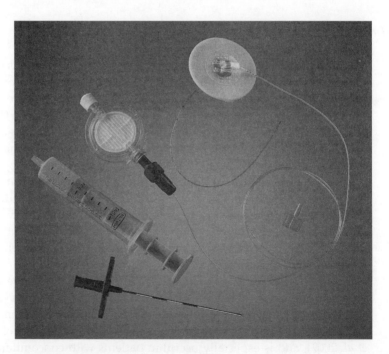

Figure 9.4 An epidural pack containing (from top to bottom) epidural catheter with fixation device, filter and connector, loss of resistance device and a Tuohy needle. (Reproduced with permission from Smiths Medical.)

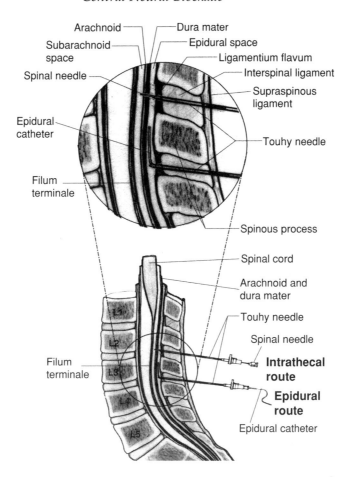

Figure 9.5 Approaches to the epidural and spinal (intrathecal) spaces.

may be used to identify the epidural space: loss of resistance (to air or saline), hanging drop and ultrasonography. The most commonly used approaches to the epidural space are midline and paramedian (Figure 9.5). The caudal approach is most commonly used in paediatrics.

To ensure that the catheter is not misplaced (subarachnoid, intravascular or subdural), a 'test dose' – 3 mL of 1.5% lidocaine with 15 mcg of epinephrine – is used, although some argue that epinephrine 15 mcg as a test dose for IV injection appears to create more problems than it solves (Dain *et al.* 1987).

Spinal (intrathecal or subarachnoid) anaesthesia

Spinal (intrathecal) anaesthesia is achieved by a single injection of local anaesthetic into the subarachnoid space to create sensory, motor and autonomic blockade of the nerve roots and spinal cord. It is indicated for surgical procedures with limited postoperative analgesic requirements below the diaphragm. Spinal anaesthesia is commonly used for total joint replacement and prostatectomy. It can benefit patients with cardiac or respiratory disease because it avoids or lessens the risk of many adverse effects associated with general anaesthesia, e.g. cardiovascular and respiratory depression, aspiration, incompetent airway and inadequate ventilatory drive resulting in hypoxaemia. Patients with a history of airway problems, difficult intubation and reactive airway disease also are good candidates for a spinal anaesthetic because of its shorter recovery time, minimal drug exposure and possibly reduced blood loss related to sympathetic blockade.

Bupivacaine is the most commonly used agent and is often combined with opioids, usually morphine or fentanyl. The opioid both hastens the onset of analgesia and prolongs analgesic effects. As the drug is given intrathecally, it comes into direct contact with the spinal cord, with its unmyelinated fibres; the drug is effective at a fraction of the dose that would be given via the epidural route.

Technique

Currently, commercially prepared, disposable spinal trays are available. Needles of different diameters and shapes have been developed for regional anaesthesia. These are shown in Figure 9.6 and include pencil-point needles (Sprotte and Whitacre) that have a rounded, non-cutting bevel with a solid tip and the Quincke, with a cutting bevel needle. The bevel of the needle should be directed longitudinally to decrease the incidence of postdural puncture headache. The

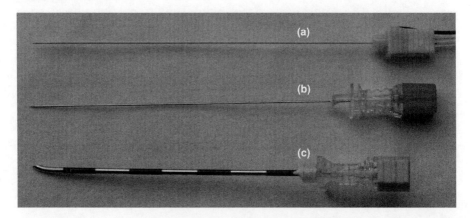

Figure 9.6 Examples of specialist needles used for regional anaesthesia: (a) insulated, short-bevel, peripheral nerve block needle for use with a nerve stimulator; (b) fine 27G needle (Quincke) used for spinal puncture; (c) larger 16G curved-ended needle (Tuohy) for epidural space identification.

L3–4 interspace or the L4–5 interspace are generally used to introduce the spinal needle. Levels above L1/L2 are avoided as the spinal cord extends down to the L1–2 level. When trying to limit the effects to the sacral/lumbar areas, a hyperbaric solution so-called *Marcain heavy* (bupivacaine 0.5% in 8% glucose) is used with the patients remaining sitting for at least 5 min to allow the drugs to settle into that region.

An indwelling catheter has been used for continuous spinal anaesthesia (especially in palliative care), but this remains a minority interest because of the fear of infection and longer term arachnoiditis. A larger gauge needle, such as a Tuohy, is used to enable the passage of the catheter. The catheter is passed 2–3 cm into the subarachnoid space and is secured to the skin surface with a transparent, sterile, semipermeable polyurethane dressing.

Duration of action

The duration of effect varies with different local anaesthetics (see Table 8.2). Opioid selection depends on the type of procedure, the expected length of time needed for pain management and the drug's lipophilic or hydrophilic characteristics. Lipid-soluble drugs such as fentanyl and sufentanil penetrate the dura mater faster than water-soluble opioids, providing a faster onset of action but a shorter duration of action. Preservative-free morphine, which is water soluble, has a slower onset of action and longer duration of action (12–24 h). For these reasons, fentanyl typically is given for immediate pain control in same-day surgery patients; morphine is a better choice for patients who need more prolonged analgesia.

Continuing care and observation

Regular continuous monitoring of heart rate, BP and pulse oximetry is required. Vital signs should be monitored every 5–15 min until stable. Patients with epidural infusions require support and explanation and the perioperative team should be aware of its planned use. This ensures that perioperative thromboprophylaxis (LMWH), anticoagulation and antiplatelet therapy can be appropriately timed. Suitable personnel should escort patients who are going for investigations, whilst the epidural or spinal catheter remains in situ.

A significant advantage of epidural catheter placement is the ability to continue analgesia into the postoperative period minimal use of systemic opioids. A continuous infusion with nurse-initiated changes or a patient-controlled infusion (PCEA) may be used. The PCEA parameters typically consist of 3–5 mL of low-dose-combination opioid and local anaesthetic (LA) patient-controlled boluses with 5- to 20-min lockout intervals, with or without a continuous infusion. These settings may require frequent self-administration of bolus doses to maintain analgesia. Alternatively, a continuous infusion rate of 10–12 mL/hr of the same combination opioid plus LA may be used, with additional bolus doses for breakthrough pain. Increasingly, larger bolus doses with longer lockout intervals, requiring fewer interventions, are used. Newer agents can increase the safety and acceptability of infusions. This includes ropivacaine, with reduced cardiac toxicity and motor blockade, and levobupivacaine, the S(−)-enantiomer from of bupivacaine, with equivalent motor blockade but less cardiotoxicity (Launo *et al.* 2003). The pharmacology of local anaesthetic agents is detailed in Chapter 6.

Larger nerve fibres recover quicker than smaller ones; i.e. motor function (which is conducted by the largest nerve fibres) returns before other functions. As sensation returns, the patient detects light touch and pressure before temperature and pain. Motor function and sensation generally return from the hip to the feet, with higher dermatome levels recovering first.

Motor function can be assessed by asking the patient to wiggle his toes or flex and extend his foot. The level of blockade should be documented according to a dermatome chart (Figure 9.7). To evaluate the level of sensory blockade, a cold object, such as an alcohol swab, can be used. Patients may believe that their legs are flexed or elevated when they are actually lying flat; i.e. they have loss of proprioception: The brain remembers the last leg position before the block took effect. Proprioception returns with the return of sensation. It is important that legs are not allowed to be placed in unphysiologic positions and kept away from radiators.

The catheter insertion site should be inspected to detect leaks, haemostasis and catheter migration. In addition to performing routine postoperative observations (respiratory rate, blood pressure and heart rate), observations specific to epidural analgesia should be made and recorded as specified on an epidural assessment chart. Observations are initially hourly for 4 hr and then 4 hourly, continuing until 8 hr after removal of the epidural catheter. The appropriateness of continuing an epidural should be reviewed daily.

Alternative analgesia should be in place prior to cessation of the epidural. The catheter should be removed at least after 8 hr have elapsed from heparin administration and 12 hr in the case of LMWH (Level II: Horlocker *et al.* 2003). Using an aseptic technique gently, in one smooth movement, the catheter should be removed. The catheter should be checked to ensure that it is intact.

Towards safer practice with neuraxial analgesia

Over a period of 3 days, more than 20 different personnel may be responsible for epidural care. Much of epidural practice can be made safer by standardising processes but must also allow for individual patient variation of response.

The concomitant administration of infusions to the epidural space and separate IV infusions can lead to disastrous confusion in inexperienced hands. The National Patient Safety Agency Patient Safety Agency published a *Patient*

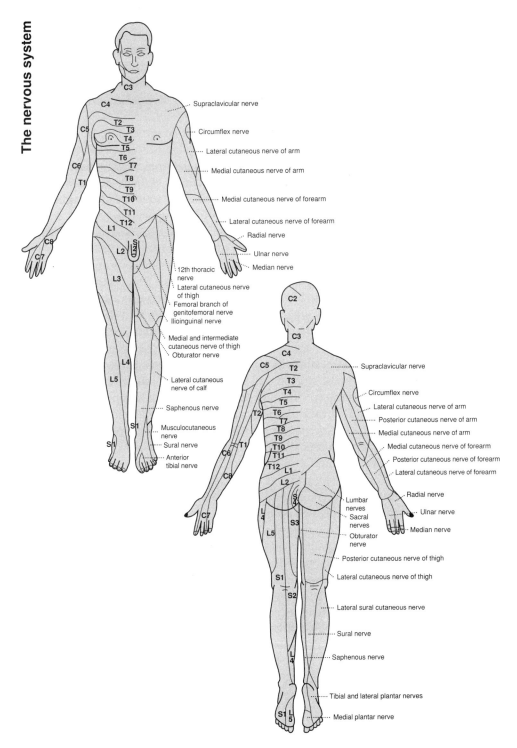

Figure 9.7 Sensory dermatomes. (© Royal Brompton & Harefield NHS Trust (2007), reproduced with permission from RBHT.)

155

Safety Alert in 2007, which focused on reducing risk associated with epidural injections and infusions (National Patient Safety Agency 2007). A number of measures are required to minimise these risks, including differentiated and dedicated epidural infusion equipment, separate storage of epidural drugs and the use of premixed bags.

The risks of infection and mechanical catheter complications and the need for escalating doses, reservoir volume, drug stability and cost are practical considerations associated with use of both external and internal infusion systems. Infusion pumps should be safe, accurate, reliable and easy to use by the patient and the health care professional and should be compatible with the drugs used. Factors to consider when comparing infusion pumps include the volume and flow rate requirements of the devices. External portable infusion devices are classified according to the mechanism of operation into three primary groups: syringe pumps, peristaltic mechanisms and elastomeric reservoir pumps. Portable patient-controlled analgesia (PCA) pumps that have syringes, flexible reservoir bags and elastomeric reservoirs have been developed. Implanted systems with flow rates that are preset at the factory make pain management more difficult when the patient requires changes or escalations in doses over time. Advantages of continuous epidural infusion include smoothing of the peaks and valleys of pain relief and the reduction of bolus injections with their risk of breakage of sterility. PCA pumps enhance the efficacy of continuous infusions by allowing the patient to administer bolus doses to control acute pain but should be clearly differentiated from regular IV PCA pumps.

Available bacterial filters (Portex/Sterifix-Braun), when perfused with reduced volumes at low injection pressures, maintain an unmodified antimicrobial function for at least 60 days (Level II: De Cicco *et al.* 1995). The giving set should be changed if there is known contamination.

Use of standard preprinted epidural analgesia prescriptions can reduce prescribing and administration errors (Level IV: Cox *et al.* 2007). The document should include patient identification label, drugs with concentration, instructions for administration (bolus doses, minimum and maximum infusion rates), instructions for treating breakthrough pain (see Figure 9.8), monitoring instructions (pain intensity, sedation level, RR, BP), instructions for treatment of side effects (Figure 9.9) and means to contact the relevant expert (anaesthetist/acute pain team).

Summary

Central neural blockade has become an established technique in obstetric practice and can significantly improve outcomes in patients with concomitant respiratory disease. Appropriate management and vigilance in the postoperative period contribute significantly to the safety and the success of its use.

Epidural Analgesia Prescription

Royal Brompton & Harefield **NHS**
NHS Trust

EPIDURAL

Patient name		Consultant surgeon
Hospital number		Procedure
Date of birth		Date of surgery
Ward		Consultant anaesthetist
Known sensitivities/allergies		Weight in kg	Pharmacy use only

Inserted at _____ to _____ depth _____ cm

EPIDURAL SOLUTION

Date	Solution	Volume	Rate range	Doctor's signature
	Levobupivacaine 0.125% + fentanyl 4mcg/ml in sodium chloride 0.9%			
	Levobupivacaine 0.125% in sodium chloride 0.9%			
	Levobupivacaine 0.125% + fentanyl _____ mcg/mL in sodium chloride 0.9%			
	Levobupivacaine 0.125% + diamorphine _____ mg in sodium chloride 0.9%			

INFUSIONS

Date	Time	Infusion type	Volume	Initial (nurse 1)	Initial (nurse 2)

BOLUS/TOP-UPS

Date	Time	Drug(s)	Volume	Anaesthetist's signature

RB100

Figure 9.8 Example of an epidural preprinted prescription chart. (© Royal Brompton & Harefield NHS Trust (2007), reproduced with permission from RBHT.)

Respiratory rate and O_2 saturation (SpO_2)	If respiratory rate <10/min, check SpO_2 and inform the patient's own doctor. If respiratory rate <8/min call the anaesthetist.
Blood pressure (BP)	If systolic BP is less than 100 mm Hg, assess whole patient. Consider fluid challenge. Contact anaesthetist if hypotension persists.
Pruritus 0 = No pruritus 1 = Pruritus 2 = Uncomfortable	Administer chlorpheniramine as first-line treatment. If no response, consider naloxone 40 µg bolus (unlicensed for this use). Contactanaesthetist if pruritus persists.
Pain intensity 0 = No pain 10 = Worst pain imaginable	If pain intensity >4–6, increase epidural infusion as prescribed. If score is still raised after 1 h contact anaesthetist. If score >7, contact anaesthetist immediately.
Nausea 0 = No nausea 10 = Severe nausea	Administer regular antiemetics. Contact anaesthetist if nausea persists.
Sedation SL = Normal sleep 0 = Fully awake 1 = Mild, occasionally drowsy, easy to rouse 2 = Moderate, constantly drowsy, easy to rouse 3 = Severe, somnolent, hard to rouse 4 = Unrousable	If patient is unrousable, stop epidural infusion. Administer oxygen via face mask, remain with patient and ask for anaesthetist to be called immediately. Consider the administration of naloxone adhering to the patient group direction.
Sensory block Level at which normal sensation returns e.g. L3 = anterior thigh, T10 = umbilicus, T4 = nipples	If block is higher than T3, sit patient up if normotensive. Reduce infusion rate or stop epidural infusion. Call anaesthetist immediately if patient is experiencing dyspnoea.
Sensation 0 = Normal sensation 1 = Altered sensation (to touch or temperature) 2 = Absence of sensation	If there is any unexpected altered sensation of upper or lower limbs, call anaesthetist.
Motor power 0 = Normal power 1 = Weakness but can lift against gravity 2 = Cannot move limb against gravity 3 = Cannot move limb	If there is any limb motor weakness, call anaesthetist.

Observations must be recorded:

- Hourly in recovery
- Hourly for the first four hours in HDU
- Four-hourly until eight hours after infusion has stopped

Neuro observations must continue for 48 hours after catheter removal.

Figure 9.9 Example of troubleshooting guidelines. (© Royal Brompton & Harefield NHS Trust (2007), reproduced with permission from RBHT.)

References

Beattie, W.S., Badner, N.H. & Choi, P. (2001) Epidural analgesia reduces postoperative myocardial infarction: a meta-analysis. *Anesthesia and Analgesia*, **93** (4), 853–858.

Ballantyne, J.C., Carr, D.B., deFerranti, S. *et al.* (1998) The comparative effects of postoperative analgesic therapies on pulmonary outcome: cumulative meta-analysis of randomized, controlled trials. *Anesthesia and Analgesia*, **86** (3), 598–612.

Ballantyne, J.C., Loach, A.B. & Carr, D.B. (1988) Itching after epidural and spinal opiates. *Pain*, **33** (2), 149–160.

Choi, P.T. (2001) Management of postdural puncture headache. *Techniques in Regional Anesthesia and Pain Management*, **5**, 41–45.

Cox, F.J., Cousins, A., Smith, A., Marwick, C. & Gullberg, C. (2007) Acute pain management after major thoracic surgery. *Nursing Times*, **103** (23), 30–31.

Dain, S.L., Rolbin, S.H. & Hew, E.M. (1987) The epidural test dose in obstetrics: is it necessary? *Canadian Journal of Anesthesia*, **34** (6), 601–605.

De Cicco, M., Matovic, M., Castellani, G.T., *et al.* (1995) Time-dependent efficacy of bacterial filters and infection risk in long-term epidural catheterization. *Anesthesiology*, **82** (3), 765–771.

Hepner, D. (2000) Neuraxial opioids and respiratory depression. *Anesthesia and Analgesia*, **91** (6), 1560–1561.

Horlocker, T.T., Wedel, D.J., Benzon, H., *et al.* (2003) Regional anesthesia in the anticoagulated patient: Defining the risks (The Second ASRA Consensus Conference on Neuraxial Anesthesia and Anticoagulation). *Regional Anesthesia and Pain Medicine*, **28** (3), 172–197. http://www.asra.com/consensus-statements/2.html. Accessed 21 October 2007.

Holte, K. & Kehlet, H. (2001) Epidural analgesia and risk of anastomotic leakage. *Regional Anesthesia and Pain Medicine*, **26** (2), 111–117.

Kawasaki, T., Ogata, M., Kawasaki, C., *et al.* (2007) Effects of epidural anaesthesia on surgical stress-induced immunosuppression during upper abdominal surgery. *British Journal of Anaesthesia*, **98** (6), 847–848.

Kovac, A.L. (2000) Prevention and treatment of postoperative nausea and vomiting. *Drugs*, **59** (2), 213–243.

Launo, C., Gastaldo, P., Piccardo, F., *et al.* (2003) Perioperative thoracic epidural analgesia in aortic surgery: role of levobupivacaine. *Minerva Anestesiologica*, **69** (10), 751–764.

Lybecker, H., Djernes, M. & Schmidt, J. (1995) Postdural puncture headache: onset, duration, severity, and associated symptoms. An analysis of 75 consecutive patients with PDPH. *Acta Anaesthesiologica Scandinavica*, **39** (5), 605–612.

Michalek, P., David, I., Adamec, M., *et al.* (2004) Cervical epidural anesthesia for combined neck and upper extremity procedures: a pilot study. *Anesthesia and Analgesia*, **99** (6), 1833–1836.

National Patient Safety Agency (2007) *Patient Safety Alert 21. Safer Practice with Epidural Injections and Infusions.* National Patient Safety Agency, London. http://www.npsa.nhs.uk/site/media/documents/2462_Epidural_alert_FINAL.pdf. Accessed 21 October 2007.

Oedit, R., van Kooten, F., Bakker, S., *et al.* (2005) Efficacy of the epidural blood patch for the treatment of the post lumbar puncture headaches. *BMC Neurology*, **5** (1), 12.

Rodgers, A., Walker, N., Schug, S., *et al.* (2000) Reduction of postoperative morbidity and mortality with epidural or spinal anesthesia: results from overview of randomised trials. *British Medical Journal*, **321** (7275), 1493.

Sand, R.P., Yarussi, A.T. & de Leon-Casasola, O.A. (1998) Complications and side effects associated with epidural bupivacaine/morphine analgesia. *Acute Pain*, **1** (2), 43–50.

Scott, N.B., Turfrey, D.J., Ray, D.A., *et al.* (2001) A prospective randomized study of the potential benefits of thoracic epidural anesthesia and analgesia in patients undergoing coronary artery bypass grafting. *Anesthesia and Analgesia*, **93** (3), 528–535.

Stritesky, M., Semrad, M., Kunstyr, J., *et al.* (2004) On pump cardiac surgery in a conscious patient using a thoracic epidural anesthesia – an ultra fast track method. *Bratislavské lekárske listy*, **105** (2), 51–55.

Vadalouca, A., Moka, E. & Sykiotis, C. (2002) Combined spinal-epidural technique for total hysterectomy in a patient with advanced, progressive multiple sclerosis. *Regional Anesthesia and Pain Medicine*, **27** (5), 540–541.

Useful websites

American Society of Regional Anesthesia: *http://www.asra.com/*.
New York School of Regional Anesthesia: *http://www.nysora.com/*.
Regional Anesthesia and Pain Medicine (journal): *http://www.rapm.org/*.

10 Patient-Controlled Analgesia

Gillian Chumbley

Key Messages

- Evidence suggests that patients are more satisfied using patient-controlled analgesia (PCA), rather than receiving conventional analgesia.
- Patients must receive an analgesic-loading dose prior to commencing PCA.
- Background infusions should be considered for patients who are taking oral opioids prior to surgery. Larger bolus doses may be required to account for tolerance.
- PCA should be discontinued only when patients have met the criteria. It should not be removed when patients are pain free, yet still require greater than 30-mg morphine (or equivalent) over a 24-h period.
- Consider the patient's views of PCA. Ensure that patients do not miss out on essential nursing care because they are receiving PCA.

Introduction

Patient-controlled analgesia (PCA) was first described by Sechzer in the 1970s (Sechzer 1971). In this work he described PCA as an 'excellent system for treating postoperative pain' and he observed that patients were generally satisfied with the results of this new technique. The original equipment used to deliver the intravenous (IV) dose of narcotic was cumbersome and was unsuitable for use in the ward environment. However, a decade later and with the advent of commercially available computerised pumps, PCA started to become an established way of treating postoperative pain.

PCA has become synonymous with giving IV narcotics, but in its broadest sense it refers to a method of pain relief, where the patient can decide how much drug they receive. It is therefore not uncommon to see patients delivering drugs via the oral, intranasal, transdermal, subcutaneous or epidural route.

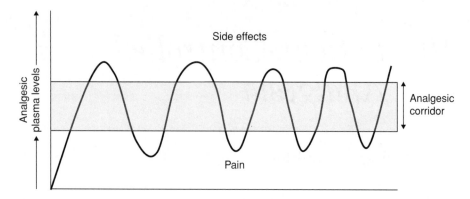

Figure 10.1 Peaks and troughs of analgesia associated with intramuscular opioids.

IV PCA has solved many of the problems associated with intramuscular injections. Patients do not have to wait or convince the nursing staff that they require pain relief; they have the potential to administer large doses of opioid and it avoids the need for frequent injections. PCA has also provided medical and nursing staff with objective documentation of how much patients vary in their need for opioids. In addition, this has given medical and nursing staff the confidence to believe patients when they say they are still in pain, having received a 'standard dose' of opioid (Lehmann 1999).

PCA is a much more efficient way of giving opioids, as it avoids the peaks and troughs in blood concentration associated with intramuscular injections (Figure 10.1). When patients start using PCA, they are loaded with opioid, until the minimum effective analgesic concentration (MEAC) in the blood is achieved (Figure 10.2). In effect this means that the patient's pain is controlled with minimal side effects. Patients will then maintain this blood level by topping themselves up with doses requested from the PCA machine, thus keeping themselves in what is known as the 'analgesic corridor'.

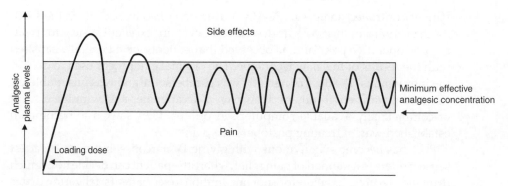

Figure 10.2 Therapeutic analgesic levels with PCA.

PCA has been readily accepted by medical and nursing staff. It has been found to save nursing time, as staff are relieved from the need to administer frequent intramuscular injections (Aitken & Kenny 1990, Koh & Thomas 1994). But some authors have speculated that the enthusiasm for PCA by nursing staff is motivated by other factors (Hall & Salmon 1997). This includes the ability to distance themselves from patients' suffering, as PCA protects ward staff from becoming too involved in the difficulties of pain management. The authors also suggest that the management of new technologies provides enhanced status for members of acute-pain teams, which are responsible for monitoring the service. The idea that technology can get in the way of the nurse/patient relationship is a subject that is discussed further in the section entitled 'Patients' views of PCA'.

The evidence for PCA versus conventional analgesia

There have now been three systematic reviews examining the evidence as to whether PCA is preferable to conventional analgesia (Level I: Ballantyne *et al.* 1993, Level I: Hudcova *et al.* 2006, Level I: Walder *et al.* 2001).

Ballantyne *et al.* (1993) conducted a meta-analysis on 15 randomised control trials with a total sample of 787 patients. They found that patients preferred PCA; there was a 42% increase in satisfaction with PCA compared with intramuscular, epidural or oral opioids, though satisfaction could only be assessed in three trials. This increase in satisfaction was not accompanied by an increase in the amount of analgesia used, or by a decrease in side effects and by only a small improvement in pain scores. The significant improvement in pain scores was only 5.6 mm on a 100-mm visual analogue scale (VAS) and it is questionable whether this small improvement is clinically relevant. The authors suggested that better designed trials were needed to establish whether PCA could produce pain relief that was clinically relevant.

Walder *et al.* (2001) analysed data from 32 randomised control trials with a total sample of 1029 patients who had received an opioid via PCA and 1082 controls who received their opioid intravenously, intramuscularly or subcutaneously. There were no significant differences between the groups in the amount of opioid used or the incidence of side effects. There were no significant differences in pain scores, though it was difficult to compare data between trials. Only pain scores at rest were analysed, as many of the trials did not report pain scores on moving. Patient satisfaction was only reported in three trials and although patients were more satisfied with PCA, this was not significant.

Hudcova *et al.* (2006) analysed data from 55 randomised control trials, with a total sample of 2023 patients who had received an opioid via PCA and 1838 controls who received their opioid intravenously, intramuscularly or subcutaneously. Patients in the PCA group reported significantly lower pain scores than those receiving conventional analgesia, though it was not stated whether these scores were at rest or moving. The difference in pain scores over the first

24 hr was 8 points on a 100-point VAS scale and it is still questionable whether such a small difference is clinically relevant.

Opioid consumption was shown to be significantly higher in the PCA group; the difference was 6.72-mg morphine equivalents in studies that reported opioid consumption from 0 to 24 h; it was found to be 23.78 mg in studies that reported opioid consumption from 0 to 72 h.

Patients were significantly more satisfied using PCA (84% PCA versus 65% controls). The incidence of side effects, such as sedation, nausea, vomiting and urinary retention, was equally distributed between both groups. Patient using PCA experienced significantly more itching than the control group.

What do the systematic reviews tell us about PCA?

It would appear from the above systematic reviews that the differences between PCA and conventional analgesia are small. The main difference still appears to be a patient preference for PCA.

Many authors have speculated as to why patients are more satisfied with PCA and some examples are shown in Table 10.1. The most dominant justification has been the control that PCA affords the patient over their pain relief.

Opioid consumption

For many professionals who work in pain management, these findings can be surprising, especially the small differences in opioid consumption between the groups. In clinical practice, intramuscular injections prescribed on a *pro re nata*

Table 10.1   Possible reasons for patient satisfaction with PCA.

Possible reasons	Reference
Immediate accessibility of analgesia	Keeri-Szanto (1979), Albert & Talbott (1988), Eisenach *et al.* (1988)
Ability to titrate analgesia against side effects	Eisenach *et al.* (1988)
Inadequate nursing care with conventional analgesia	McGrath *et al.* (1989)
Control that PCA gives the patient over their pain relief	Keeri-Szanto (1979), Albert & Talbott (1988), Wheatley *et al.* (1991)

PCA, patient-controlled analgesia.

(prn) basis do not get given. One survey found that patients received only 2.7 injections in the first 24 hr after surgery (Owen *et al.* 1990). Recent unpublished audits at my own institution have revealed that patients receive only one or two injections of morphine in a 24-h period. As there is little disparity in the amount of analgesia consumed between the groups in the research studies, it can only be concluded that in research situations, patients do receive their intramuscular pain relief.

Patient control

Chumbley *et al.* (1999) found, in a survey of patients' views, that feelings of control were not important to patients. When patients referred to control, they were merely repeating the professional's view or commenting on how successful they had been in accessing pain relief, rather than an irreducible manifestation of personal autonomy. The study found three factors that did predict patients having a positive experience with PCA and these factors are discussed in section entitled 'Patients' views of PCA'.

Satisfaction

There is one final consideration to be taken into account when trying to interpret these data from the systematic reviews and that is the issue of satisfaction. As stated earlier, patients appear to be more satisfied when using PCA, as opposed to having intramuscular injections (Ballantyne *et al.* 1993, Hudcova *et al.* 2006). This finding is curious, as patients do not appear to use more analgesic medicine and pain intensity scores are not dramatically improved. Just how accurate these measurements of satisfaction are is difficult to evaluate.

Satisfaction scores have been found to produce spurious results. Coleman & Booker-Milburn (1996) conducted an audit of postoperative pain and found that 93% patients had moderate-to-severe pain on movement, but despite high levels of uncontrolled pain, 69% patients were satisfied with their care. So it would appear that patients would say that they are satisfied with their care, even when their pain control is far from adequate. Similarly, Wheatley *et al.* (1991) found that 37% patients using PCA had moderate-to-severe pain, with 45% patients experiencing nausea, but 96% patients reported being satisfied.

There is obviously an underlying problem with measuring satisfaction, as surveys tend to produce positive results, because patients are reluctant to criticise their treatment (Fitzpatrick 1993, Fitzpatrick & Hopkins 1983). Fitzpatrick & Hopkins found that what appeared to be most important to patients was the outcome of their treatment, rather than the process that brought them to this outcome. Patients generally express satisfaction unless an extreme departure from normal practice causes them to feel dissatisfied (Williams 1994).

In conclusion, what has the evidence shown us about PCA? In test situations, where patients receive their conventional analgesia on a regular basis, there is little to choose between PCA and conventional analgesia. However, in clinical practice we know that this is far from the norm. Therefore, PCA is superior to conventional analgesia in clinical practice, as patients have immediate access to their analgesia and PCA allows them to have larger amounts of opioid than a fixed dosing regimen. This allows for the fivefold variation between patients in their need for opioids (Royal College of Surgeons of England 1990).

It is unsurprising that patients prefer PCA, as they don't have to convince nurses of their need for analgesia and don't have to experience painful injections. In terms of side effects, patients using PCA will experience the same level of side effects, with the exception of pruritus, which occurs more often in patients using PCA.

Standard prescriptions for PCA

For opioid naive patients, the examples of standard prescriptions of PCA are as follows:

- IV morphine PCA, 1-mg bolus, 5-min lockout
- IV fentanyl PCA, 10-mcg bolus, 3-min lockout
- IV oxycodone PCA, 2-mg bolus, 5-min lockout

Prescriptions may vary from centre to centre, so please refer to your local policies and procedures. Some centres prescribe PCA on self-adhesive labels that can be attached to the patient's drug chart. The anaesthetist just has to complete the prescription for the bolus dose and lockout for the individual patient. This system obviously allows for fewer prescribing errors. Preprinted labels can also include a prescription for an anti-emetic or for naloxone, the antidote of opioid agonists, to be given if respiratory depression occurs.

Standard prescriptions do not take account of conditions such as renal failure, which would require a reduction in dose. Fentanyl and oxycodone are preferred in patients with renal impairment, as they have less metabolites (see Chapter 12 for further reading on this topic).

Patient selection and contraindications for using PCA

The most important consideration in patient selection is the willingness of the patient to administer their own analgesia. This fact should not be taken for granted. Patients can find the task of administering opioids daunting. Patients are being asked to perform a task that most nurses have trained for 3 years to gain competence in. Patients are expected to perform this task, usually having had very little preoperative information; it is therefore not surprising that many are worried about taking responsibility for administration (Chumbley *et al.* 1999).

Apart from consent, it is essential for patients to understand the concept of PCA. If the patient is confused or has language difficulties, other forms of analgesia should be considered in preference. Patients must be physically able to press the button. Therefore patients who have had a stroke, arthritis or trauma to the hands may not be physically able to demand analgesia. In my own clinical practice, I came across a patient who had been attacked and received multiple lacerations to both arms. After surgery, both arms were elevated in roller towels and the patient was given PCA for pain relief. He could not even reach the button, let alone press it. You cannot therefore assume that sensible decisions are always made in theatre about postoperative pain relief.

PCA programmes and definitions

When nurses are caring for patients receiving PCA, it is extremely important that they understand the programme parameters and can check that the PCA programme matches what is prescribed on the drug chart. Each nurse should take responsibility for checking the PCA programme and checking against the prescription, when they start their shift.

Loading dose

As mentioned previously, the loading dose is the amount given to the patient to ensure that their pain is controlled, prior to starting PCA. Patients are loaded with opioid, until the MEAC in the blood is achieved, which means that the patient's pain is controlled with minimal side effects.

It is unfair for a patient to be handed the button to start PCA when they are experiencing moderate, severe or unbearable pain, as this would require the patient to press the button very regularly to effectively 'load' themselves. Most recovery or intensive care units would normally load the patient with up to 10 mg of morphine if the patient was opioid naive. As most standard PCA prescriptions start with a 1-mg bolus dose and 5-min lockout, this may require the patient to press up to ten times to achieve a comfortable state and would take a minimum of 50 min. Most patients will stop trying after three or more presses and assume that the system does not work.

Bolus dose

This is the amount of drug that the patient receives when they press the button. For most patients this is usually 1 mg of morphine. There is minimal evidence to suggest what size the bolus dose should be. Too low a dose may result in inadequate analgesia; too high a dose may result in side effects. One study found that the optimal bolus dose was 1 mg of morphine (Level II: Owen *et al.* 1989a). Another study either randomised patients to receive a standard 1-mg morphine bolus dose or offered patients a choice of doses of either 0.5-, 1.0- or 1.5-mg morphine (Level II: Love *et al.* 1996). The authors found no differences between the groups in terms of total morphine consumption, time spent with mild or severe oxyhaemoglobin desaturation, ease of controlling pain, satisfaction of pain control, experience of pain on movement or the severity of nausea. When given a choice of morphine doses, patients chose the high dose (1.5 mg) on 59% occasions. They concluded that variable-dose PCA offered no advantage over a standard-dose PCA.

Dose duration

The dose duration is the amount of time that it takes to deliver the bolus dose. Most PCA machines allow for the bolus duration to be altered. In practice, most doses are given over approximately 30–45 s. One study investigated whether prolonging the time over which the bolus dose was delivered would reduce the incidence of nausea and vomiting (Level II: Woodhouse & Mather 1998). Patients received the dose either over 40 s or over 5 min. There were no significant difference in the incidence of nausea or vomiting between the groups, but patients in the 5-min group reported more emetic episodes. So contrary to their hypothesis, prolonging the dose duration had a detrimental effect on emesis.

Lockout interval

This is the minimal time interval before another bolus dose can be requested. The main purpose of this interval is to allow time for the drug to start to work, though peak concentration of most opioids following IV administration can take up to 15 min. The lockout interval for IV PCA morphine is usually 5 min, for subcutaneous morphine 10 min and for IV fentanyl 3 min.

The lockout interval does limit the total amount of drug that the patient can request, but it should not be viewed as a method of preventing overdose. For example an IV morphine PCA with a standard dose of 1 mg and a 5-min lockout would allow the patient to receive a possible 12 mg/hr. For many patients this would be a sedating and possibly a respiratory depressing dose. The main method of preventing overdose with PCA is that the patient will fall asleep when they have had too high a dose for their individual requirements. The patient cannot press the button and request a further dose when they are asleep and so prevent themselves from overdosing. For more information about safety issues, please refer to the section on safety.

Dose limits

Dose limits can be programmed on most PCA devices, though in practice many centres do not use this facility. Dose limits will limit the amount of drug that patients can request over a 1- or 4-hr period. For example a standard programme of 1-mg morphine, with a 5-min lockout interval, will allow a patient a maximum of 12 mg/hr, or 48 mg over 4 hr. A dose limit could restrict these maximum doses to perhaps 8 mg/hr. In effect, the machine would alarm if the patient used 8 mg/hr and then requested a further dose. In practice, this often confuses ward staff, as they cannot understand why the machine is alarming. There is also a school of thought that would suggest that if the patient has used 8 mg and is still requesting analgesia, then their bolus dose and hourly limit should be increased, rather than restricted. There is no good scientific evidence to support the beneficial use of dose limits.

Background infusion

PCA devices will allow for a concurrent background infusion in addition to allowing the patient to request a bolus dose. This facility is not used for routine patients, as there is evidence to suggest that there is a greater incidence of respiratory depression (Hagle *et al.* 2004). One study comparing PCA and PCA with a background infusion found no difference in pain relief (Level II: Owen *et al.* 1989b). The group with the background infusion used twice as much drug and the background infusion did not alter the amount of drug requested.

The use of a background infusion is useful in patients who are receiving long-term opioids prior to surgery. These would include patients who have malignant disease, sickle-cell disease or are IV drug misusers. For these patients there is a risk of poor pain control and even withdrawal, should they have long periods without requesting a bolus dose. The reason for surgery may have nothing to do with their long-term opioid usage. For example patients may take long-term opioid medications for chronic painful conditions, such as arthritis. After surgery, they will still need their medication for arthritic pain, but will also require additional analgesia for surgical pain. These patients will have a tolerance to opioids and will therefore require larger doses.

It is useful to have a system of converting patients from their normal dose of opioid to an appropriate PCA programme that will account for the above. At Imperial College Healthcare NHS Trust, half of their normal opioid dose, converted to IV morphine equivalents, is run as a background infusion over 24 h. The oral dose is halved to ascertain the IV equivalent dose. Their normal oral opioids are discontinued and only PCA used until surgical pain settles and their 24-h requirements stabilise and a new oral dose is established. An example is shown in Box 10.1.

Box 10.1   An example of converting an opioid-dependent patient into PCA.

Patient A

On admission takes:

   Morphine sulphate modified release (MST Continus) 40 mg bd

   Morphine sulphate immediate release oral solution 20 mg (one dose daily)

Therefore:

   Total daily dose of oral morphine (40 + 40 + 20) = 100 mg

   Total daily dose of intravenous morphine (100/2) = 50 mg

   Half of the daily intravenous dose = 25 mg

   Run as a background infusion over 24 hr = approximately 1 mg/hr

The bolus dose should be started at 2-mg morphine, with a 5-min lockout, to allow for tolerance[a]

[a]But bolus doses may need to be increased further if pain is not controlled.
   On average, patients will press the PCA button about three times per hour and so this should be accounted for in the size of the bolus dose.

Monitoring and documentation of PCA

The monitoring of patients whilst they are using PCA is essential and Box 10.2 lists those that require recording. The frequency of observations is a matter for local agreement and should be well documented in policies and procedures. Suffice to say that patients are monitored more closely when they first start using PCA.

Respiratory rate

The major life-threatening complication of using IV opioids is respiratory depression. Respiratory depression is usually defined as a respiratory rate of

Box 10.2   Observations for patients receiving PCA.

The type of observations that should be recorded are:

(1)   Respiratory rate
(2)   Sedation scores
(3)   Blood pressure
(4)   Pain score
(5)   Location of pain
(6)   Amount of drug used
(7)   Side effects of PCA

Box 10.3 Management of opioid-induced respiratory depression.

- Take the PCA button away from the patient and stop any background infusion
- Apply oxygen therapy if the patient is not already receiving it
- Monitor the patient's respiratory rate and oxyhaemoglobin
- Stay with the patient
- Ask for a member of the patient's medical team to urgently review
- Make the patient sit in a upright position to allow for chest expansion
- Stimulate the patient
- Continue to monitor the patient, including respiratory rate and oxyhaemoglobin saturation
- Give naloxone if prescribed, as per local guidelines

$\leq$8 breaths per minute. Respiratory rates must be counted for the full minute, as breathing patterns may be abnormal and irregular in nature. If the patient is found to have respiratory depression, the actions to be taken are as outlined in Box 10.3.

Naloxone is a pure opioid antagonist that reverses the effects of pure agonists such as morphine at the μ, κ and δ opioid receptors. Naloxone will not only reverse respiratory depression, but also reverse the pain-relieving effects of this drug. Patients will often be woken from a sedated condition into a state of agonising pain. If there is time, it is better to give incremental doses of naloxone in order to reverse the respiratory depression, but not the pain relief. This can be achieved by giving 50-mcg naloxone, every 5 min, until normal breathing rates are achieved. As naloxone is supplied as 400 mcg in 1 mL, this requires the ampoule contents to be diluted with sodium chloride 7 mL, thus producing a final volume of 8 mL with naloxone 50 mcg/mL.

It is important to remember that the onset of action of naloxone is 1–2 min but that the duration of action is around 30 min, so the patient must continue to be closely monitored, as they may require further doses. If further frequent doses are required, then an infusion of naloxone should be considered. Rates as low as 50 mcg of naloxone per hour may be sufficient.

In a recent review of respiratory depression in adult patients receiving IV PCA, it was stated that the incidence ranges from 0.19 to 5.2% (Hagle *et al.* 2004). Contributing factors were found to be the use of a continuous infusion with PCA, increasing age, obesity, impaired renal/hepatic/cardiac function, upper abdominal surgery, sleep apnoea and concurrent use of sedatives or hypnotics.

Sedation scores

Sedation is an important observation, as it is a forewarning of respiratory depression. Patients will become sedated prior to respiratory depression and it is therefore best to start to treat the sedated patient, rather than wait for

Box 10.4   Example of a sedation-scoring tool.

0. Awake
1. Dozing
2. Asleep, but rousable
3. Unrousable

respiratory depression. Various scores are used to measure sedation; a standard example is given in Box 10.4.

Blood pressure

Opioids can cause hypotension due to the release of histamine. It is therefore important to monitor blood pressure and assess the patient for hypovolaemia and treat hypotension according to local policy.

Pain score

A standard verbal pain-rating score is given below. Patients can find pain scoring difficult, so it is best to keep scoring as simple as possible. Chapter 2 describes the principles of pain assessment. On the whole, patients tend to find verbal pain-rating scores (as given in Box 10.5) easier to understand than visual analogue scales.

It is perhaps stating the obvious, but pain intensity scores should continue to be monitored not just when patients are having PCA, but for all patients regardless of their analgesic regimen. Only pain scores on movement or coughing should be recorded; patients will usually report the pain scores at rest, which can be misleading. The minimum frequency that pain scores should be monitored is with routine observations; after taking the four routine observations of temperature, pulse, blood pressure and respiratory rate, pain scoring should be seen as the fifth vital sign (Royal College of Surgeons of England 1990). The reason for continual monitoring is to assess the effectiveness of the current regimen and if ineffective, to get the regimen changed. Most centres would accept a pain score of none or mild pain on movement. Pain scores above mild pain should be treated.

When monitoring pain scores of patients using PCA, it is also important to know how much drug they have used in the preceding few hours. For example

Box 10.5   Example of a verbal pain intensity rating score.

0 = None
1 = Mild
2 = Moderate
3 = Severe

if a patient complains of moderate pain at rest and severe pain on movement, they have used 8 mg of morphine PCA over the past 4 h; then their pain is due to insufficient demands for morphine. It is important to establish why the patient is reluctant to use PCA. This may be due to worries or anxieties about the use of opioids. The patient should be reassured and the importance of pain relief and the risks of complications of uncontrolled pain discussed. It would also be helpful for the patient to be reloaded with opioid.

If however the patient complains of moderate pain at rest and severe pain on movement, having used 36 mg of morphine PCA over the past 4 h, then they need to have their bolus dose increased, to allow for their individual requirements.

Location of pain

It is very easy to assume that you know where the patient is feeling their pain. There is an expectation after surgery that a patient should feel pain in the operative site. But patients can experience pain in other areas after surgery, which may be an indication of a serious complication. Morphine can be very good at relieving pain associated with serious complications.

For example it is not uncommon for patients to have a myocardial infarction after surgery. They may experience pain in their central chest, which radiates down their left arm or up into their neck. This pain is relieved by morphine. From the patient's point of view, this pain was not present before surgery and so must be related. They may not understand that this is a complication of surgery and volunteer information about this new site of pain to their nurse. It is vitally important, therefore, that we ask this question in order to detect possible life-threatening complications.

Patients may be using PCA to treat pain from deep-vein thrombosis, from pulmonary embolism or from more minor conditions such as a sore throat. Commonly, patients can use PCA to treat painful colic after abdominal surgery. Colic is often experienced as the postoperative ileus resolves and the bowel starts to peristalse. Using an opioid will slow down the return of peristalsis and the patient should be encouraged not to use PCA at this point, but to mobilise to help the passage of air through the gut.

Amount of drug used (analgesic consumption)

This is an important observation, as it is one of the measures to be taken into account when assessing whether a patient is ready to stop PCA and step down to weaker oral analgesia. For further information, please see the section below.

Side effects of PCA

It is important to monitor and treat the side effects of PCA, as if left un-treated, patients tend to restrict their use of PCA and pain is left uncontrolled

(Chumbley *et al.* 1998). There are numerous side effects associated with morphine and these adverse effects are usually dose related. Therefore, the higher the consumption, the more likely patients are to experience side effects. Chumbley *et al.* asked patients about five common side effects of PCA: nausea, vomiting, feeling sleepy, feeling itchy and feeling peculiar in the head (Chumbley *et al.* 1998, 2004). Feeling 'peculiar in the head' covered symptoms such as feeling dizzy, hallucinations and nightmares. These side effects are discussed below, but are not the only side effects to be attributed to morphine.

Nausea and vomiting

The treatment of nausea and vomiting is essential to maintaining patients' willingness to continue to use this method of pain relief. Studies have found that 57% patients can experience nausea and 37–38% can vomit when using IV morphine (Chumbley *et al.* 1998, 2004). Patients should be given an anti-emetic and if this is ineffective, then an alternative anti-emetic, with a different action, should be prescribed. Most centres choose cyclizine first line and 5-HT$_3$ receptor antagonists, e.g. ondansetron second line. Care should be taken when using medicines such as ondansetron as they are extremely constipating.

Those patients at high risk for developing nausea and vomiting should receive their anti-emetics regularly, rather than on a prn basis. Apfel *et al.* (1999) have produced an easy tool for assessing high-risk patients (Box 10.6). Patients are deemed high risk if they score 3 or 4 points out of a 4-point score; these patients should be prescribed prophylactic anti-emetics.

Statistically, women are more likely to vomit after surgery then are men. Non-smokers are at higher risk, as nicotine is an emetogenic substance. Smokers expose themselves to a nausea-inducing drug every time they have a cigarette; therefore, when another nausea-producing substance, such as morphine, is given to them, they have accommodated to the stimulus.

One study investigated whether nausea and vomiting with PCA could be reduced by the addition of droperidol or ondansetron to the opioid reservoir (Alexander *et al.* 1995). Seventy-two per cent of patients in the ondansetron

Box 10.6 A simplified risk score for predicting postoperative nausea and vomiting.

> Patients score a point if they answer 'yes' to the following four questions:
>
> (1) Is the patient female?
> (2) Do they have a history of postoperative nausea and vomiting or motion sickness?
> (3) Are they having opioids?
> (4) Are they non-smokers?
>
> Apfel *et al.* (1999).

group and 45% in the droperidol group were asymptomatic, compared to 20% in the control group. Other authors have found little benefit to adding anti-emetic to opioid reservoirs (Chumbley *et al.* 2004, Woodhouse & Mather 1997). Of note is that droperidol has since been withdrawn due to association with long QT syndrome.

Hallucinations and nightmares

Studies have found that between 33 and 46% patients complain of feeling 'peculiar' using PCA (Chumbley *et al.* 1998, 2004). Treating these adverse effects is difficult, as they are often dose related. Opioid-sparing drugs, such as paracetamol and non-steroidal anti-inflammatory drugs (NSAIDs), can be useful for reducing consumption. Often the only way of reducing these effects is to switch to another opioid, such as fentanyl or oxycodone.

Pruritus

Studies have found that between 27 and 32% patients complain of feeling itchy using PCA (Chumbley *et al.* 1998, 2004). Treatments such as antihistamines are routinely employed to treat this side effect. But anti-emetics that block 5-HT$_3$ (ondansetron, granisetron) can also be effective. As with other side effects, if the above measures are ineffective then switching opioid can be helpful.

When to stop PCA?

PCA should be discontinued and patients stepped down to oral analgesia only when they are ready to do so. To assess whether the time is correct, the following criteria should be met:

- The patient should have an oral route.
- The patient should have no more than mild pain on movement.
- The patient should have used less than 30 mg of IV morphine or equivalents in the past 24 hr.

There is little point in stopping PCA if the patient does not have an oral route, as this would require changing from PCA to intramuscular or subcutaneous injections. The evidence shows that patients find PCA preferable to injections. Therefore changing to a regimen that patients deem to be less satisfactory would not be logical.

The patient should have none or mild pain on movement. If the patient has more than mild pain on movement, it would suggest that they require more opioid, which may affect the third criterion of using less than 30 mg in the past 24 hr.

Thirty milligrams of IV morphine is equivalent to 60 mg of oral morphine. This equates to giving 10-mg oral morphine solution, every 4 h. Full-dose

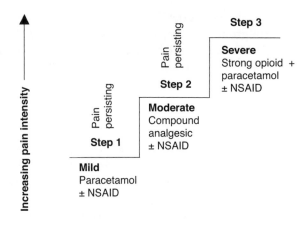

Figure 10.3 An adaptation of the WHO analgesic ladder NSAID, non-steroidal anti-inflammatory, compound analgesic, paracetamol combined with a mild opioid, (e.g. codeine or tramadol).

tramadol or codeine is not as potent. Therefore, if the patient requires this level or more of analgesia, they are not ready to step down the analgesic ladder to step 2 analgesia. Step 2 analgesia, such as tramadol or codeine, is usually given in conjunction with step 1 analgesia (paracetamol), as this improves the potency of these drugs (Moore *et al.* 2003; See Figure 10.3).

It is obviously good practice to have the step-down analgesia prescribed regularly, but oral doses should be reviewed to check whether the patient is ready to step down further. Patients should also be prescribed a stronger analgesic prn to cover possible painful conditions, such as drain removal or a sudden worsening of their pain. A typical step-down prescription would be as follows:

- Paracetamol 1 g, 4 times daily
- Tramadol 100 mg, 4 times daily
- Oral morphine solution 10 mg, 4 hourly, as required (prn)

If the patient has been using much less than 30-mg IV morphine in 24 h, then the following prescription may be more appropriate:

- Paracetamol 1 g, 4 times daily
- Tramadol 50 mg, 4 times daily
- Tramadol 50 mg, 6 hourly, as required (prn)
- Oral morphine solution 10 mg, 4 hourly, as required (prn)

This prescription allows for the patient to have the full dose of step 2 analgesia, should they experience more pain, perhaps due to increased mobilisation, but also allows for opioid pain relief for the removal of drains etc. It should be noted that tramadol cannot be given to epileptics, as it lowers the fit threshold. In this instance, it should be changed to dihydrocodeine 30 or 60 mg.

Some centres will stop PCA and step down immediately once the patient has met the above criteria. Other centres may start step 2 analgesia and keep the PCA, in situ, for a further 24 h. Patients are normally given instruction to use the PCA only if the regular analgesia is insufficient. In effect, this allows the patient to use PCA as 'prn' analgesia for a further 24 hr and gives them confidence that their oral regimen is sufficient to meet their analgesic requirements.

Maintaining the patient's safety when using PCA

Maintaining the patient's safety is obviously the primary objective for any nurse in any situation. PCA devices do have safety features built in to reduce the risk to the patient. But safety features alone cannot reduce the risk of human error. In order to avoid human error, hospital staff are asked to work within policies and procedures to keep risks to a minimum. All centres that use PCA must have policies and procedures that the staff can follow. If you work within the policies and procedures, then the institution will protect you should something untoward occur. It is the responsibility of each member of the staff to make themselves familiar with these documents and to follow them.

Patient to press

PCA is meant to be a safe method of giving patients large doses of opioids, as the patient will fall asleep when they have had too much. Once sedated, they can no longer press the button and therefore avoid respiratory depression. The first rule of safety with PCA is that it should only be the patient who presses the button, *never* the nurse or the patient's relative.

Staff education

In order to maintain safety, all staff that care for patients receiving PCA should have attended additional training on the principles of PCA, how to monitor patients and how to care and manage the PCA pump. At my institution, a minimum of 75% of staff on wards that run a PCA service have been trained and have been assessed as competent. In order to reduce risks when programming PCA machines, most centres will allow only a small select group of staff to perform this task. These tend to be members of the pain service, recovery staff and senior staff in intensive care or high-dependency areas. All of these staff should have received additional training on programming and have been certified as proficient at programming the machine.

Standardisation of PCA solutions

Standard solutions of PCA infusions should be sourced by the pharmacy department. Ward staff should not be making up infusion bags, as there is a huge risk for human error. As mentioned previously, the use of preprinted prescription labels also reduces the risk of prescription errors.

Dedicated IV access

PCA is normally administered via a dedicated IV line. In effect, this means that only PCA and no other solution is attached to the patient's cannula. If PCA or another infusion is run concurrently through the same IV line, then an extra piece of equipment called a 'one-way valve' must be inserted in the infusion line. If this valve is absent, then it will allow the PCA to pump the bolus dose into the giving set of the infusion if the IV cannula occludes. It will continue to do this every time the patient presses the PCA button. When the nurse comes to unblock the cannula and run the infusion to flush the line, the patient could receive numerous doses of opioid instantly and stop breathing.

PCA giving sets should also have an antisiphon valve (Figure 10.4). This valve stops opioid solution from being sucked out of the machine by the negative pressure exerted in the venous system. This is especially a risk if the PCA machine is positioned much higher than the patient.

Device malfunction

Local policy at my institution does not allow patients to leave the ward unattended when they are receiving PCA. There have been reports of devices malfunctioning (Macintyre 2001) and the qualified nurse who accompanies the patient should be able to maintain airway, breathing and circulation, should an adverse event occur.

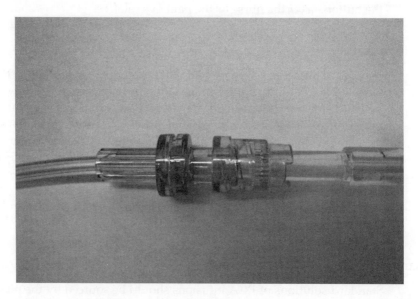

Figure 10.4 PCA antisyphon valve in line.

Patients' views of PCA

Much time and energy have been expanded investigating the PCA machine itself. What type of drug to use; what size of bolus is most effective; how long should the length of the lockout be? But the successful use of PCA depends on two factors, the device and the patient. You can have the most efficacious device ever invented, but if the patient is reluctant to press the button because of worries or because they are experiencing side effects, then this technique is not going to work.

Fear of addiction and overdose

One study has provided a detailed investigation of patients' experiences of PCA (Chumbley *et al.* 1998). The overall evaluation of PCA was favourable; the majority of patients felt positive about it and experienced good pain relief, but there were underlying fears about addiction and overdose. These worries affected over a third of patients and restricted the use of PCA in a quarter of patients. The incidence of side effects was a major feature of the patients' experience and many were unaware of the adverse effects of morphine and did not seek help to alleviate them. These misconceptions effectively deterred many patients from obtaining analgesia and left them anxious and in pain. This study also revealed that 43% patients failed to receive preoperative instruction and 39% patients felt that the information they had received whilst using PCA was inadequate.

As mentioned previously, three factors were found to predict a positive experience with PCA; these were having good pain relief, feeling safe and having a lack of side effects (Chumbley *et al.* 1999). The primary side effect that caused problems was feeling 'peculiar in the head'. This phrase covered symptoms such as feeling drowsy, hallucinations and nightmares. Feeling safe referred to issues such as overdose and addiction. Safety had not hitherto been regarded as an important component of the patient's experience of PCA, as with conventional analgesia, the nurse had administered the opioid. Now we are asking patients to take on this responsibility; it is unsurprising that safety is important in determining their perceptions of PCA.

It could be argued that if we want to ensure that patients have a good experience with PCA, then we should strive to create an environment where these positive effects happen.

Information about the device

For patients to have good pain relief, we have to ensure that they have been informed about how to use the PCA machine. This is covered in the section below, entitled 'What do patients want to know about PCA'. But for good pain relief to be sustained, it is vital that we maintain the instant accessibility of

PCA. When IV access is lost, or nurses take time to change the opioid reservoir on the machine, their ability to demand analgesia is lost. Many patients limit their opioid use and ration themselves if they fear that nursing staff will not change the opioid reservoir quickly enough.

Opioid side effects

Side effects of opioids can be distressing for patients. Focus groups of patients who commented on the experience of PCA were most likely to discuss side effects as their first concern (Chumbley *et al.* 2002). A wide range of side effects were discussed and, in some cases, they were the cause of patients wanting to stop using PCA. They would rather experience pain than vomit and have hallucinations or nightmares. Often patients do not attribute side effects to opioids; nausea, vomiting and drowsiness are blamed on the anaesthetic and deemed an inevitable consequence of surgery (Chumbley *et al.* 1998, 1999).

Snell *et al.* (1997) found no differences in the incidence of nausea when comparing patients having intramuscular injections or PCA, but noted that patients receiving intramuscular injections were given three times the amount of anti-emetic drug as those in the PCA group (Snell *et al.* 1997). This effect of increased anti-emetic administration has been noted by others (Woodhouse & Mather 1997) and is possibly due to nursing staff routinely giving an anti-emetic with an intramuscular injection, whereas patients receiving PCA may only be given an anti-emetic sporadically.

Most centres ask nurses to use a score to record nausea, but it is unusual for nurses to monitor side effects such as hallucinations and nightmares. These side effects are most distressing for patients and one study found that nightmares was the single best predictor of patients' dissatisfaction with PCA (Jamison *et al.* 1993).

Alleviating worries about overdose and addiction can be difficult. Patients have long been known to overestimate the incidence of addition associated with postoperative analgesia (Laing *et al.* 1993). One study found that 38% patients were worried about overdose and addiction when using PCA (Chumbley *et al.* 1998). This could mean that patients are not using PCA due to these worries.

Other concerns: alarms and attention from nurses

Apart from overdose and addiction, patients also have worries about issues that professionals may not have considered a problem. Patients are concerned when the machine alarms, as they associate this with something going drastically wrong, as opposed to the machine alerting staff that it needs attention, such as the reservoir being empty. If machines continue to alarm, due to problems such as a vein occluding, then patients will ration their analgesia in an attempt not to upset their fellow patients with irritating alarms.

Patients also become concerned about nurses paying more attention to the machine, rather than to them. Just a simple question such as 'have you used your PCA machine?' can make them feel that the nurse is more concerned with the machine. A better question to ask would be 'how is your pain' and then ask the patient if they are finding the machine helpful.

It is very easy in a busy ward environment for nurses to concentrate on observations and recording information from the PCA machine and forget to pay as much attention to the patient. In this respect, there were advantages for patients having intramuscular injections. Nurses would firstly talk to the patient when they requested analgesia, to establish where the pain was located and its severity. Having established that pain relief was required, they selected the appropriate drugs from the cupboard and two nurses would normally return to the bedside, drawing the curtains in order to ensure privacy. The patient knowing that they had the undivided attention of two nurses would normally choose this time to pass on information or make other requests. In the process of giving the injection, the nurses would be careful to move the patient into the most comfortable position, smoothing sheets and plumping pillows. Mouth care may have been undertaken at this time and other needs met, before drawing back the curtains, ensuring that the patient had the nurse-call buzzer. In addition, there would have been a lot of touching, and human touch can be very reassuring in times of illness. The question is, do patient using PCA get lavished with the same level of care and attention? If we are honest, the answer is probably *no*. So we have to work harder to ensure that patient using PCA do not miss out on essential nursing care.

What do patients want to know about PCA?

Chumbley *et al.* (2002) employed the use of focus groups to identify what patients wanted to know about PCA. Various topics were identified, these being the dangers of morphine, side effects of morphine, alternative pain relief, support from staff, how to use PCA and when to receive information.

Dangers of morphine

Patients want to be informed that the drug used in PCA is an opioid, such as morphine. The layperson associates morphine with dying or drug abuse; therefore, they want to be reassured that this drug is safe. They want to know that this is a drug, which is routinely used in hospital, and that they will not overdose or become addicted to it. I often explain to patients that if this drug was so addictive, then we would never empty our hospital beds, as patients would be reluctant to go home.

Side effects of morphine

Patients want to be told about the common side effects of morphine, so that they can recognise them and ask for help to alleviate them. The following list identifies side effects that patients would like to be informed about. They included feeling sleepy, feeling dizzy, hallucinations, nightmares, nausea, vomiting, feeling itchy and constipation. In my practice, I usually ask patients if they have seen anything strange or had any strange dreams, rather than make suggestions of hallucinations and nightmares, which can have negative connotations.

Alternative pain relief

Patients want to know that if there are alternative methods of controlling their pain, other than PCA. If they find they dislike administering their own pain relief, or are having uncontrolled side effects, then a member of the pain service will be made available to assess them and suggest alternatives.

Support from staff

Patients want to receive support from staff when they are using PCA. They may require further explanation or reinforcement on how to use the machine. They may want to discuss side effects. They do not appreciate contradictory information, such as staff telling them that they are using the machine too much or not enough. They prefer staff to ask 'how is their pain', rather than 'have you used your machine'.

How to use PCA and when to receive information

Patients prefer not to be 'told' how to use their machine, rather that we 'suggest' the best ways to use it. They would like to receive information in a leaflet, which they can study and then be given the opportunity to ask questions of anaesthetic or medical staff. The leaflet should contain diagrams of the machine, give detailed information about how PCA works and when to press the button to request analgesia. Patients want to receive information preoperatively, preferable at preassessment. The patient's first experience of PCA should not occur in the recovery room, having just had major surgery and an anaesthetic.

Summary

PCA has provided medical and nursing staff with an alternative method of controlling the patient's pain after surgery. It has solved many of the problems associated with conventional analgesia, such as the need for frequent injections. It allows the patients immediate access to analgesia, without having to convince medical or nursing staff that they are in pain. But PCA has brought along a new set of problems that we now have to consider and if we fail to resolve these issues, patients will not use it. Therefore, if we want the patients to have a positive experience with PCA, then we have to ensure that we maintain access; we monitor and treat side effects; we allay patients' worries about safety; and we give patients information on how to use it.

References

Aitken, H.A. & Kenny, G.N. (1990) Use of patient controlled analgesia in postoperative cardiac surgical patients – a survey of ward staff attitudes. *Intensive Care Nursing*, **6** (2), 74–78.

Albert, J.M. & Talbott, T.M. (1988) Patient-controlled analgesia vs. conventional intramuscular analgesia following colon surgery. *Diseases of the Colon and Rectum*, **31** (2), 83–86.

Alexander, R., Lovell, A.T., Seingry, D., *et al.* (1995) Comparison of ondansetron and droperidol in reducing postoperative nausea and vomiting associated with patient-controlled analgesia. *Anaesthesia*, **50** (12), 1086–1088.

Apfel, C.C., Laara, E., Koivuranta, M., *et al.* (1999) A simplified risk score for predicting postoperative nausea and vomiting between two centers. *Anesthesiology*, **91** (3), 694–700.

Ballantyne, J.C., Carr, D.B., Chalmers, T.C., *et al.* (1993) Postoperative patient-controlled analgesia: meta-analyses of initial randomized control trials. *Journal of Clinical Anesthesia*, **5** (3), 182–193.

Chumbley, G.M., Hall, G.M. & Salmon, P. (1998) Patient-controlled analgesia: an assessment by 200 patients. *Anaesthesia*, **53** (3), 216–221.

Chumbley, G.M., Hall, G.M. & Salmon, P. (1999) Why do patients feel positive about patient-controlled analgesia? *Anaesthesia*, **54** (4), 386–389.

Chumbley, G.M., Hall, G.M. & Salmon, P. (2002) Patient-controlled analgesia: what information does the patient want? *Journal of Advanced Nursing*, **39** (5), 459–471.

Chumbley, G.M., Ward, L., Hall, G.M., *et al.* (2004) Pre-operative information and patient-controlled analgesia: much ado about nothing. *Anaesthesia*, **59** (4), 354–358.

Coleman, S.A. & Booker-Milburn, J. (1996) Audit of postoperative pain control. Influence of a dedicated acute pain nurse. *Anaesthesia*, **51** (12), 1093–1096.

Eisenach, J.C., Grice, S.C. & Dewan, D.M. (1988) Patient-controlled analgesia following cesarean section: a comparison with epidural and intramuscular narcotics. *Anesthesiology*, **68** (3), 444–448.

Fitzpatrick, R. (1993) Scope and measurement of patient satisfaction. In: *Measurement of Patients' Satisfaction with their Care* (eds R. Fitzpatrick & A. Hopkins). Royal College of Physicians of London, London, pp. 1–17.

Fitzpatrick, R. & Hopkins, A. (1983) Problems in the conceptual framework of patient satisfaction research: an empirical exploration. *Sociology of Health and Illness*, **5** (3), 297–311.

Hagle, M.E., Lehr, V.T., Brubakken, K., *et al.* (2004) Respiratory depression in adult patients with intravenous patient-controlled analgesia. *Orthopedic Nursing*, **23** (1), 18–27; quiz 28–29.

Hall, G.M. & Salmon, P. (1997) Patient-controlled analgesia – who benefits? *Anaesthesia*, **52** (5), 401–402.

Hudcova, J., McNicol, E. & Quah, C., *et al.* (2006) Patient controlled opioid analgesia versus conventional opioid analgesia for postoperative pain. *Cochrane Database of Systematic Reviews*, Issue 4, Art No CD003348.

Jamison, R.N., Taft, K., O'Hara, J.P., *et al.* (1993) Psychosocial and pharmacologic predictors of satisfaction with intravenous patient-controlled analgesia. *Anesthesia and Analgesia*, **77** (1), 121–125.

Keeri-Szanto, M. (1979) Drugs or drums: what relieves postoperative pain? *Pain*, **6** (2), 217–230.

Koh, P. & Thomas, V.J. (1994) Patient-controlled analgesia (PCA): does time saved by PCA improve patient satisfaction with nursing care? *Journal of Advanced Nursing*, **20** (1), 61–70.

Laing, R., Lam, M., Owen, H., *et al.* (1993) Perceived risks of postoperative analgesia. *Australian and New Zealand Journal of Surgery*, **63** (10), 760–765.

Lehmann, K.A. (1999) Patient-controlled analgesia: an efficient therapeutic tool in the postoperative setting. *European Surgical Research*, **31** (2), 112–121.

Love, D.R., Owen, H. Ilsley, A.H., *et al.* (1996) A comparison of variable-dose patient-controlled analgesia with fixed-dose patient-controlled analgesia. *Anesthesia and Analgesia*, **83** (5), 1060–1064.

Macintyre, P.E. (2001) Safety and efficacy of patient-controlled analgesia. *British Journal of Anaesthesia*, **87** (1), 36–46.

McGrath, D., Thurston, N., Wright, D., *et al.* (1989) Comparison of one technique of patient-controlled postoperative analgesia with intramuscular meperidine. *Pain*, **37** (3), 265–270.

Moore, A., Edwards, J., Barden, J., *et al.* (2003) *Bandolier's Little Book of Pain.* Oxford University Press, Oxford.

Owen, H., McMillan, V. & Rogowski, D. (1990) Postoperative pain therapy: a survey of patients' expectations and their experiences. *Pain*, **41** (3), 303–307.

Owen, H., Plummer, J.L., Armstrong, I., *et al.* (1989a) Variables of patient-controlled analgesia. 1. Bolus size. *Anaesthesia*, **44** (1), 7–10.

Owen, H., Szekely, S.M., Plummer, J.L., *et al.* (1989b) Variables of patient-controlled analgesia. 2. Concurrent infusion. *Anaesthesia*, **44** (1), 11–13.

Royal College of Surgeons of England, Faculty of Anaesthetists (1990). *Commission on the Provision of Surgical Services. Report of the Working Party on Pain after Surgery.* Royal College of Surgeons, London.

Sechzer, P.H. (1971) Studies in pain with the analgesic-demand system. *Anesthesia and Analgesia*, **50** (1), 1–10.

Snell, C.C., Fothergill-Bourbonnais, F. & Durocher-Hendriks, S. (1997) Patient controlled analgesia and intramuscular injections: a comparisons of patient pain experiences and postoperative outcomes. *Journal of Advanced Nursing*, **25** (4), 681–690.

Walder, B., Schafer, M., Henzi, I., *et al.* (2001) Efficacy and safety of patient-controlled opioid analgesia for acute postoperative pain. A quantitative systematic review. *Acta Anaesthesiologica Scandinavica*, **45** (7), 795–804.

Wheatley, R.G., Madej, T.H., Jackson, I.J., *et al.* (1991) The first year's experience of an acute pain service. *British Journal of Anaesthesia*, **67** (3), 353–359.

Williams, B. (1994) Patient satisfaction: a valid concept? *Social Science and Medicine*, **38** (4), 509–516.

Woodhouse, A. & Mather, L.E. (1997) Nausea and vomiting in the postoperative patient-controlled analgesia environment. *Anaesthesia*, **52** (8), 770–775.

Woodhouse, A. & Mather, L.E. (1998) The effect of duration of dose delivery with patient-controlled analgesia on the incidence of nausea and vomiting after hysterectomy. *British Journal of Clinical Pharmacology*, **45** (1), 57–62.

Useful websites

Bandolier: *http://www.jr2.ox.ac.uk/bandolier/booth/painpag/Acutrev/Other/PCAup.html.*

The Institute for Safe Medication Practices: *http://www.ismp.org/profdevelopment/ PCAMonograph.pdf.*

The Royal College of Anaesthetists – 'Raising the Standard' Acute Pain chapter: *http://www.rcoa.ac.uk/docs/ARB-section11.pdf.*

11 Other Routes of Opioid Administration

Ian McGovern

Key Messages

- The oral route should be considered the route of choice in most acute postoperative pain situations.
- Intramuscular injections of opioid medications are less effective than either intravenous patient-controlled analgesia or subcutaneous injections, are less acceptable to patients and cannot be recommended.
- Continuous intravenous opioid infusions are associated with an unacceptably high incidence of respiratory depression and are not recommended for most postoperative settings.
- Intermittent intravenous bolus administration is the most effective means of titrating opioid analgesia in the acute severe pain setting.
- Innovative drug delivery systems such as the fentanyl iontophoretic transdermal system have a significant and increasing role in the management of acute severe postoperative pain.

Introduction

Opioid analgesic medicines can be delivered to the systemic circulation by a number of alternative routes. The route selected will be influenced by the nature, site and severity of the pain requiring treatment; the patient's physiological condition and willingness or ability to tolerate or comply with the suggested treatment; pharmacological factors; the setting, equipment and staffing suitability; and of course costs.

Pharmacological factors that must be considered include absorption and bioavailability, speed of onset of analgesia, efficacy, duration of action and side effects both systemic and related to the route of administration.

Not every opioid analgesic medicine is suitable or licensed for administration by every route, so careful consideration must be given to each individual patient's analgesic requirement when selecting a regimen in the perioperative setting.

Common to all routes of administration is the desire to rapidly achieve and maintain plasma levels within the therapeutic range while avoiding periods of either subtherapeutic or toxic levels. In most cases, rapid achievement of therapeutic plasma levels of the medicine is achieved by means of a loading dose. Steady-state therapeutic levels must then be maintained either by means of a continuous infusion, a slow or controlled release preparation or by intermittent fast-acting supplementation.

Intravenous route

Medicines given by the intravenous (IV) route enter directly into the systemic circulation and therapeutic plasma levels can be reached more rapidly than by most other routes of administration. Limitations to absorption encountered by other routes of administration are avoided. This rapid achievement of analgesic effect makes this an ideal route for titration of opioid analgesia in situations where acute severe pain is encountered. High doses and volumes of injectate can be administered into a peripheral vein with little danger of irritation or discomfort at the site of injection. Venous access is required and this may be difficult to achieve and maintain particularly in children or patients requiring analgesia for prolonged periods.

Medicine, equipment and disposable costs are considerable. Sterility must be maintained and highly skilled trained personnel and facilities are required to store and prepare the injections/infusions, to administer IV medications into existing indwelling cannulae and to monitor the patients in a safe environment. These costs are even greater when sophisticated patient-controlled analgesia (PCA) equipment is included.

Opioid analgesic drugs can be administered intravenously in the following ways.

Intermittent intravenous bolus administration

While onset of analgesic effect is rapid for the reasons mentioned, offset of action is also rapid after IV administration and more prolonged analgesic management requires the consideration of a continuous infusion, patient- or nurse-controlled top-up strategies or an alternative route of administration. PCA is described in Chapter 10.

Toxic levels can be achieved very quickly when large boluses are given. This risk can be reduced by giving smaller, more frequent boluses or by using continuous infusions titrated to effect while monitoring the patient closely for side effects and signs of toxicity.

Continuous intravenous infusion

In the absence of a loading or bolus dose of opioid analgesic drug, steady-state plasma concentrations are achieved in approximately four half-lives of the drug used. Stable steady-state plasma levels can be reliably maintained. Potential problems arise as analgesic requirements differ between patients and over time in the same patient. Even with frequent rate adjustment, the lag time between any change and effect may result in either inadequate pain relief or adverse effects due to excessive plasma levels. The significantly higher incidence of respiratory depression associated with continuous IV opioid infusions compared with PCA (Schug & Torrie 1993) makes this an unsuitable method of postoperative pain control in most situations.

PCA techniques

The most commonly used opioids for IV PCA in the UK are morphine, fentanyl and oxycodone.

Some of the limitations of nurse-controlled infusions and intermittent or as required (*pro re nata*, prn) bolus administration can be avoided by means of PCA systems. After a suitable loading dose of opioid analgesia, patients are able to titrate supplemental doses within preset limits to maintain therapeutic plasma levels and good analgesic effect. Supplemental boluses can be delivered in isolation or in addition to a fixed-rate background infusion.

Despite the wealth of evidence to support the use of epidural or regional techniques for postoperative pain management, the role of parenteral opioids should not be underestimated. Epidural analgesia, despite producing improved analgesia compared to parenteral opioids, has some adverse effects and has been shown not to shorten the duration of hospital stay after colorectal surgery (Level I: Marret *et al.* 2007).

Numerous studies have demonstrated the benefits of PCA when compared with conventional opioid analgesia. PCA provides better pain control and greater patient satisfaction than conventional parenteral analgesia for postoperative pain (Hudcova *et al.* 2006, Level I: Walder *et al.* 2001).

In postcardiac surgical patients, PCA increases morphine consumption and improves analgesia as measured by visual analogue scale compared with a nurse-controlled analgesia regime (Level I: Bainbridge *et al.* 2006).

While tramadol is effective when administered by IV PCA, large boluses are associated with a high incidence of nausea and vomiting. The incidence and severity of the nausea and vomiting can be reduced and the effectiveness of the pain relief increased by administering the loading dose of tramadol during the surgery (Level II: Pang *et al.* 2000). Co-administration of metoclopramide has also been shown to reduce the incidence and severity of these symptoms but the combination was associated with an increase in sedation over tramadol alone (Level II: Pang *et al.* 2002).

Intramuscular and subcutaneous routes

Medicines that do not reliably produce adequate plasma concentrations when given enterally may be given by alternate routes. In situations where oral administration is undesirable or impracticable, parenteral administration should be considered.

Morphine is usually well absorbed from both intramuscular and subcutaneous sites where vascularity is good and produces plasma levels equal to those achieved after IV administration. Absorption is relatively rapid and maximal plasma concentrations are usually achieved 15–60 min after injection. The peak effect is achieved after 30–60 min being limited by the permeability of the blood–brain barrier more than by absorption from the injection site.

Absorption is adversely affected by peripheral vasoconstriction and will therefore be prolonged in the presence of pain, hypovolaemia, hypotension or hypothermia. In these situations a reservoir of drug can remain at the injection site, causing inadequate analgesia and risking unpredictable absorption when normal peripheral circulation recovers.

Absorption is also dependent on the formulation of the medicine concerned. Precipitation at the site of injection can occur if the solvent is absorbed faster than the drug. Inadequate analgesia would result.

Injections are painful and the volumes of drug it is possible to give are limited. Approximately 2 mL is the maximum volume tolerated subcutaneously by most adult patients. Slightly larger volumes can be given via the intramuscular route. Local tissue damage can occur, though this is uncommon with opioid analgesics.

The site of injection is important both to ensure adequacy of absorption and to avoid damage to neighbouring structures. Subcutaneous fat over the gluteus maximus muscle in adults can be as thick as 3.5 cm and has a very poor blood supply. Absorption of any drug delivered into this tissue will be limited, so it is important to ensure that a needle of appropriate length is used. Care must be taken to avoid causing damage to the sciatic nerve in the gluteal region; therefore, the upper outer quadrant of the buttock is recommended.

Extra care must be taken to avoid haematoma formation in patients with thrombocytopenia or other bleeding diathesis. Intramuscular injection should be avoided in these groups. Intramuscular injections should also be avoided in patients who are neutropenic because of the risk of infection.

In most cases, trained personnel are required to administer the injections and to maintain the sterility of drugs and equipment.

For ongoing acute pain or more chronic pain situations where analgesia is required for weeks or months and in situations where oral opioid medication is not appropriate, the subcutaneous route can be used to provide continuous therapy. Indwelling subcutaneous cannulae can be sited to provide access for continuous subcutaneous opioid infusion, a technique that can be utilised for patients in whom IV access is either difficult or undesirable. Continuous subcutaneous infusions are widely used to treat chronic pain associated with malignancy and with appropriate training of patients and their carers can be safely managed in the community. The cannula site should be rotated to reduce local irritation and patient discomfort.

Individual agents

Intramuscular morphine and pethidine have both been shown to be effective when compared to placebo in the initial treatment of moderate-to-severe postoperative pain (McQuay *et al.* 1999, Level I: Smith *et al.* 2000).

Intramuscular pethidine provides similar, but variable, quality analgesia compared with ketorolac after caesarean section (Level II: Gin *et al.* 1993).

Despite encouraging results when compared with placebo morphine, pethidine and nalbuphine have all been shown to be less effective when given intramuscularly than when administered by an IV PCA regime (Level I: Walder *et al.* 2001).

Subcutaneous bolus injection of morphine produces as effective analgesia, has a similar side-effect profile and has a greater patient acceptance than intramuscular morphine (Level II: Cooper 1996).

Continuous subcutaneous infusion of morphine provides as effective postoperative analgesia as regular intramuscular injections after upper abdominal surgery (Level II: Goudie *et al.* 1985).

In keeping with the trends towards PCA in the postoperative setting, trials of subcutaneous PCA systems have been undertaken with encouraging results. Tramadol, when given by PCA via the subcutaneous route, provides effective analgesia following major orthopaedic surgery and has a similar side-effect profile to that of morphine (Level II: Hopkins *et al.* 1998).

Oxycodone given either by intermittent subcutaneous injection or by continuous subcutaneous infusion is now used more widely in palliative care than is diamorphine. This may be due to both efficacy and the ongoing shortage of opium poppy crops.

Enteral routes

Oral route

The oral route is the most widely used route of drug administration across the world. It is simple, convenient, relatively safe, inexpensive and well tolerated by most patients. Assuming that patients are able and willing to swallow oral preparations, it remains the route of choice in most situations.

Medicines taken via the oral route pass into the stomach where some are unstable in the presence of gastric acid, may irritate the stomach, or may cause nausea and vomiting.

Before absorption from the gastrointestinal tract can take place, the drug must be present in solution. Drug dissolution usually takes place in the stomach where it is affected by gastric pH, the presence and nature of gastric contents, and the pharmaceutical preparation of the medicine concerned.

Absorption

Absorption from the stomach and small intestine is usually dependent on the medicine's ability to penetrate lipid cell membranes. The lipid solubility, extent of ionisation and molecular weight of the medicine determine the rate and extent of its absorption. More lipid-soluble, predominantly non-ionised and low-molecular-weight drugs pass more easily into the plasma. Weakly basic drugs will tend to be less ionised and more lipid soluble in an alkaline environment and will be more readily absorbed from the small intestine than the stomach. The converse is true of weakly acidic medicines. Most opioid analgesics are weak bases and have high pK_a values. They are mainly present in the acidic environment of the stomach as ionised compounds and are largely not available for absorption by the gastric mucosa. Once these medicines have passed into the more alkaline environment of the small intestine they are mostly present in their unionised form and are readily absorbed.

Patients with delayed gastric emptying (common in the postoperative setting) may accumulate orally administered opioids in the stomach, resulting in poor absorption and inadequate analgesia. There is a further risk that these accumulated medicines reach and are absorbed from the small intestine in large quantities when normal gastric emptying is resumed. This is known as dumping. The resulting high plasma levels may produce unpredicted and unacceptable adverse effects. Opioid analgesics themselves may contribute to the reduced gastric motility.

Clinical situations associated with a low splanchnic blood flow such as hypotension or hypovolaemia may result in reduced absorption from the gastrointestinal tract. The oral route is unlikely to be suitable following major surgery, immediately after gastrointestinal surgery or after significant trauma.

Nausea and vomiting are commonly experienced side effects associated with almost all opioid analgesics and may limit the ability of patients to take medications orally.

Medicines taken orally usually reach peak plasma concentration and produce clinical effects after about 30–120 min. Because of this slow rate of onset of analgesic effect, the ability to titrate orally administered opioid analgesics to response is limited. Other routes may be more suitable in the immediate postoperative period.

Modified (sustained or prolonged)-release preparations

A number of opioid analgesic agents are available in both immediate-release and modified-release oral preparations. Most modified-release preparations are enteric coated and thus pass undissolved from the stomach into the small intestine where absorption takes place over a prolonged period. Peak plasma levels may not be reached after controlled- or modified-release oral dosing for a number of hours, limiting their role in the management of acute postoperative analgesia. Patients taking modified-release preparations should avoid all alcohol, as consumption will impair the release of the active constituents.

The prolonged-release preparation of oxycodone (oxycodone CR) has biphasic absorption – combining the controlled- and immediate-release components to achieve more rapid onset of action and longer lasting effect. OxyContin® (Napp Pharmaceuticals) is a crush-resistant film-coated preparation of a tamper-resistant design to reduce the potential for abuse as the particle size is unsuitable for injection when crushed.

Individual agents

Morphine can be administered orally but undergoes extensive first-pass metabolism with only 10–30% of the given dose reaching the systemic circulation (see Box 11.1). The main metabolites produced are morphine-3-glucuronide and morphine-6-glucuronide. Morphine-3-glucuronide is partly excreted in bile but can be broken down by intestinal bacteria to release morphine that can then be reabsorbed and metabolised by enterohepatic recirculation. Morphine-6-glucuronide is pharmacologically active and may accumulate after prolonged administration of morphine or in the presence of renal impairment. Despite this limitation, oral therapy with oral solutions and sustained-release preparations are used extensively in the management of chronic pain associated with malignancy.

Routes of administration of morphine which avoid first-pass metabolism (intravenous, transdermal, rectal, intramuscular, epidural and intrathecal) result in lower production of either metabolite than oral, buccal or sublingual (SL) routes (Level I: Faura *et al.* 1998). Regularly dosed oral morphine can produce comparable or even superior analgesia to on-demand intramuscular regimes in some postoperative settings (Level II: McCormack *et al.* 1993).

Codeine (methylmorphine) is less susceptible to hepatic first-pass metabolism and has a higher availability than morphine. However, in isolation it has limited usefulness in the postoperative setting (Level I: Moore & McQuay 1997). The same is true of dihydrocodeine (Level I: Edwards *et al.* 2000a).

The effectiveness of a number opioid analgesic medicines has been shown to be improved when combined with other agents. Codeine when combined with paracetamol slightly increases the analgesic effects of paracetamol but causes more side effects (Level I: Moore *et al.* 2000, Zhang & Li Wan Po 1996).

Tramadol, although effective alone (Level I: Moore & McQuay 1997), when combined with paracetamol produces greater analgesic effect than either of its components alone without additional toxicity (Edwards *et al.* 2002). The combination is also superior in terms of time to onset and duration of analgesic effect (Level I: Medve *et al.* 2001).

Box 11.1   Bioavailability and first-pass effect.

The bioavailability of a medicine is that fraction of the dose that reaches the systemic circulation still pharmacologically active after absorption from the given route compared with that achieved after intravenous administration

Oral administration
Medicines administered by the oral route pass into the systemic circulation from the gastrointestinal tract via the liver and are exposed to first-pass metabolism. Drugs that undergo more extensive hepatic metabolism (i.e. have a high hepatic extraction ratio) will thus have a more reduced bioavailability than those less extensively metabolised. Most opioid analgesics undergo significant first-pass metabolism either in the intestinal mucosa or in the liver and thus have low oral bioavailability. Doses need to be adjusted accordingly

Rectal administration
Medicines given rectally are absorbed into the systemic circulation via the superior, middle and inferior rectal veins. With the exception of the superior rectal vein, these veins lead directly into the inferior vena cava, avoiding the portal circulation and exposure of the absorbed medicine to hepatic first-pass metabolism. This absorption pattern is, however, variable and first-pass metabolism may still be significant

Transdermal administration
Medicines absorbed through the skin pass directly into the systemic circulation, avoiding exposure to hepatic first-pass metabolism. The use of iontophoresis also bypasses first-pass metabolism

Transmucosal routes
Medicines administered by intranasal, sublingual, buccal and pulmonary routes are rapidly absorbed by the vascular mucosa directly into the systemic circulation and are not subject to hepatic first-pass metabolism

There is little evidence to support prescribing the combination of dextropropoxyphene and paracetamol in preference to paracetamol alone for the treatment of postoperative pain (Level I: Li Wan Po & Zhang 1997). Of note is that the combination of dextropropoxyphene and paracetamol (65 and 650 mg respectively) has a higher NNT (number needed to treat) (is less effective) than has ibuprofen (400 mg) alone (Level I: Collins *et al.* 2000).

Single-dose oral oxycodone appears to be of comparable efficacy to intramuscular morphine and non-steroidal anti-inflammatory drugs for acute postoperative pain (Level I: Edwards *et al.* 2000b). Combining oxycodone with paracetamol improves its efficacy (Level I: McQuay & Edwards 2003).

Some combination analgesic formulations can provide an effective means of delivering pain relief particularly when other groups of analgesics such as non-steroidal anti-inflammatory drugs are undesirable. The effectiveness of compound (co-analgesics) is described further in Chapter 7.

A number of studies have demonstrated a role for the regular administration of controlled- or sustained-release opioid preparations in the management of acute postoperative pain. Single-dose preoperative controlled-release oral morphine reduces postoperative IV morphine requirement following abdominal hysterectomy (Level II: Cruikshank *et al.* 1996).

Regular dosing of controlled-release oxycodone prevents pain and halves postoperative IV PCA opioid consumption after breast surgery (Kampe *et al.* 2004) and provides superior analgesia to IV tramadol/metamizol after retinal surgery (Kaufmann *et al.* 2004) with fewer adverse effects and greater patient satisfaction in both groups. Similar results have been found following abdominal and gynaecological surgery (Level II: Reuben *et al.* 2002, Sunshine *et al.* 1996).

Rectal route

The rectal route can be very useful in patients unable or unwilling to take oral medications and is widely used in younger children. The management of perioperative pain in children is described in Chapter 12.

Medicines given rectally are absorbed into the systemic circulation via the superior, middle and inferior rectal veins. With the exception of the superior rectal vein these veins lead directly into the inferior vena cava, avoiding the portal circulation and exposure of the absorbed drug to hepatic first-pass metabolism (see Box 11.1). This absorption pattern is, however, variable and first-pass metabolism may still be significant.

Rectal administration of medication avoids the need for sterilisation and specialist equipment and thus represents a cost-effective option when compared with other routes of administration. The rectal route should be avoided in neutropenic patients due to the risk of infection.

Although side effects such as rectal irritation are uncommon, patient acceptability is a factor and prior informed consent from the patient or their guardian where appropriate is essential before administering medications via this route. This is especially important if the drug is to be given to a patient under anaesthesia.

A study comparing rectally administered paracetamol and codeine with the same medication given orally following adenotonsillectomy in children aged 1–5 years found that the suppositories achieved equivalent pain control as the oral medication with few side effects and good tolerance. Of note is that many of the parents preferred the suppositories to the oral medication because of the ease of administration (Level II: Owczarzak & Haddad 2006).

Transdermal route (reservoirs and matrix)

Potentially, the skin represents a remarkable vector through which to administer medicines. Despite the fact that the stratum corneum of the epidermis represents a significant barrier, some opioid analgesic drugs are available as transdermal preparations. Any medicine that is absorbed through the skin passes directly into the systemic circulation, avoiding exposure to hepatic first-pass metabolism (see Box 11.1).

Transdermal fentanyl reservoir patches

Transdermal fentanyl delivery systems consist of either a drug-containing reservoir or a matrix patch (Durogesic®, DTrans®, Janssen Cilag) applied to the skin. The amount of fentanyl released is proportional to the surface area of the skin exposed to the medicine and thus that of the patch applied. Patches are available in different sizes to deliver different doses but are unlicensed for postoperative or acute pain.

The fentanyl initially accumulates as a depot in the superficial skin layers before being absorbed into the systemic circulation. The time from application to initial effect can be from 1 to 40 hr, with maximum plasma concentrations not being achieved for between 12 and 48 hr. Steady-state concentrations are reached after about 72 hr and can be maintained by repeated application of patches. The site of application should be rotated. Serum concentrations start to fall after 48 hr if the patch is not reapplied, but fentanyl continues to be absorbed from the cutaneous depot after the patch has been removed. These pharmacokinetics and the wide interpatient variation in maximum plasma levels achieved means that transdermal fentanyl delivery systems are unsuitable for use in the management of acute postoperative pain. This is because therapeutic levels cannot be reached rapidly and the effects then outlast the analgesic requirement in most cases exposing patients to unnecessary side effects.

Transdermal fentanyl is used successfully in the management of chronic pain and the pain associated with malignancy. It provides improved pain relief when compared with sustained-release oral morphine and is associated with reduced constipation and somnolence (Level I: Clark *et al.* 2004).

Other transdermal opioids are available in a matrix-patch presentation, e.g. buprenorphine (BuTrans®, Napp Pharmaceuticals), but are indicated only for the treatment of severe opioid responsive pain conditions which are not adequately responding to non-opioid analgesics. Although not an opioid, of note is that lidocaine (lignocaine) is now available as a medicated plaster (Versatis®, Grunenthal) and is indicated for the management of neuropathic pain associated with previous herpes zoster infection.

Iontophoretic transdermal delivery systems

The passage of ionised medicines through the epidermis and particularly the stratum corneum of the epidermis is limited and slow. Opioid medicines such as fentanyl are usually highly ionised.

Iontophoresis is the facilitated movement of ions across a membrane under the influence of an externally applied small electrical potential difference.

The technology has been successfully applied to the delivery of a number of medicines with poor absorption profiles across the skin (including fentanyl). Absorption into the systemic circulation is achieved without delay.

Iontophoresis provides all the advantages of the transdermal route in that it is needle-free, bypasses first-pass metabolism (see Box 11.1) and avoids the variability of absorption associated with orally administered drugs. In addition, the system can reduce dose variation by providing programmable delivery of the drug. Rapid therapeutic levels are achieved and drug delivery can be rapidly terminated by turning off the iontophoretic system in contrast to the passive transdermal system.

The analgesic effect achieved by the delivery system can be further enhanced by enabling the patient to control the frequency of administration of the programmed dose.

The fentanyl iontophoretic transdermal system (ITS) uses an imperceptible current of 170 mA to actively deliver into the vasculature a dose of fentanyl of 40 mcg over 10 min. The unit is programmed to lock out further doses after either 80 doses or 24 hr, whichever is arrived at first (Herndon 2007).

This patient-controlled iontophorectic system provides an easy-to-use, compact, needle-free, reliable and safe way to deliver preprogrammed doses of fentanyl into the patient's systemic circulation on demand. Such systems are superior to placebo (Chelly *et al.* 2004, Level II: Viscusi *et al.* 2006) and are as safe and effective as IV morphine PCA for managing acute postoperative pain (Grond *et al.* 2007, Level II: Viscusi *et al.* 2004). Patients, nurses and physiotherapists rated the fentanyl transdermal iontophoretic system higher than an IV morphine system in terms of ease of care (Level II: Grond *et al.* 2007).

Recent analysis of pooled data from three multicentre, randomised, active-controlled trials ($n = 1941$) suggest that fentanyl ITS is effective and has a consistent safety and efficacy profile for postoperative pain management (Level I: Viscusi *et al.* 2007).

Transmucosal routes

During the perioperative period, the use of oral analgesia is limited by the effects of gastric emptying and hepatic first-pass metabolism.

Drugs administered by intranasal, sublingual, buccal and pulmonary routes are rapidly absorbed by the vascular mucosa directly into the systemic circulation and are not subject to hepatic first-pass metabolism (see Box 11.1). The bioavailability of transmucosal opioids is greater than that when administered orally. The rapid absorption enables effective titration of effective analgesia in the acute pain setting.

Intranasal route

The nasal mucosa is very vascular and permits rapid absorption of drugs into the bloodstream. The maximum volume that can be administered by this route is limited to 150 mcL to prevent run-off into the pharynx. Any swallowed component will be absorbed from the stomach or small intestine and be subject to first-pass metabolism. Patient acceptability may be limited by the bitter taste often experienced (Dale *et al.* 2002).

Sufentanil has been used successfully in low dosage as a premedicant for children administered by nasal spray (Level II: Bayrak *et al.* 2007) and as a patient-controlled intranasal system for acute postoperative pain management in adults (Level II: Mathieu *et al.* 2006).

As an alternative to intramuscular morphine in the paediatric population, patient-controlled intranasal diamorphine seems to provide a well-tolerated, rapid, effective and safe method of providing analgesia (Level II: Kendall *et al.* 2001). The intranasal method of administration was preferred by patients, parents and staff.

A number of studies have found intranasal fentanyl to be as effective for postoperative analgesia as IV fentanyl in adult (Striebel *et al.* 1992, 1996, Level II: Toussaint *et al.* 2000) and paediatric patient groups (Level II: Manjushree *et al.* 2002).

Sublingual and buccal routes

Medicines may be administered by placing a tablet or lozenge under the tongue or against the buccal mucosa (cheek) where it is permitted to dissolve.

Holding the drug in the mouth requires patient cooperation and may not be possible in all situations. Any portion of the drug that is swallowed and absorbed from the stomach or small intestine will be exposed to first-pass metabolism and adequate plasma levels may not be achieved. Analyses of morphine metabolites after administration by various routes show that first-pass metabolism after sublingual and buccal administration is not inconsiderable (Level I: Faura *et al.* 1998).

The doses of analgesics deliverable by these routes are limited by the physical size of the preparation that can be comfortably held in the mouth and by the often bitter or unpleasant taste experienced in many cases.

Fentanyl is available as a flavoured solid lozenge on a stick (oral transmucosal fentanyl citrate, OTFC). Oral transmucosal fentanyl provides a rapid onset of pain relief and is appropriate for treating episodes of breakthrough pain (Mercadante & Fulfaro 1999). Rather than resting the lozenge against the mucosa, the patient should be advised to 'paint' all inside surfaces of the mouth (cheeks and tongue) for a period of up to 15 min. This action may be quite difficult if the patient is weak or has a dry or ulcerated mouth.

OTFC has been shown to provide effective postoperative analgesia following orthopaedic (Level II: Ashburn *et al.* 1993) and abdominal surgery (Level II: Lichtor *et al.* 1999).

OTFC can be useful for patients who require analgesia with a short onset and duration and has been successfully used for burns and wound dressings in a number of population settings (including non-opioid naïve adolescents), providing a palatable alternative route of opioid administration without IV access (Level II: Sharar *et al.* 1998).

SL buprenorphine is licensed as a strong analgesic for the relief of moderate-to-severe pain. Buprenorphine is a µ (mu) opioid partial agonist and a κ (kappa) antagonist. It is a strong analgesic of the partial agonist (mixed agonist/antagonist) class. The bioavailability of SL buprenorphine is 30–35% and that of OTFC about 52%. Buprenorphine undergoes first-pass hepatic metabolism with *N*-dealkylation and glucuroconjugation in the small intestine. The use of this medication by the oral route is therefore inappropriate.

Pulmonary route

Absorption of medication from the pulmonary route is dependent on the size of the molecule concerned with only solids and liquids smaller than 20 µm being absorbed. Substances larger than this tend to impact in the mouth and throat (Calvey & Williams 2001).

Administration of morphine using standard nebulisers results in bioavailability of only 5% (Masood & Thomas 1996). Newer drug delivery systems can increase the bioavailability of morphine up to 59–100% (Mather *et al.* 1998, Ward *et al.* 1997) and that of fentanyl up to 100% (Mather *et al.* 1998, Ward *et al.* 1997).

Locally administered opioids

Much effort has been made to demonstrate that peripherally administered opioids might have an effect on opioid receptors locally with avoidance of central or systemic adverse effects. Much of the work has concentrated on intra-articular administration or on opioid supplementation of IV regional anaesthetic for joint replacement surgery. Large-scale studies have not been undertaken and meta-analysis of those studies that have been done has found no evidence to support the use of peripherally administered opioids (Level I: Kalso *et al.* 1997).

Summary

In the acute pain setting, the aim is to achieve rapidly, and to maintain, therapeutic plasma levels of opioid analgesic medication while avoiding periods of subtherapeutic levels or levels associated with toxicity or unacceptable side effects. The route chosen must be influenced by the nature and severity of the pain, availability of suitable opioid formulations and their increasingly sophisticated delivery systems, and the acceptability of the suggested regime to the patient and their carers.

While traditional routes of administration still have a role to play in some settings, there is a significant body of evidence to support the rejection of intermittent intramuscular regimes or of inflexible regular analgesia regimes in favour of more patient-centred and directed strategies for opioid delivery by intravenous, subcutaneous, transmucosal or transdermal routes. Routes previously considered unsuitable for titration in the acute postoperative pain setting are becoming more applicable with the development of effective PCA systems able to deliver appropriate preprogrammed doses of opioid medication rapidly and safely into the systemic circulation.

References

Ashburn, M.A., Lind, G.H., Gillie, M.H., *et al.* (1993) Oral transmucosal fentanyl citrate (OTFC) for the treatment of postoperative pain. *Anesthesia and Analgesia*, **76** (2), 377–381.

Bainbridge, D., Martin, J.E. & Cheng, D.C. (2006) Patient-controlled versus nurse-controlled analgesia after cardiac surgery – a meta-analysis. *Canadian Journal of Anaesthesia*, **53** (5), 492–499.

Bayrak, F., Gunday, I., Memis, D. & Turan, A. (2007) A comparison of oral midazolam, oral tramadol, and intranasal sufentanil premedication in pediatric patients. *Journal of Opioid Management*, **3** (2), 74–78.

Calvey, T.N. & Williams, N.E. (2001) *Principles and Practices of Pharmacology for Anaesthetists*, 4th edn. Blackwell Science, Oxford.

Chelly, J.E., Grass, J., Houseman, T.W., *et al.* (2004) The safety and efficacy of a fentanyl patient-controlled transdermal system for acute postoperative analgesia: a multicenter, placebo-controlled trial. *Anesthesia and Analgesia*, **98** (2), 427–433.

Clark, A.J., Ahmedzai, S.H., Allan, L.G., *et al.* (2004) Efficacy and safety of transdermal fentanyl and sustained-release oral morphine in patients with cancer and chronic non-cancer pain. *Current Medical Research and Opinion*, **20** (9), 1419–1428.

Collins, S.L., Edwards, J.E., Moore, R.A. & McQuay, H.J. (2000) Single dose dextropropoxyphene, alone and with paracetamol (acetaminophen), for postoperative pain. *Cochrane Database of Systematic Reviews*, Issue 2, Art No CD001440.

Cooper, I.M. (1996) Morphine for postoperative analgesia. A comparison of intramuscular and subcutaneous routes of administration. *Anaesthesia and Intensive Care*, **24** (5), 574–578.

Cruikshank, R.H., Spencer, A. & Ellis, F.R. (1996) Pretreatment with controlled-release morphine for pain after hysterectomy. *Anaesthesia*, **51** (12), 1097–1101.

Dale, O., Hjortkjaer, R. & Kharasch, E.D. (2002) Nasal administration of opioids for pain management in adults. *Acta Anaesthesiologica Scandinavica*, **46** (7), 759–770.

Edwards, J.E., McQuay, H.J. & Moore, R.A. (2000a) Single dose dihydrocodeine for acute postoperative pain. *Cochrane Database of Systematic Reviews*, Issue 4, Art No CD002760.

Edwards, J.E., McQuay, H.J. & Moore, R.A. (2002) Combination analgesic efficacy: individual patient data meta-analysis of single-dose oral tramadol plus acetaminophen in acute postoperative pain. *Journal of Pain and Symptom Management*, **23** (2), 121–130.

Edwards, J.E., Moore, R.A. & McQuay, H.J. (2000b) Single dose oxycodone and oxycodone plus paracetamol (acetominophen) for acute postoperative pain. *Cochrane Database of Systematic Reviews*, Issue 4, Art No CD002763.

Faura, C.C., Collins, S.L., Moore, R.A. & McQuay, H.J. (1998) Systematic review of factors affecting the ratios of morphine and its major metabolites. *Pain*, **74** (1), 43–53.

Gin, T., Kan, A.F., Lam, K.K. & O'Meara, M.E. (1993) Analgesia after caesarean section with intramuscular ketorolac or pethidine. *Anaesthesia and Intensive Care*, **21** (4), 420–423.

Goudie, T.A., Allan, M.W., Lonsdale, M., *et al.* (1985) Continuous subcutaneous infusion of morphine for postoperative pain relief. *Anaesthesia*, **40** (11), 1086–1092.

Grond, S., Hall, J., Spacek, A., *et al.* (2007) Iontophoretic transdermal system using fentanyl compared with patient-controlled intravenous analgesia using morphine for postoperative pain management. *British Journal of Anaesthesia*, **98** (6), 806–815.

Herndon, C.M. (2007) Iontophoretic drug delivery system: focus on fentanyl. *Pharmacotherapy*, **27** (5), 745–754.

Hopkins, D., Shipton, E.A., Potgieter, D., *et al.* (1998) Comparison of tramadol and morphine via subcutaneous PCA following major orthopaedic surgery. *Canadian Journal of Anaesthesia*, **45** (5 Part 1), 435–442.

Hudcova, J., McNicol, E., Quah, C., *et al.* (2006) Patient controlled opioid analgesia versus conventional opioid analgesia for postoperative pain. *Cochrane Database of Systematic Reviews*, Issue 4, Art No CD003348.

Kalso, E., Tramér, M.R., Carroll, D., *et al.* (1997) Pain relief from intra-articular morphine after knee surgery: a qualitative systematic review. *Pain*, **71** (2), 127–134.

Kampe, S., Warm, M., Kauffman, J., *et al.* (2004) Clinical efficacy of controlled-release oxycodone 20 mg administered on a 12-h dosing schedule on the management of postoperative pain after breast surgery for cancer. *Current Medical and Research Opinion*, **20** (2), 199–202.

Kaufmann, J., Yesiloglu, S., Patermann, B., *et al.* (2004) Controlled-release oxycodone is better tolerated than intravenous tramadol/metamizol for postoperative analgesia after retinal-surgery. *Current Eye Research*, **28** (4), 271–275.

Kendall, J.M., Reeves, B.C. & Latter, V.S. (2001) Multicentre randomised controlled trial of nasal diamorphine for analgesia in children and teenagers with clinical fractures. *British Medical Journal*, **322** (7281), 261–265.

Lichtor, J.L., Sevarino, F.B., Joshi, G.P., *et al.* (1999) The relative potency of oral transmucosal fentanyl citrate compared with intravenous morphine in the treatment of moderate to severe postoperative pain. *Anesthesia and Analgesia*, **89** (3), 732–738.

Li Wan Po, A. & Zhang, W.Y. (1997) Systematic overview of co-proxamol to assess analgesic effects of addition of dextropropoxyphene to paracetamol. *British Medical Journal*, **315** (7122), 1565–1571.

Manjushree, R., Lahiri, A., Ghosh, B.R., *et al.* (2002) Intranasal fentanyl provides adequate postoperative analgesia in pediatric patients. *Canadian Journal of Anaesthesia*, **49** (2), 190–193.

Marret, E., Remy, C. & Bonnet, F. (2007) Meta-analysis of epidural analgesia versus parenteral opioid analgesia after colorectal surgery. *British Journal of Surgery*, **94** (6), 665–673.

Masood, A.R. & Thomas, S.H. (1996) Systemic absorption of nebulized morphine compared with oral morphine in healthy subjects. *British Journal of Clinical Pharmacology*, **41** (3), 250–252.

Mather, L.E., Woodhouse, A., Ward, M.E., *et al.* (1998) Pulmonary administration of aerosolised fentanyl: pharmacokinetic analysis of systemic delivery. *British Journal of Clinical Pharmacology*, **46** (1), 37–43.

Mathieu, N., Cnudde, N., Engelmann, E. & Barvais, L. (2006) Intranasal sufentanil is effective for postoperative analgesia in adults. *Canadian Journal of Anaesthesia*, **53** (1), 60–66.

McCormack, J.P., Warriner, C.B., Levine, M. & Glick, N. (1993) A comparison of regularly dosed oral morphine and on-demand intramuscular morphine in the treatment of postsurgical pain. *Canadian Journal of Anaesthesia*, **40** (9), 819–824.

McQuay, H. & Edwards, J. (2003) Meta-analysis of single dose oral tramadol plus acetaminophen in acute postoperative pain. *European Journal of Anaesthesiology*, **28** (Suppl), 19–22.

McQuay, H.J., Carroll, D. & Moore, R.A. (1999) Injected morphine in postoperative pain: a quantitative systematic review. *Journal of Pain and Symptom Management*, **17** (3), 164–174.

Medve, R.A., Wang, J. & Karim, R. (2001) Tramadol and acetaminophen tablets for dental pain. *Anesthesia Progress*, **48** (3), 79–81.

Mercadante, S. & Fulfaro, F. (1999) Alternatives to oral opioids for cancer pain. *Oncology (Williston Park)*, **13** (2), 215–220, 225; discussion 226–229.

Moore, A., Collins, S., Carroll, D., *et al.* (2000) Single dose paracetamol (acetaminophen), with and without codeine, for postoperative pain. *Cochrane Database of Systematic Reviews*, Issue 2, Art No CD001547.

Moore, R.A. & McQuay, H.J. (1997) Single-patient data meta-analysis of 3453 postoperative patients: oral tramadol versus placebo, codeine and combination analgesics. *Pain*, **69** (3), 287–294.

Owczarzak, V. & Haddad, J. (2006) Comparison of oral versus rectal administration of acetaminophen with codeine in postoperative pediatric adenotonsillectomy patients. *Laryngoscope*, **116** (8), 1485–1488.

Pang, W.W., Mok, M.S., Huang, S., *et al.* (2000) Intraoperative loading attenuates nausea and vomiting of tramadol patient-controlled analgesia. *Canadian Journal of Anaesthesia*, **47** (10), 968–973.

Pang, W.W., Wu, H.S., Lin, C.H., *et al.* (2002) Metoclopramide decreases emesis but increases sedation in tramadol patient-controlled analgesia. *Canadian Journal of Anaesthesia*, **49** (10), 1029–1033.

Reuben, S.S., Steinberg, R.B., Maciolek, H. & Joshi, W. (2002) Preoperative administration of controlled-release oxycodone for the management of pain after ambulatory laparoscopic tubal ligation surgery. *Journal of Clinical Anesthesiology*, **14** (3), 223–227.

Schug, S.A. & Torrie, J.J. (1993) Safety assessment of postoperative pain management by an acute pain service. *Pain*, **55** (3), 387–391.

Sharar, S.R., Bratton, S.L., Carrougher, G.J., *et al.* (1998) A comparison of oral transmucosal fentanyl citrate and oral hydromorphone for inpatient pediatric burn wound care analgesia. *The Journal of Burn Care and Rehabilitation*, **19** (6), 516–521.

Smith, L.A., Carroll, D., Edwards, J.E., *et al.* (2000) Single-dose ketorolac and pethidine in acute postoperative pain: systematic review with meta-analysis. *British Journal of Anaesthesia*, **84** (1), 48–58.

Striebel, H.W., Koenigs, D. & Kramer, J. (1992) Postoperative pain management by intranasal demand-adapted fentanyl titration. *Anesthesiology*, **77** (2), 281–285.

Striebel, H.W., Oelmann, T., Spies, C., *et al.* (1996) Patient-controlled intranasal analgesia: a method for noninvasive postoperative pain management. *Anesthesia and Analgesia*, **83** (3), 548–551.

Sunshine, A., Olson, N.Z., Colon, A., *et al.* (1996) Analgesic efficacy of controlled-release oxycodone in postoperative pain. *Journal of Clinical Pharmacology*, **36** (7), 595–603.

Toussaint, S., Maidl, J., Schwagmeier, R. & Striebel, H.W. (2000) Patient-controlled intranasal analgesia: effective alternative to intravenous PCA for postoperative pain relief. *Canadian Journal of Anaesthesia*, **47** (4), 299–302.

Viscusi, E.R., Reynolds, L., Chung, F., *et al.* (2004) Patient-controlled transdermal fentanyl hydrochloride vs intravenous morphine pump for postoperative pain: a randomized controlled trial. *Journal of the American Medical Association*, **291** (11), 1333–1341.

Viscusi, E.R., Reynolds, L., Tait, S., *et al.* (2006) An iontophoretic fentanyl patient-activated analgesic delivery system for postoperative pain: a double-blind, placebo-controlled trial. *Anesthesia and Analgesia*, **102** (1), 188–194.

Viscusi, E.R., Siccardi, M., Damaraju, C.V., *et al.* (2007) The safety and efficacy of fentanyl iontophoretic transdermal system compared with morphine intravenous patient-controlled analgesia for postoperative pain management: an analysis of pooled data from three randomized, active-controlled clinical studies. *Anesthesia and Analgesia*, **105** (5), 1428–1436.

Walder, B., Schafer, M., Henzi, I. & Tramér, M.R. (2001) Efficacy and safety of patient-controlled opioid analgesia for acute postoperative pain. A quantitative systematic review. *Acta Anaesthesiologica Scandinavica*, **45** (7), 795–804.

Ward, M.E., Woodhouse, A., Mather, L.E., *et al.* (1997) Morphine pharmacokinetics after pulmonary administration from a novel aerosol delivery system. *Clinical Pharmacology and Therapeutics*, **62** (6), 596–609.

Zhang, W.Y. & Li Wan Po, A. (1996) Analgesic efficacy of paracetamol and its combination with codeine and caffeine in surgical pain – a meta-analysis. *Journal of Clinical Pharmacy and Therapeutics*, **21** (4), 261–282.

Useful websites

Association of British Pharmaceutical Industries: *http://www.abpi.org.uk/*.
Current Controlled Trials Register: *http://www.controlled-trials.com/mrct/search.html*.
Medicines and Healthcare products Regulatory Agency (MHRA): *http://www.mhra.gov.uk/home*.
The Wellcome Trust: *http://www.wellcome.ac.uk/*.

12 *Managing Perioperative Pain in Special Circumstances*

PAEDIATRIC PAIN MANAGEMENT
Elizabeth M.C. Ashley

Key Messages

- A multimodal approach using oral analgesics, local anaesthetic infiltration or blocks is effective and safe in children.
- More sophisticated techniques, such as patient-controlled analgesia, nurse-controlled analgesia and epidurals, require appropriately trained personnel, monitoring and the support of a paediatric acute pain team.
- Chronic pain can develop in children who undergo surgery or painful procedures, and is an area of expanding interest and research.

Introduction

Historically, pain has been poorly managed in paediatric practice for various reasons; the extent to which neonates and babies feel pain has not been widely studied together with anaesthetists and paediatricians inexperienced in pain management in children. Fears concerning side effects of analgesic techniques and drugs have resulted in a reluctance to use neuraxial blocks, for example, or prescribe therapeutically efficacious doses of analgesia. Many new drugs have not undergone clinical trials in paediatrics and therefore have to be prescribed 'off-licence'. This means that paediatric pain prescribing lags behind adult practice.

However, this has now been addressed and there are many proponents of paediatric pain management, from major paediatric surgical centres that publish widely in the anaesthetic and pain literature who have set up comprehensive paediatric pain services in their own institutions. The impetus for this has been the wish for humane treatment of children, the recognition that good analgesia prevents complications post-surgery, the prevention of the development of chronic pain, economic pressures to decrease hospital stay and the increase in day-case surgery. Other paediatric patient groups have also benefited, such as children with sickle cell disease. Children now benefit from patient-controlled opioid analgesia, nurse-controlled analgesia or epidural infusions. The approach to paediatric analgesia is multimodal and it is managed by a multidisciplinary paediatric pain team, consisting of anaesthetists, specialist pain nurses, trained ward nurses and pharmacists (Lloyd-Thomas 1999).

Licensing of analgesic medicines in paediatric practice

Many medicines have been used 'off-licence' in paediatric pain because pharma companies have been unwilling to carry out the necessary research in children to obtain a paediatric licence. This has inevitably slowed down the evolution of paediatric pain management. Recently, however, the FDA in America has made it mandatory for the pharmaceutical industry to carry out research in children as part of the licensing process. Prior to this many drugs were, and still are, used in an 'unapproved' way. This did not imply an improper or illegal use, but left the physician with increased responsibility regarding the decision to use a particular analgesic and the appropriate dose of the drug in a child (Coté 1997).

Routes of drug delivery

Traditional routes of postoperative analgesia, such as intramuscular injections, have been replaced by intravenous or subcutaneous infusions or patient-controlled analgesia (PCA) in paediatric practice based on paediatric pharmacokinetics (Table 12.1). Neuraxial blockade in the form of epidural analgesia and

Table 12.1 Paediatric pharmacokinetics.

Absorption	Reduced muscle blood flow and poor contraction delays intramuscular absorption
Distribution	High extracellular fluid volume and total body water. Smaller fat deposits. Reduced protein binding increases the concentration of free drug. More permeable blood–brain barrier. Possibly increased sensitivity of opioid receptors in the brain
Detoxification	Immature oxidation and glucuronidation leads to variably prolonged half-life of analgesics, including opioids and paracetamol
Excretion	Immature renal function and reduced glomerular filtration rate leads to reduced clearance

local anaesthetic infiltration and blocks are popular. Local anaesthetic creams are used prior to venepuncture or cannulation. Inhaled nitrous oxide has been used as an analgesic for short painful procedures, such as the change of burns dressings. A multimodal approach using oral analgesics with different pharmacodynamics or modes of action is an important concept in paediatric pain relief. Transmucosal and transdermal drug delivery systems show potential for simple, elegant paediatric pain management in the future (Gaukroger 1991). They avoid first-pass metabolism and large variations in plasma concentration, as well as avoiding needles and cannulation (Margettes & Sawyer 2007).

Pain management in neonates and children

Foetal pain

Foetal pain has been widely debated in the context of late abortion or fetal surgery. Pain is defined as 'an unpleasant sensory and emotional experience associated with actual or potential tissue damage'. It requires experience related to past injury. Before 26 weeks' gestation, the thalamocortical pain fibres have not penetrated the neural plate and therefore it is impossible for any higher cortical process to be involved in the perception of pain. Any response to pain prior to 26 weeks' gestation is reflex withdrawal at a spinal cord level. After 26 weeks' gestation, premature infants grimace in response to heel prick and also mount a biochemical stress reaction in response to needle insertion to an intrahepatic vein. The connection between a biochemical or hormonal response and the perception of pain remains unclear. The foetal nervous system mounts responses to noxious stimuli to prevent tissue injury, but probably does not feel pain according to the conventional definition until the last trimester. However, exposure to painful stimuli in utero may influence neural development and the development of chronic pain in adult life (Derbyshire & Furedi 1996).

Neonatal pain

Until the late 1980s, neonates and infants were assumed to be incapable of perceiving pain and were seldom given analgesia for surgery. This has been partially attributed to concerns about complications, especially in neonates with immature physiology including immature renal function and glomerular filtration rate (GFR), reduced plasma protein binding and increased free drug concentration and immature hepatic enzyme systems for drug conjugation and metabolism (Marsh *et al.* 1997). There is, however, overwhelming clinical evidence that neonates react to noxious stimuli, but analgesic pathways are anatomically and functionally different in the neonatal rat compared with the adult. There are numerous afferent terminations, in addition to a lack of local and ascending inhibitory controls, paradoxically causing exaggerated pain responses. In addition, the use of opioids has increased in neonates, but knowledge of their effects is incomplete, in particular, analgesic potency and the effects of opioids on the development of immature pain pathways (Marsh *et al.* 1997).

Pain in children

Providing good pain relief in children requires a pre-emptive, pro-active, preventive approach; the intramuscular route should be avoided by using intravenous, subcutaneous in-dwelling cannulae or rectal or oral routes of administration. Topical local anaesthetic creams (EMLA, Ametop) should be used prior to painful needle procedures. Local anaesthetic – infiltration or regional – techniques should be carried out intraoperatively, in addition to loading with opioids, non-steroidal anti-inflammatory drugs (NSAIDs) and paracetamol as indicated during surgery. This multimodal approach should be continued in the postoperative period with regularly prescribed analgesia, as opposed to 'as required' regimens. Adequate rescue analgesia for breakthrough pain must be prescribed. Extra analgesia should be administered in anticipation of painful procedures such as physiotherapy, dressing changes or drain removal.

Stress response

At 23 weeks' gestation, a biochemical stress response can be measured in response to a noxious stimulus. Young infants can mount a massive stress response to surgery, which can be reduced by inhalational anaesthesia and opiates (Aynsley-Green 1996).

Pain assessment

There are seven dimensions of the pain experience that should be considered when assessing a child's pain. These include cognitive, physiological, sensory, behavioural, affective, sociocultural and environmental factors. Additional information on these factors can be found in Chapters 2–4. Pain scores are limited in that they assign a numerical value to only one dimension (Morton 1997). A pain assessment system should:

(1) Detect the presence of pain
(2) Estimate its severity
(3) Determine the effectiveness of interventions

Pre-verbal children and those with learning difficulties are the most difficult to assess.

Neonates (up to 1 month; or ex-premature up to 60 weeks' post-conceptual age)

A variety of assessment tools are available, based on observation of facial expression, body position and mobility, crying and heart rate, blood pressure, skin colour, oxygen saturation, respiratory rate and sleeplessness. These are subjective, however, depending on the maturity of the neonate and the severity of illness. They include the objective pain score (OPS), CRIES, NIPS, COMFORT and CHEOPS. CRIES for example is an acronym based on five physiological and behavioural variables: C, crying; R, requires increased oxygen administration; I, increased vital signs; E, expression; S, sleeplessness (Level III-2: Krechel & Bildner 1995). CHEOPS stands for Children's Hospital of Eastern Ontario Pain Scale. It considers six elements: cry, facial, child verbal, torso, touch and legs. A score greater than 4 indicates pain. NIPS, the Neonatal or Infant Pain Score, considers facial expression, cry, breathing patterns, arm position, leg position and state of arousal. It is used in neonates and children under 1 year and a score of 3 or greater indicates pain.

Infants and toddlers (1 month–3 years)

Similar assessment tools are used as in neonates, remembering that the very sick or ventilated and sedated infant will not exhibit the same behaviour as the healthy baby. Toddlers may demonstrate a vigorous response, grabbing at the operation site. Information from parents and experienced paediatric nurses are usually helpful and accurate.

Children (3–7 years)

Most children over the age of 3 years can explain where they feel pain and how bad it is. The 'Oucher' Faces scale consisting of a series of faces in varying degrees of discomfort is useful in those more than 4 years of age, as is the Poker Chip tool, which involves 'pieces of hurt'. A visual analogue scale can be understood by children over the age of 7 years. Previous pain experience will influence older children; those who have undergone multiple painful procedures and surgery may be highly sensitised and have very low pain thresholds.

Older children and adolescents (7 years plus)

Older children can use visual analogue scales as well as describe the intensity, location and quality of pain. Clinical signs such as heart rate, blood pressure and response to movement remain important adjuncts in sedated and ventilated children and those with learning difficulties.

With all children, pain assessment must be carried out, analgesia titrated to control pain and then pain reassessed at regular intervals.

A pain service for children

The report 'Pain after Surgery' (Royal College of Surgeons 1990) recommended the establishment of an acute pain service in hospitals carrying out paediatric surgery. The service provides clear protocols for pain assessment, patient medication and patient observation, which can be applied consistently throughout the institution.

The acute pain service aims to:

- Provide safe and successful analgesia
- Train staff
- Carry out research and development

The elements of the service include:

(a) *Staffing*
  - Trained ward nurses
  - Anaesthetists
  - Physiotherapists
  - Pharmacists
  - Acute pain nurses

(b) *Nursing areas*
  Although Level 2 (HDU) or 3 (ICU/ITU) facilities may be safer, an acute pain service needs to establish acceptable, practical standards of observation and treatment, thereby enabling patients to be managed on surgical wards.

(c) *Equipment*
  Epidural and PCA infusion devices should be standardised throughout the hospital to reduce programming errors. Standards of monitoring including saturation monitoring and apnoea mattresses must be established.

(d) *Funding*
  - Capital costs for equipment
  - Ongoing staff costs, i.e. staff salaries
  - Audit to show improved patient outcomes and decreased length of hospital stay (Lloyd-Thomas & Howard 1994)

A multimodal approach to pain relief in children

A multimodal approach to analgesia aims to reduce nociceptive activity by different therapeutic interventions at various points in the pain pathway, thereby reducing the dose and consequently the side effects of any single drug (Lloyd-Thomas 1997).

Local anaesthetic infiltration and peripheral nerve blocks

Topical local anaesthetic gels can be used prior to cannulation or painful procedures on the ITU.

Simple wound infiltration with local anaesthetic by the surgeons is a useful adjunct as long as toxic dose limits are not exceeded. Commonly performed regional nerve blocks in children are detailed in Table 12.2.

Table 12.2 Paediatric regional blockade.

Local block	Nerves anaesthetised	Surgical procedures
Inguinal	Ilioinguinal and iliohypogastric	Inguinal hernia repair, orchidopexy
Penile	Dorsal nerve of penis	Circumcision
Axillary	Brachial plexus	Arm and hand surgery
Femoral	Femoral nerve	Surgery to femur and thigh

Simple analgesics

Paracetamol

Paracetamol is a mild analgesic that has a synergistic effect when used with other drugs. It acts in the central nervous system by inhibition of COX-4 receptors, serotonergic pathway activation, or inhibition of substance P or nitric oxide or by NMDA antagonism. It is predominantly metabolised in the liver by glucuronidation or sulphation, but a small amount is metabolised by the cytochrome P450 enzyme system to the potentially hepatotoxic metabolite *N*-acetyl-*p*-amino-benzoquinone imine (NAPQI). Paracetamol toxicity is more likely to occur in chronic paracetamol therapy, malnutrition (reduced glutathione stores) or P450 enzyme induction.

Toxicity in children is associated with doses in excess of 150 mg/kg, especially if continued for more than 5 days. The P450 enzyme has lower activity in the neonate, which confers protection against hepatotoxicity due to decreased production of NAPQI. Previously, paracetamol has been administered to children in subtherapeutic doses. Therefore, to achieve therapeutic plasma concentrations, rectal loading dose of 40 mg/kg is followed by oral or rectal doses of 20 mg/kg 6-hourly. This rectal loading dose has been shown to be safe in children with liver disease (Level IV: Cormack *et al.* 2006).

Non-steroidal anti-inflammatory drugs

Non-steroidal anti-inflammatory drugs (NSAIDs) provide effective analgesia for moderate postoperative pain and have an opioid-sparing effect. Aspirin is not used in children due to its association with Reye's syndrome. Ibuprofen and diclofenac are the most commonly prescribed NSAIDS in children over 6 months of age. In younger children, there are concerns about their effects on cerebral and renal perfusion. NSAIDs inhibit cyclooxygenase, which reduces prostaglandin-mediated peripheral nociception. Side effects include platelet dysfunction, gastrointestinal bleeding, renal dysfunction and exacerbation of asthma. They have also been implicated in the failure of spinal fusion surgery due to inhibition of osteoblast activity. They should be avoided therefore in children with renal dysfunction, liver disease, severe asthma or those at risk of significant bleeding. Some anaesthetists would avoid them post-tonsillectomy for example (Howard 2002, Romsing & Walther-Larsen 1997). It is important never to cut suppositories as the active drug is not evenly distributed within the suppository.

Codeine phosphate

Codeine is safe and can be used by the oral or rectal route for mild to moderate pain in children. It can be given as an intramuscular injection in anaesthetised children, but causes severe hypotension if given intravenously. Codeine is metabolised to morphine, but 10% of the population lack the appropriate enzyme and therefore do not benefit from the analgesic effects of the drug (Tremlett 1999, Zacharias & Watts 1998).

Morphine

Morphine is the drug of choice for severe pain in infants and children. It can be given orally, by subcutaneous or intravenous routes and via nurse-controlled or patient-controlled analgesia. Prolonged elimination in neonates implies that the maintenance dose should be reduced and the dosing interval increased.

Oral morphine

Immediate-release suspensions (Oromorph) and slow-release morphine sulphate continus (MST) are available for paediatric use. Morphine is well absorbed orally if the gastrointestinal tract is functioning.

Intravenous morphine infusions

Dosage regimens are illustrated in Table 12.3. The body weight of the child in milligrams of morphine is diluted in 50 mL of 5% dextrose. Then 1 mL of diluted morphine solution always equals 20 mcg/kg/mL. The infusion should

Table 12.3 Morphine infusions for patient-controlled and nurse-controlled analgesia.

IV or SC	Standard morphine infusions	Maximum 4-hourly dose
IV up to 50 kg	Morphine sulphate 1 mg/kg in 50 mL 5% dextrose = 20 mcg/kg/mL	400 mcg/kg = 20 mL
SC up to 50 kg	Morphine sulphate 1 mg/kg in 20 mL of normal saline = 50 mcg/kg/mL	400 mcg/kg = 8 mL

be on a dedicated IV cannula with an antisyphon valve in the infusion line. If this is impossible and the morphine infusion has to run with IV fluids, an antireflux valve must also be included in the infusion line. A suitable loading dose is 50–100 mcg/kg, with an infusion running at 10–30 mcg/kg/hr.

Subcutaneous morphine infusions

A cannula, e.g. 23 gauge, can be inserted into the subcutaneous tissue over the deltoid muscle and firmly secured with a clear dressing. The child's weight in milligrams of morphine is dissolved in 20 mL of sodium chloride 0.9% for a subcutaneous infusion. The solution is necessarily more concentrated to decrease the bolus volume and therefore decrease pain on administration.

Morphine PCA

PCA is suitable for children over the age of 5 years (GOS 2000). In fact most adapt to it more readily than the technophobic elderly population. For safe PCA, it is important to educate those involved that it is the child that must press the button, not the parents or the nursing staff. A bolus dose of 20 mcg/kg has been shown to be optimal in achieving lower pain scores with fewer side effects (particularly, hypoxaemic episodes) (Level III-2: Doyle *et al.* 1994). Contrary to adult practice, a small background infusion is often used in paediatrics to prevent a child waking up in pain and becoming disillusioned and distrustful of the technique. A low-dose background infusion has been shown to be associated with a better sleep pattern, and less hypoxaemia compared with no background infusion (Level III-2: Doyle *et al.* 1993). PCA can be carried out using intravenous or subcutaneous routes of administration, and indeed the subcutaneous route may result in lower morphine consumption, less hypoxic episodes and equivalent pain scores to IV PCA because of positive feedback when a valid demand is administered (Doyle *et al.* 1994).

Morphine NCA

Nurse-controlled analgesia (NCA) uses the principles of PCA but allows the nurses flexibility in managing breakthrough pain in neonates, infants, children under 5 years and children unable to manage PCA. A continuous background infusion is prescribed, with the availability of extra bolus doses to manage breakthrough pain, procedural pain, anticipated physiotherapy etc. The lockout period is long to protect the patient from excessive sedation. In premature or sick infants, the NCA can be used to administer morphine boluses in a controlled way. The background infusion can be omitted (GOS 2000). Suggested PCA regimens can be found in Table 12.4.

All children over 50 kg should be given an adult regimen, e.g. morphine sulphate 100 mg in sodium chloride made up to a total volume of 100 mL = 1 mg/mL (GOS 2000).

Table 12.4 Suggested nurse-controlled analgesia and patient-controlled analgesia programming.

	Loading dose (mcg/kg)	Background infusion (mcg/kg/hr)	Bolus dose (mcg/kg)	Lockout (min)
PCA	50–100	4	10 or 20	5 or 10
NCA 5–50 kg	50–100	0, 4, 10 or 20	10 or 20	20
NCA neonates and infants <5 kg in ICU	20–100	0–20	10 or 20	20

PCA, patient-controlled analgesia; NCA, nurse-controlled analgesia; ICU, intensive care unit.

Epidural analgesia

Epidural analgesia can be achieved by the lumbar or caudal route in babies and children. It is an invasive technique that is reserved for major surgery and requires parental consent. Epidural catheters are inserted under full aseptic conditions using a loss of resistance technique, preferably to saline. The technique is described in Chapter 9. The epidural space can be very superficial in neonates (0.5 cm) and may only be 1 or 2 cm from the skin in older children. Therefore, continuous pressure must be applied to the loss of resistance device to prevent neurological damage or accidental dural puncture. The smallest Tuohy needles that are available are 19 gauge, through which a 23-gauge epidural catheter can be threaded. About 4 cm of the catheter should remain in the epidural space to prevent displacement and leakage in the postoperative period. The catheter should be clearly identified and securely taped to the patient's back with a clear dressing that allows for inspection of the insertion site.

The epidural block is established using 0.75 mL/kg of 0.25% bupivacaine. A suitable infusion solution is bupivacaine 0.125% with 10 mcg/mL of preservative-free morphine. This should run at 0.1–0.4 mL/(kg/hr) according to block height, pain scores and level of sedation (Rowney & Doyle 1998). Alternatively levobupivacaine, the S-(−)-isomer of bupivacaine, is less likely to cause myocardial depression and fatal arrhythmias and is also less toxic to the central nervous system than racemic bupivacaine. Levobupivacaine 0.125% 0.5–0.75 mL/kg can be used to establish the epidural block intraoperatively. This is followed by an infusion consisting of levobupivacaine 0.125% and preservative-free morphine 0.001% at 0.1–0.4 mL/kg/hr (Great Ormond Street Hospital, Department of Anaesthesia and Pain Management Guidelines 2005). Ropivacaine has also been used in paediatric epidural analgesia.

Ropivacaine has a higher therapeutic index and at low concentrations, may produce less motor block and comparable analgesia when compared to bupivacaine with decreased incidence of cardiac and central nervous system toxicity. Due to its possible vasoconstricting properties, ropivacaine may undergo slower systemic absorption than bupivacaine. This may have clinical implications when a prolonged local anaesthetic infusion is used in children with hepatic dysfunction. For a single-shot caudal or epidural block, a bolus of 1 mL/kg of 0.2% ropivacaine is recommended. An infusion of 0.2 mg/kg/hr of 0.1% ropivacaine in infants and 0.4 mg/kg/hr in older children lasting no longer than 48 hr has also been shown to be effective and safe (Tsui *et al.* 2006).

Fentanyl can also be used instead of preservative-free morphine.

Ketamine

Ketamine is an NMDA receptor antagonist and has an analgesic effect at low dosage. NMDA receptors are found in greater numbers at birth and therefore ketamine may have greater efficacy in the young. Hallucinations and bizarre dreams are very rare at low analgesic dosages, compared with anaesthetic doses. Ketamine has been used for analgesia and sedation on the paediatric ICU (Howard 2002).

Clonidine

Clonidine, an α_2-adrenoreceptor antagonist, acts on adrenoreceptors in the dorsal horn of the spinal cord. It can be used orally, intravenously or epidurally in combination with local anaesthesia in children. Side effects include hypotension and sedation (Howard 2002).

Monitoring and complications

Complex analgesic techniques require appropriate nursing ratios, expertise and equipment. The ward staff must be supported, educated and assessed by the acute pain team. A trained anaesthetist must be on site to deal with analgesic problems especially from epidurals, NCA and PCA. Observations should be carried out at hourly intervals, and comprise of conscious level, respiratory rate, analgesic efficacy and the settings on the infusion system. Apnoea mattresses and pulse oximeters are adjuncts to, but not substitutes for, regularly recorded nursing observations. Oxygen and naloxone must be prescribed (Morton 1999).

Paediatric day-case surgery

With the expansion in paediatric day-case surgery, pain management is essential for satisfactory patient outcomes. Regional analgesia that lasts past discharge, optimal dosing regimes for simple analgesics, a multimodal pharmacological approach and parental education to assess pain and administer effective analgesia are important aspects. Topical local anaesthetic gel can be supplied to place on wounds when regional blockade has worn off. Regional block duration can be prolonged with the use of adjuncts, such as ketamine and clonidine. Regular prescribing and administration of therapeutic doses of paracetamol and non-steroidal anti-inflammatory drugs are effective in prevention of breakthrough pain. Parents tend to undertreat a child's pain and therefore simple clear instructions are required, with phone calls from the daycase unit to reinforce the advice that has been given prior to discharge (Morris 1992, Wolf 1999).

Pain on the paediatric ICU

Paediatric intensive care units (PICUs) have been slower to adopt concepts of acute pain management in children, including postoperative pain and pain due to the presenting condition (including burns, meningitis etc.), procedural pain from line insertion, physiotherapy, tracheal suction, chest-drain insertion and removal, catheterisation and nasogastric tubes. Simple topical local anaesthetic creams such as Ametop® and EMLA are useful in addition to non-pharmacological methods; these include parental presence, day/night lighting schemes, toys, music, play therapists and nasal as opposed to oral intubation.

A multimodal pharmacological approach to analgesia is equally applicable on the intensive care unit, with the use of simple analgesics such as paracetamol in conjunction with opioid analgesia. NSAIDs tend to be avoided on the PICU due to concerns regarding renal and cerebral perfusion. Opioids have been shown to decrease surges in blood pressure and decrease heart rate, oxygen consumption and carbon dioxide production. Catecholamines, growth hormone and glucagon are also reduced. Therefore, a detrimental catabolic state may be avoided and physiological stability conferred by effective analgesia. Ketamine and remifentanil also have a role on PICU. Sedation is not equivalent to analgesia and most sedatives do not have analgesic properties. Similarly, paralysis must be used in conjunction with adequate sedation *and* analgesia (Townsend *et al.* 1998).

Postoperative nausea and vomiting in children

Postoperative nausea and vomiting in children has not been widely studied. Concerns include dehydration and electrolyte imbalance, unpleasant patient and parental experience and delayed discharge after day-case surgery. Young children below the age of 2 years are less likely to vomit after surgery. Tonsillectomy, strabismus surgery and ear surgery are more emetic than other procedures. Side effects from anti-emetic agents, such as dystonic reactions, are thought to be more common in children, which has led to a reluctance to prescribe older agents such as metoclopramide in paediatrics. However, the 5-HT$_3$ receptor antagonists are widely prescribed by paediatric anaesthetists (Baines 1996).

Chronic pain development in children

Experience of pain in early life may lead to long-term behavioural changes and/or the development of chronic or neuropathic pain. Behavioural changes can extend far beyond what would be considered normal for a period of post-injury recovery. Timing, the extent of tissue injury and analgesia and its nature may be important in the development of chronic pain states in infants and children. Chronic pain in children has been largely disregarded, but is an area of expanding future interest and research (Howard 2003).

References

Aynsley-Green, A. (1996) Pain and stress in infancy and childhood – where to now? *Paediatric Anaesthesia,* **6** (3), 167–172.

Baines, D. (1996) Postoperative nausea and vomiting in children. *Paediatric Anaesthesia,* **6** (1), 7–14.

Cormack, C.R., Sudan, S., Addison, R., *et al.* (2006) The pharmacokinetics of a single rectal dose of paracetamol 40 mg/kg in children with liver disease. *Paediatric Anaesthesia,* **16** (4), 417–423.

Coté, C.J. (1997) Unapproved uses of approved drugs. *Paediatric Anaesthesia,* **7** (2), 91–92.

Derbyshire, S.W. & Furedi, A. (1996) Do foetuses feel pain? For debate. *British Medical Journal,* **313** (760), 795–799.

Doyle, E., Harper, I. & Morton, N.S. (1993) Patient-controlled analgesia with low dose background infusions after lower abdominal surgery in children. *British Journal of Anaesthesia,* **71** (6), 818–822.

Doyle, E., Morton, N.S. & McNicol, L.R. (1994) Comparison of patient-controlled analgesia in children by i.v. and s.c routes of administration. *British Journal of Anaesthesia,* **72** (5), 533–536.

Doyle, E., Mottart, K.J., Marshall, C. & Morton, N.S. (1994) Comparison of different bolus doses of morphine for patient-controlled analgesia in children. *British Journal of Anaesthesia,* **72** (2), 160–163.

Gaukroger, P.B. (1991) Paediatric analgesia. Which drug? Which dose? *Drugs,* **41** (1), 52–59.

Howard, R.F. (2002) Pain management in infants: systemic analgesics. *British Journal of Anaesthesia CEPD Reviews,* **2** (2), 37–40.

Howard, R.F. (2003) Current status of pain management in children. *Journal of the American Medical Association,* **290** (18), 2464–2469.

Krechel, S.W. & Bildner, J. (1995) CRIES: a new neonatal postoperative pain measurement score. Initial testing of validity and reliability. *Paediatric Anaesthesia,* **5** (1), 53–61.

Lloyd-Thomas, A.R. (1997) Paediatric pain management – the next step? *Paediatric Anaesthesia,* **7,** 487–493.

Lloyd-Thomas, A.R. (1999) Modern concepts of paediatric analgesia. *Pharmacology and Therapeutics,* **83** (1), 1–20.

Lloyd-Thomas, A.R. & Howard, R.F. (1994) A pain service for children *Paediatric Anaesthesia,* **4,** 3–15.

Margettes, L. & Sawyer, R. (2007) Transdermal drug delivery: principles and opioid therapy. *Continuing Education in Anaesthesia, Critical Care and Pain,* **7** (5), 171–176.

Marsh, D.F., Hatch, D.J. & Fitzgerald, M. (1997) Opioid systems and the newborn. *British Journal of Anaesthesia,* **79,** 787–795.

Morris, P. (1992) Paediatric day-case surgery. *British Journal of Anaesthesia,* **68** (1), 3–4.

Morton, N.S. (1997) Pain assessment in children. *Paediatric Anaesthesia,* **7** (4), 267–272.

Morton, N.S. (1999) Prevention and control of pain in children. *British Journal of Anaesthesia*, **83** (1), 118–129.

Peutrell, J. & Millar, S. (1999) Regional analgesia in children: extending the blocks in the lower limb. *CPD Anaesthesia*, **1** (3), 132–140.

Romsing, J. & Walther-Larsen, S. (1997) Peri-operative use of non-steroidal anti-inflammatory drugs in children: analgesic efficacy and bleeding. *Anaesthesia*, **52** (7), 673–683.

Rowney, D.A. & Doyle, E. (1998) Epidural and subarachnoid blockade in children. *Anaesthesia*, **53** (10), 980–1001.

Royal College of Surgeons of England and the Faculty of Anaesthetists (1990) *Report of the Working Party on Pain after Surgery*. The Royal College of Surgeons of England and the College of Anaesthetists, London.

The Hospital for Sick Children. (2000) *Drug Administration Guidelines: Department of Anaesthesia and Pain Control Service*, 8th edn. Great Ormond Street Hospital for Children, London.

Townsend, P., Moriarty, A. & Bagshaw, O. (1998) Pain control on the paediatric intensive care unit. *British Journal of Intensive Care*, **8** (6), 186–193.

Tremlett, M.R. (1999) Paediatric pain relief: improving analgesia in the district general hospital. *CPD Anaesthesia*, **1** (1), 8–12.

Tsui, B.C.H., Fredrickson, M. & Suresh, S. (2006) Paediatric epidural and caudal anaesthesia in children. www.nysora.com. Accessed 31 December 2007.

Wolf, A.R. (1999) Tears at bedtime: a pitfall of extending paediatric day-case surgery without extending analgesia. *British Journal of Anaesthesia*, **82** (3), 319–320.

Zacharias, M. & Watts, D. (1998) Pain relief in children – doing simple things better. *British Medical Journal*, **316** (7144), 1552.

Useful websites

IASP Special Interest Group for Paediatrics: *http://childpain.org/*.
Paediatric Pain Letter: *http://pediatric-pain.ca/ppl/*.
The UCL Institute for Child Health: *http://www.ich.ucl.ac.uk*.

THE OLDER PERSON
Lesley Bromley

Key Messages

- Increasing age produces a decline in cardiovascular and renal function.
- Cognitive function may be impaired and this may reduce the patient's involvement in pain assessment.
- A reduction in prostaglandin production in the gastric mucosa in the elderly makes them particularly vulnerable to the effects of non-steroidal anti-inflammatory drugs.

The elderly population represents a particular challenge in acute pain management. Elderly people have altered physiological and pharmacokinetic responses to pain and to analgesics. Evidence suggests that their pain is frequently undertreated and they may be reluctant to report pain or have cognitive impairment that reduces their ability to report their pain.

Physiological changes of aging

With advancing age, cardiovascular and renal function declines, hepatic function tends to be maintained and neurological function is altered. Cardiac output declines by 1% per year from the age of 30, and GFR declines by 1.0–1.5% per year from the age of 20. Elderly people tend to have a reduced muscle bulk, this makes creatinine an unreliable marker of renal function; however, many labs now provide an estimated GFR, which is a reasonably reliable indicator. Both of these factors contribute to a reduction in renal clearance of drugs.

Hepatic function is maintained despite a reduction in liver blood flow and a reduction in liver bulk; this reflects the enormous reserve of liver function in adults. Elderly people tend to have a reduction in prostaglandins in the gastric mucosa, and *Helicobacter pylori* infection is common. In the nervous system, there is a general trend with age for reduction of sympathetic tone, autonomic function generally and C- and Aδ-fibre deterioration. This results in an exaggerated hypotensive response to epidural and spinal analgesia, and a slower response to painful stimuli.

Pharmacokinetic changes in the elderly

Absorption

The oral route remains effective as transit time in the gut is slowed, but blood flow is also reduced. The buccal route may be a problem if production of saliva falls. Transdermal routes work well, despite the reduction in subcutaneous fat in some elderly people. Transbronchial routes also work well. Intramuscular routes should be avoided in any age group but are particularly unreliable in the elderly due to reduction in muscle bulk and muscle-to-fat ratios.

Distribution

Elderly people tend to have less muscle mass and less total body water, their ratio of muscle to fat is altered and so lipophilic drugs may have a prolonged action. Water-soluble drugs such as morphine may achieve higher than normal plasma levels and thus demonstrate more side effects. If the patient has been chronically undernourished, serum albumin may be low, allowing high levels of free drug for those drugs that are normally highly protein bound.

Elimination

The major element in reduction of drug clearance in the elderly is the effects of reduced renal function. This may be compounded by hypovolaemia, use of nephrotoxic drugs and illness.

Pharmacodynamic changes

The populations of receptors at which drugs act is altered in old age, in particular μ (mu)-opioid receptors are reduced in older people, and as already discussed autonomic function is reduced, which may lead to more side effects.

Cognitive impairment

Many elderly people suffer from some form of cognitive impairment. Evidence suggests that those with dementia are less likely to be prescribed analgesia, and even if it is prescribed they still may not receive their medication. Health care professionals are reluctant to give analgesia to those with cognitive impairment. Whether this is due to fears of addiction or not considering pain as a possibility in such patients is not clear. Patients with dementia tend to express pain by increased agitation, screaming and verbal and physical abuse. This is often treated with antipsychotic drugs, which mask the effects of the pain.

Pain assessment tools can be used for those with mild dementia, but scoring systems more akin to those used in preverbal children have been developed for the elderly with severe cognitive impairment, for example the Assessment of Discomfort in Dementia Protocol (Kovach *et al.* 1999). Chapter 2 provides additional guidance. The views of relatives and carers are also important in assessing pain in these patients.

Where pain is an element of disease in elderly people, it is important to prescribe analgesia regularly, rather than as required. In general, those elderly patients who do not have any cognitive impairment can use the standard tools for pain assessment; however, it is important to give the older person time to think about his or her response, as reaction times are slower with aging.

Management of pain with analgesic drugs should follow the World Health Organization Analgesic Ladder, as for younger patients. Further information on pain assessment in the elderly is available in Chapter 2 and also in the comprehensive document 'Assessment of Pain in Older People' (Royal College of Physicians *et al.* 2007).

Specific medicines in the older person

Opioids

Opioid medicines provide effective pain relief in elderly people with acute pain. They may also be used in chronic pain conditions. The major drawback is the higher incidence of side effects in this group.

Nausea and vomiting occurs in 25% of patients and concomitant anti-emetics are often required. These should be given regularly, and rotated if they become ineffective.

Constipation is also a common problem in the elderly, and if opioids are to be used for any length of time, laxatives should also be regularly prescribed.

Itching can be troublesome and the use of antihistamines in response can be sedating. Tolerance can be a problem due to smaller populations of receptors, and a multimodal approach to pain management is recommended.

Where renal impairment is present, reduced dosing may be necessary, to prevent high plasma levels occurring. Renal function should be assessed before prescribing.

Paracetamol

Paracetamol is commonly used in the older person. Hepatic function is well preserved in older people and they are at risk only if they have specific liver disease. It is the first-line medicine in the management of osteoarthritis (Level II: Nikles *et al.* 2005) and is very effective when given intravenously (Level II: Moller *et al.* 2005). It is of particular value in this group, because it has very few interactions with other drugs, and many patients are taking multiple medicines for cardiac and other morbidities.

Tramadol

Tramadol has a mixed action, binding to opioid receptors and to 5-hydroxytryptamine (5-HT) receptors. It is rapidly absorbed and peak serum concentrations are attained about 2 hr after oral ingestion. It has an elimination half-life of 6.3 hr and is poorly bound to plasma proteins (20%). Tramadol is extensively metabolised, with only 1 of its 11 metabolites possessing anti-nociceptive activity in animals. Tramadol is indicated for the management of moderate to moderately severe pain and the usual dose is 50–100 mg every 4–6 h, as needed. Immediate- and sustained-release tramadol were generally well tolerated in a study with age group controls. Patients >75 years of age used 20% less tramadol than patients <65 years but experienced similar analgesia (Level II: Likar *et al.* 2006). The maximum dosage of tramadol should not exceed 400 mg daily or 100 mg/dose, and patients older than 75 years of age should not receive more than 300 mg daily. In patients with a creatinine clearance less than 30 mL/min, the dosing interval should be increased to every 12 hr and the total dose should not exceed 200 mg daily. Patients with cirrhosis of the liver should not receive more than 50 mg of tramadol every 12 h.

Local anaesthetics

Local anaesthetic blocks can be used to good effect in elderly people. Epidural and spinal analgesia can be used, but care must be taken as the decrease in sympathetic tone may result in an exaggerated hypotensive response to extradural or intrathecal local anaesthetics.

NSAIDs

NSAIDs should be used with caution in the older person because of their widespread unwanted effects.

Gastrointestinal effects: The reduction in prostaglandin production in the gastric mucosa in the elderly makes them particularly vulnerable to the effects of NSAIDs, which will further reduce the prostaglandin protection. Acute gastrointestinal haemorrhage with no preceding pain or dyspepsia can occur. Proton pump inhibitors may be protective, but they can also mask symptoms relating to mucosal damage.

Renal effects fall into two categories. First, renal blood flow is maintained by prostaglandins and falls when NSAIDS are given. Second, renal sodium reabsorption increases in the presence of NSAIDs and this can lead to water retention and precipitation of heart failure.

Platelet dysfunction occurs with NSAIDS and may be significant if the patient is already receiving aspirin or anticoagulants.

Other effects of NSAIDs that are less commonly appreciated include central nervous system disturbance such as sedation, confusion, cognitive dysfunction, psychosis and personality changes.

The choice of agent is mostly dependent on cost, duration of action and route of administration. In the elderly, it is advisable to use the lowest dose for the shortest possible time, monitoring closely for adverse effects. Dose reduction is required in patients with liver disease as most NSAIDs are metabolised by the liver.

References

Kovach, C.R., Weissman, D.E., Griffie, J., *et al*. (1999) Assessment and treatment of discomfort for people with late-stage dementia. *Journal of Pain and Symptom Management*, **18** (6), 412–419.

Likar, R., Wittels, M., Molnar, M., Kager, I., Ziervogel, G. & Sittl, R. (2006) Pharmacokinetic and pharmacodynamic properties of tramadol IR and SR in elderly patients: a prospective, age-group-controlled study. *Clinical Therapeutics*, **28** (12), 2022–2039.

Moller, P.L., Juhl, G.I., Payen-Champenois, C. & Skoglund, L.A. (2005) Intravenous acetaminophen (paracetamol): comparable analgesic efficacy, but better local safety than its prodrug, propacetamol, for postoperative pain after third molar surgery. *Anesthesia and Analgesia*, **101** (1), 90–96.

Nikles, C.J., Yelland, M., Del Mar, C. & Wilkinson, D. (2005) The role of paracetamol in chronic pain: an evidence-based approach. *American Journal of Therapeutics*, **12** (1), 80–91.

The Royal College of Physicians, British Geriatrics Society & British Pain Society (2007) *The Assessment of Pain in Older People*. The Royal College of Physicians, London.

http://www.britishpainsociety.org/book_pain_older_people.pdf. Accessed 7 December 2007.

Further reading

Aubrun, F. (2005) Management of postoperative analgesia in elderly patients. *Regional Anesthesia and Pain Medicine*, **30** (4), 363–379.

Cunningham, C. (2006) Managing pain in patients with dementia in hospital. *Nursing Standard*, **20** (46), 54–58.

Schnitzer, T.J. (1999) Managing chronic pain with tramadol in elderly patients. *Clinical Geriatrics*, **7** (8), 35–45. www.clinicalgeriatrics.com/article/184. Accessed 27 November 2007.

Useful websites

WHO Cancer Pain Release: *http://www.whocancerpain.wisc.edu/eng/17_1-2/17_1-2.html*.
The Merck Manual of Geriatrics: *http://www.merck.com/mkgr/mmg/sec6/ch43/ch43a.jsp*.

RENAL DYSFUNCTION
Lesley Bromley

Key Messages

- Renal dysfunction can lead to reduced clearance of medicines.
- Metabolites may accumulate leading to an increase in side effects.
- Non-steroidal anti-inflammatory drugs should be avoided.
- Fentanyl and oxycodone are the opioids of choice.

Renal dysfunction leads to reduced clearance of drugs and their metabolites, resulting in their accumulation in the body. They may then have a prolonged action and increased incidence of side effects. Drugs that depend on renal excretion and those with active metabolites are most affected. Some analgesics fall into these categories.

Creatinine clearance is the best indicator of reduced GFR. In mild to moderate impairment, drugs dependent on renal excretion may be used in reduced doses, but in severe renal impairment they should be avoided.

As renal function deteriorates, urea will accumulate in the blood. This alters the degree of protein binding, reducing the amount of plasma protein available for binding and displacing drugs that are normally highly protein bound, thus increasing the fraction of drug available in the plasma. This results in increased activity and side effects for a given dosage. NSAIDS are likely to be affected by this.

In renal failure, morphine and its active metabolites will accumulate. It is therefore important to use an opioid that does not have active metabolites (such as oxycodone) in these patients.

Specific drugs in renal failure

Paracetamol

This is the drug of choice for simple analgesia in renal failure. It can very rarely cause nephropathy in very high doses. It is not dependent on renal clearance and can be used safely.

NSAIDs

NSAIDS are generally avoided in patients with renal dysfunction. They reduce renal blood flow and alter sodium balance. These effects are compounded by hypovolaemia.

Opioids

Codeine and dihydrocodeine should be avoided as they are metabolised to morphine, which may accumulate. Morphine and its metabolite morphine 3-glucuronide and morphine 6-glucuronide will accumulate in patients with renal impairment. The commonest effect is a delayed onset of sedation; this often results from high loading doses used in the perioperative period followed by onset of profound sedation in the ward on return from the theatre. This can be avoided by using opioids with no active metabolites.

Fentanyl and oxycodone are recommended for use in patients with renal dysfunction. These drugs do not have active metabolites and have relatively short half-lives, and so can be titrated more easily. Fentanyl PCA can be used in the immediate postoperative period and oxycodone can be used intravenously or orally as a step-down. In using these drugs in PCA, a strict titration of dose is needed as there will be large individual variations in response. Lockout times are traditionally lengthened to increase safety. Bolus doses may also be decreased, but it must be remembered that the goal is still to produce analgesia.

Tramadol

Tramadol is metabolised in the liver and its metabolites are dependent on renal excretion. However, none of them are active, and so tramadol can be used with caution in patients with renal dysfunction. The manufacturers recommend an increased dosing interval of 12 hr in renal dysfunction as a precaution.

Further reading

Murphy, E.J. (2005) Acute pain management pharmacology for the patient with concurrent renal or hepatic disease. *Anaesthesia and Intensive Care*, **33** (3), 311–322.

Useful website

Pain topic: *http://pain-topics.org/pdf/Opioids-Renal-Hepatic-Dysfunction.pdf.*

DAY SURGERY SETTING

Lesley Bromley

Key Messages

- Unresolved pain is one of the commonest reasons for readmission after day surgery.
- A multimodal approach to analgesia should be used.
- The patient should be comfortable on discharge and have an appropriate supply of analgesia and anti-emetics.

The Department of Health is working towards having 75% of all elective surgery performed as day cases. Therefore, analgesia is a key component of the day-case package. Research has shown that 30–50% of patients do not take their analgesia regularly as instructed after leaving the day surgery unit, and 30% reported moderate to severe pain after their day-case surgery. This commonly is worse on the second postoperative day when they start to mobilise. This underlines the fact that education of the patient about how to take their analgesic drugs is almost as important as the choice of drugs.

Analgesic drugs for use after day-case surgery need to be effective and to have minimal side effects. Unfortunately, there is a large individual variation in the response and incidence of side effects with analgesic drugs.

The objective of day-case analgesia is to provide good long-lasting intraoperative analgesia, using a multimodal approach. Thus, pre-emptive use of modern, shorter acting opioids during the surgery accompanied by paracetamol and diclofenac, often given intravenously and supplemented whenever possible by regional or local analgesia with long-lasting local anaesthetic agents, forms the basis of day-case anaesthesia and analgesia (Russon & Thomas 2007, White *et al.* 2007).

In the early recovery phase, analgesia needs to be established so that the patient is pain free on discharge. Short-acting strong opioids such as fentanyl have the advantage of less concomitant nausea than morphine and are preferred.

On discharge, combination packs of mild opioid (dihydrocodeine, codeine or tramadol), an NSAID (commonly diclofenac) and paracetamol are commonly given (Townsend & Cox 2007). A 5-day supply, with instructions to take the medicines regularly, is usually given. If tramadol is to be used, the first dose should be given during anaesthesia as it can cause marked nausea if given intravenously in recovery.

At every stage of the day-case surgery experience, the need for regular analgesia must be re-enforced. The instructions given at pre-assessment should include emphasis on the need for regular analgesia after the surgery. Clear instructions on what type of pain to expect and when to call for assistance is also very important.

References

Russon, K. & Thomas, A. (2007) Anaesthesia for day surgery. *Journal of Perioperative Practice*, **17** (7), 302–307.

Townsend, R. & Cox, F. (2007) Standardised analgesia packs after day case orthopaedic surgery. *Journal of Perioperative Practice*, **17** (7), 340–346.

White, P.F., Kehlet, H., Neal, J.M., *et al.* (2007) The role of the anesthesiologist in fast-track surgery: from multimodal analgesia to perioperative medical care. *Anesthesia and Analgesia*, **104** (6), 1380–1396.

Further reading

Crews, J.C. (2002) Multi-modal pain management strategies for office based and ambulatory procedures. *Journal of the American Medical Association*, **288** (5), 629–663.

McGrath, B., Elgendy, H., Chung, F., *et al.* (2004) Thirty percent of patients have moderate to severe pain 24 hr after ambulatory surgery: a survey of 5,703 patients. *Canadian Journal of Anaesthesia*, **51** (9), 886–891.

Rawal, N. (2001) Analgesia for day-case surgery. *British Journal of Anaesthesia*, **87** (1), 73–87.

White, P.F., Kehlet, H., Neal, J.M., *et al.* (2007) The role of the anesthesiologist in fast-track surgery: from multimodal analgesia to perioperative medical care. *Anesthesia and Analgesia*, **104** (6), 1380–1396.

Useful website

The British Association of Day Surgery (BADS): *http://www.daysurgeryuk.org/content/default.asp*.

THE KNOWN OR SUSPECTED SUBSTANCE MISUSER

Brigitta Brandner and Julia Cambitzi

Key Messages

- Addiction is a chronic relapsing disease.
- Acute pain management can be rewarding as long as the high opioid requirements in these patients are taken into account and replaced.
- Good communication is essential.
- Discharge planning is successful only if the psychosocial background of the patient is considered.

Introduction

Pain in patients with addiction can be challenging in the acute setting such as after trauma or surgery. The fear of exacerbating addiction and insufficient knowledge leads to inadequate pain relief and poor standards of care (Portenoy *et al.* 1997). A consensus document has recently been published that aims to improve the patient's experience of pain management (British Pain Society *et al.* 2007). Pain is a potent trigger to cause a relapse in patients who have been addicted to opioids and related drugs. Addiction is a unique drug reinforcement behaviour of binge, loss of control and withdrawal. The disease of addiction affects approximately 10% of the population. In the United Kingdom, the government is advising on strategies to reduce drug-related harm (Department of Health, National Treatment Agency for Substance Misuse 2007). The National Institute for Clinical Excellence (NICE) has issued guidelines regarding maintenance therapy (Level I: National Institute for Health and Clinical Excellence 2007), opioid detoxification (Level I: National Collaborating Centre for Mental Health 2007a) and psychosocial support (Level I: National Collaborating Centre for Mental Health 2007b). Methadone is the recommended first-line opioid (National Institute for Health and Clinical Excellence 2007) although buprenorphine has also been shown to be effective. Addiction can be seen as a chronic disease where recovery is a long process involving many relapses into drug misuse. Only very motivated patients abstinent from opioids or alcohol should be treated with naltrexone.

Definition of addiction

Addiction is a compulsive drug-seeking behaviour that results from recurring drug intoxification. It is modulated by genetic, experiential, psychological

225

and environmental factors. Craving is recognised as a central driving force in ongoing substance abuse as well as for relapse following abstinence. It is a neurobiological disorder within the limbic reward system, with the mesocorticolimbic dopamine system being central; all drugs abused by humans have been shown in animals to interact with this system. Permanent alteration in neuropathways persists even in long-term abstinence.

Common treatments for addiction

Relapse prevention strategies range from maintenance therapy, by substituting with a safe alternative with the aim of reduction of harm to the patient and society to abstinence via detoxification. Psychological support is essential for long-term success.

Methadone maintenance

Methadone is a synthetic opioid agonist with a long half-life of 12–100 h; it has slow onset and no 'rush'. It is an effective treatment in doses of 10–20 mg twice daily to block craving, ideation and withdrawal for 24–36 h. Opioid tolerance does not eliminate the possibility of methadone overdose, iatrogenic or otherwise. Deaths have been reported during conversion to methadone from chronic, high-dose treatment with other opioid agonists and during initiation of methadone treatment of addiction in subjects previously abusing high doses of other agonists. Methadone is an effective analgesic in acute and chronic pain. It is a racemic mixture that includes an NMDA antagonist and can therefore have an unexpectedly high potency. Its analgesic effect lasts 4–8 hr and a steady-state plateau is reached in days to weeks.

Methadone for maintenance therapy (MMT) is typically dosed between 60 and 120 mg/day, fixed or flexible dosing. The success of therapy is dependent on correct dosing and psychosocial support.

Buprenorphine

Buprenorphine is a thebaine derivative used for maintenance therapy (BMT). It is prescribed in either fixed or flexible dosing of 8–32 mg orally (Schering-Plough 2006, data from SPC). Its analgesic effect is due to partial agonist activity at μ-opioid receptors. An overdose cannot be easily reversed although overdose is unlikely in substance misusers or people with tolerance to opioids. This therapy has a higher relapse rate than high MMT (Level I: National Institute for Health and Clinical Excellence 2007). People who are less opioid dependent are more likely to achieve successful abstinence with this therapy. However, for the pain clinician buprenorphine poses a problem due to the unpredictability in its interaction with other opioid therapies and with an elimination half-life of 20–37 h.

Naltrexone

Naltrexone, an opioid receptor antagonist, is used for abstinence therapy for alcohol and opioids. When given orally, its action is between 24 and 48 hr (Bristol-Myers Squibb 2006, data from SPC) and as a depot injection 1 month. In the United Kingdom, there is little experience in treating patients on this therapy, who require acute pain management. In emergencies, such as cases of acute severe pain, higher doses of opioid analgesics may be used with extreme caution to override the blockade produced by naltrexone. The narcotic dose needs to be carefully titrated to achieve adequate pain relief without oversedation or respiratory suppression. If a patient is taken off naltrexone and put on an opioid analgesic, he or she should be abstinent from the narcotic for at least 3–5 days before resuming naltrexone treatment.

Perioperative pain management in the substance misuse patients

Pain management in substance misuse patients is often inadequate due to fear of exacerbating addiction, regulatory sanctions and lack of respect for these patients. This is compounded by poor knowledge in prescribing analgesia.

Physiologically, the thermal and nociceptive thresholds are lowered due to central sensitisation (Level III-2: Doverty *et al.* 2001). The depletion of endogenous opioids with downregulation of secondary messenger systems increases substance misuser's opioid requirements.

The stress response in these patients is impaired even after long abstinence (Level IV: Sinha *et al.* 2007). As pain is one of the most important triggers of the stress response, it is essential to treat pain promptly and effectively; this also helps to facilitate a therapeutic relationship.

The main goals in treating perioperative pain are effective analgesia and prevention of withdrawal (Jage & Bey 2000). Withdrawal can occur within few hours of drug use with restlessness, muscle and bone pain. Insomnia, diarrhoea, vomiting and cold flashes (cold rush, cold turkey) are typical, peaking at 24–48 hr. Withdrawal is unlikely to be life threatening; however, the perioperative period is not an appropriate time to initiate abstinence therapy.

Preoperative patient assessment

Ideally, the initial consultation should include a physical (HIV, hepatitis B and C) and mental health assessment as anxiety, depression and personality disorders are common. Previous and current medical records should be attained wherever possible. Establishing the social circumstances with current health care providers will facilitate treatment and discharge. Particular attention has to be paid to the drug history, and urine toxicology is mandatory.

Patients who are on maintenance therapy under the care of drug dependency services or general practitioners have to have their doses confirmed. An accepted local code of practice in patients either unknown to health care providers or prior to dose confirmation is to commence on 10 mg of methadone BD to prevent withdrawal, although only after positive urine toxicology for opioids, as overdose may occur.

Perioperative pain management

Perioperative pain management in this high-risk group is ideally delivered via a multidisciplinary framework. This will reduce the risk of withdrawal or relapse whilst treating acute pain. Reasons for hospital admissions are frequently trauma and infection manifesting in endocarditis and abscesses. Inadvertent intra-arterial injection causing severe ischaemic pain may lead to amputation of the affected limb. Phantom limb pain is not uncommon as pre-amputation pain may be severe.

Maintenance medication should be administered as long as the enteral route is possible. This is most commonly methadone; however, buprenorphine may be used and care will need to be taken when titrating strong opioids. Despite the partial agonistic effect of buprenorphine, pure μ (mu)-agonists will be effective. Depending on the estimated duration of the acute pain, BMT may be discontinued during acute pain therapy with opioids.

There is little in the literature on the effects of opioids given for the management of acute pain whilst on naltrexone depot therapy.

Acute pain is best treated in a multimodal fashion with paracetamol and NSAIDs as baseline if not contraindicated. Clinical experience shows that it is often best to use a single full opioid receptor agonist with little euphoric effect such as morphine. As codeine, tramadol, oxycodone, pethidine and diamorphine have potential to be abused, it is best to avoid their use in a clinical situation.

For severe pain, opioids are still the mainstay with the oral route preferred. However, parenteral administration can be via a PCA system, intravenous or subcutaneous, with the background opioid analgesia taken into account. The PCA setting may have to be tailored to the patient's opioid requirements. Conversion of methadone to morphine can be difficult (Ayonrinde & Bridge 2000).

Non-opioid analgesia via epidural, plexus or nerve blockade is effective; however, withdrawal can occur if the underlying dependency to opioids is not addressed. The increased risk of infection in this group can limit the duration of this form of pain relief.

Depending on the nature of pain such as after amputation, adjuvant agents such as gabapentin can be useful.

Some patients will have excruciating uncontrolled pain, which will need more invasive treatment such as sedation, ketamine (Haller *et al.* 2002) or lidocaine (lignocaine) infusions. Treating anxiety and sleep disorders can reduce escalating opioid requirements. In this scenario, the patient should be in a monitored area such as high dependency as the effect can be unpredictable.

The opioid requirements are much larger than those of an opioid-naïve patient and pain is often prolonged. Once pain is controlled, it is useful to discuss and agree a discharge plan with the patient. This requires clear documentation. Planning for the patient's discharge with the local drug action team or the GP is essential as there is often a reluctance to prescribe opioids other than methadone; in prisons even methadone may be unavailable.

Discharge planning

It is essential to establish a therapeutic trustful relationship with the patient to address the issue of opioid reduction. However, once the acute pain has settled, the patients are often more motivated to return home. This is dependant on social factors. A multidisciplinary meeting with nurses, medical team, acute pain team, drug misuse keyworker, physiotherapist, occupational therapist and social worker, and occasionally a psychiatrist, is useful to establish progress.

In practice, intravenous opioids are converted to a slow-release opioid preparation such as slow-release morphine, as this has less euphoric effects. The reduction of the oral opioids is negotiated with the patient according to their pain. The amount of methadone can be increased temporarily for its analgesic effects; this is liaised with the drug dependency unit. However, patients on MMT programs can be reluctant to increase their MMT dose.

References

Ayonrinde, O.T. & Bridge, D.T. (2000) The rediscovery of methadone for cancer pain management. *Medical Journal of Australia*, **174** (10), 547–548.

Bristol-Myers Squibb (2005) Nalorex Special Product Characteristics. www.medicines. org.uk/. Accessed 6 July 2008.

British Pain Society, Royal College of Psychiatrists, The Royal College of General Practitioners (2007) *Pain and Substance Misuse: Improving the Patient Experience*. British Pain Society, London. http://www.britishpainsociety.org/book_drug_misuse_main.pdf. Accessed 7 December 2007.

Department of Health, National Treatment Agency for Substance Misuse (2007) *Reducing Drug-Related Harm: An Action Plan*. Department of Health, London. http://www. dh.gov.uk/en/Publicationsandstatistics/Publications/PublicationsPolicyAnd Guidance/DH_074850. Accessed 1 October 2007.

Doverty, M., White, J.M. & Somogyi, A.A., *et al.* (2001) Hyperalgesic responses in methadone maintenance patients. *Pain*, **90** (1–2), 91–96.

Haller, G., Waeber, J.-L., Infante, N.K. & Clergue, F. (2002) Ketamine combined with morphine for the management of pain in an opioid addict. *Anesthesiology*, **96** (5), 1265–1266.

Jage, J. & Bey, T. (2000) Postoperative analgesia in patients with substance abuse disorders. Part 1. *Acute Pain*, **3**, 141–156.

National Institute for Health and Clinical Excellence (2007) *Methadone and buprenorphine for the management of opioid dependence* (NICE Technology Appraisal Guidance 114). National Institute for Health and Clinical Excellence, London. www.nice.org.uk/TA114. Accessed 1 October 2007.

National Collaborating Centre for Mental Health (2007a) *Drug Misuse – Opioid Detoxification* (National Clinical Practice Guideline 52). National Institute for Health and Clinical Excellence, London. www.nice.org.uk/CG052fullguideline. Accessed 1 October 2007.

National Collaborating Centre for Mental Health. (2007b) *Drug Misuse – Psychosocial Interventions* (National Clinical Practice Guideline 51). National Institute for Health and Clinical Excellence, London. www.nice.org.uk/CG051fullguideline. Accessed 1 October 2007.

Portenoy, R.K., Dole, V., Joseph, H., *et al.* (1997) Pain management and chemical dependency. Evolving perspectives. *Journal of the American Medical Association*, **278** (7), 592–593.

Schering-Plough Ltd (2006) *Subutex Special Produce Characteristics*. www.medicines.org.uk. Accessed 6 July 2008.

Sinha, R., Fox, H., Hong, K.I., *et al.* (2007) Sex steroid hormones, stress response, and drug craving in cocaine-dependent women: implications for relapse susceptibility. *Experimental and Clinical Psychopharmacology*, **15** (5), 445–452.

THE OPIOID-DEPENDENT PATIENT

Brigitta Brandner and Julia Cambitzi

Key Messages

- Pain relief in the opioid-dependent patient is complex.
- Good knowledge of physiological changes is necessary to adjust opioid therapy in the acute situation.
- A pain plan should be formulated and agreed with the patient.
- Opioid requirements can be multifold higher than expected.
- On discharge, liaison with the practitioner is important.

Pain relief in opioid-dependent patients is considered to be difficult and challenging. It is well recognized that opioid-dependent patients use significantly more morphine postoperatively than opioid-naïve patients, with reported pain scores being higher (Level III-2: Rapp *et al.* 1995). Patients often find themselves in a vicious circle, resulting in repeated hospital admission and sometimes

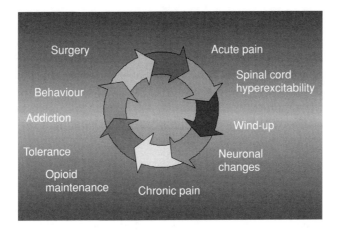

Figure 12.1   Pain strategies: the vicious cycle of pain.

surgery (Figure 12.1). In severe acute pain, opioid therapy remains a corner-stone; however, exploring non-opioid options to treat pain can reduce escalating opioid requirements. By following the World Health Organization (1996) pain ladder, adjuvants such as antidepressants and antiepileptics may be incorporated into the drug regime depending on the nature of pain. Non-pharmacological options should be encouraged such as transcutaneous electrical nerve stimulation (TENS), acupuncture and hypnosis. Psychological support can help to reduce stress and anxiety.

Opioid use for non-malignant pain is acceptable within the recommendations of the British Pain Society (2005), which describes the appropriate use of opioids for persistent non-cancer pain and further that opioids should only be prescribed to relieve pain and improve rehabilitation.

Definitions

A clear understanding of the differences of physical dependence, tolerance, abuse, addiction and pseudoaddiction are crucial to set up appropriate treatment plans.

Addiction

Addiction is a compulsive drug-seeking behaviour that results from recurring drug intoxification. Physical dependence and the emergence of withdrawal symptoms were once believed to be the key features of addiction, but craving and relapse can occur weeks and months after withdrawal symptoms have long passed.

Physical dependence

Physical dependence may develop within days and is an expected consequence of drug use and is not an addiction. It is characterised by the compulsion to take the drug in order to experience its physical effects, due to downregulation and proliferation of opioid receptors. On cessation of the drug or administration of an antagonist, intense withdrawal symptoms may occur. Patients who use opioids for pain relief may be physically dependent on them, although few may be psychologically dependent.

Tolerance

Tolerance is a progressively decreasing response to repeated dosage of a drug. This has been demonstrated in animals and volunteer studies. It classically occurs with all opioids. The adaptive changes can be explained by a right shift of the opioid response curve through progressive loss of receptor site action, and functional uncoupling of opioid receptors from the GTP subunit decreases agonist-binding affinity and loss of receptors from cell surface. In chronic pain, once a dose has been established, tolerance is seldom a problem. Acute opioid tolerance is a new concept described in animal models; it is more likely to occur with large doses of short-acting drugs (Level II: Guignard *et al.* 2000). Tolerance can also occur when different opioid agonists are used and is called cross tolerance.

Pseudoaddiction

This is described as a drug-seeking behaviour in patients in severe pain and is due to the pharmacokinetics of a short-acting opioid such as pethidine with a short onset and offset of action.

Maladaption

Care needs to be taken if the patient shows loss of control demonstrated by overuse, craving or pre-occupation despite adequate pain relief and continued use despite ill effect. Behaviours such as seeking premature prescription, unsanctioned dose escalation, request of specific drugs, polypharmacy from several prescribers and coexistence of illicit drug use should prompt concern.

Opioid rotation

There are numerous reports describing improvement of analgesia or reduction of adverse effects from opioids after switching to an alternative opioid. Switching the opioid, 'opioid rotation', allows the metabolites to be eliminated while maintaining analgesia with a strong opioid. This strategy can be particularly

Table 12.5   Equianalgesic doses.

Oral/rectal dose (mg)	Analgesic	Parenteral dose (mg)
30–60	Morphine	10
7.5–8	Hydromorphone	1.5
20	Oxycodone	(Not available)
See below	Methadone	See below
(Not available)	Fentanyl	0.1 (100 mcg)
See below	Fentanyl (transdermal)	See below
300	Pethidine (not recommended)	75
200	Codeine (not recommended)	120
20	Hydrocodone	(Not available)

Adapted from American Pain Society (1999). Note that morphine is the reference drug against which other opioids are compared.

useful when the toxicity is severe and/or pain is not well controlled. Switching the opioid requires the use of equianalgesic doses as outlined in Table 12.5. To correctly calculate the appropriate equivalent dose, the equianalgesic table should be employed. Given the inter-individual variability in response to various opioids, these should be viewed as guidelines and close patient monitoring is essential. There is no sound evidence to suggest superiority of one opioid over another.

Treatment plan

The main goal for treating acute pain in opioid-dependent patients is satisfactory pain relief, prevention of withdrawal and provision of psychological support. Patients on chronic opioid therapy often have a background of chronic illness or malignancy. It is important to understand the medical history. The general practitioner, palliative care practitioner or pain management consultant will be able to confirm opioid medication on admission for surgery.

Satisfactory pain relief

Patients can have unrealistic expectations about the outcome of a new treatment or surgery, and it is crucial to state that complete pain relief may not be achieved. The patient should be made aware of the nature of their exaggerated pain response (Level III-2: Rapp *et al.* 1995) and also be informed of the available techniques before surgery. Ideally, this should occur in a pre-assessment clinic, thus reducing anxieties and fear and improving coping.

A treatment plan for acute pain in drug-dependent patients guides the health care providers involved. Patients are identified as early as possible and referred to the specialist acute pain team to formulate an individualised plan that is discussed with the patient, agreed and then liaised with all care workers involved.

Suitable techniques

All regular pain medication should be continued as long as possible orally as often inadvertent discontinuation can lead to severe exacerbation and withdrawal symptoms. There is occasionally a misconception that all opioids should be withdrawn before surgery.

If only the parenteral route is available, all opioids should be converted into a parenteral dose (Table 12.5) with morphine as the reference drug. Conversion to intravenous opioids requires clinical experience to convert opioids safely. There is no hard evidence that one opioid is better than another; however, some patients seem to tolerate one better than another (Woodhouse *et al*. 1999). Oral opioids need to be converted to parenteral administration according to their bioavailability, i.e. 10-mg oral morphine equates to 5-mg intravenous morphine. Conversion of methadone can be difficult as the morphine/methadone ratio does not have a linear correlation (Ayonrinde & Bridge 2000). Transdermal fentanyl (Durogesic® DTrans matrix patch) can be converted to parenteral morphine, for example a 50-mcg/hr patch is equivalent to oral morphine up to approximately 190-mg oral morphine over 24 hr according to the SPC or up to 85 mg intravenous morphine.

PCA is a safe method of delivering parenteral opioids. Morphine is often the first-line opioid used in conjunction with non-opioid medication. Patients who are opioid tolerant require multifold higher doses and are less likely to suffer side effects such as respiratory depression. A background infusion can address the underlying requirement with an altered bolus setting (Figure 12.2). Ultra-short-acting opioids such as remifentanil may lead to acute tolerance and worsen pain in the opioid-dependent patient.

If regional blockade or local anaesthetic limb blocks are used, the underlying dependency has to be addressed to avoid withdrawal.

As soon as oral intake is possible, the patient should be converted to all-oral medication. The discharge planning will be in conjunction with the general practitioner and the patient reviewed in a follow-up clinic as an escalation in opioid requirement from preoperative levels is of serious concern.

Some patients will suffer 'excruciating pain' despite high opioid use. Alternative agents such as sedatives, antipsychotic agents or NMDA antagonists (Haller *et al*. 2002) can be prescribed. The response can be unpredictable and respiratory depression is likely, and the patient should be transferred to a high dependency unit for monitoring. This structured approach has led to good patient satisfaction and raised the awareness within clinicians involved in ongoing patient care (Brandner *et al*. 2001).

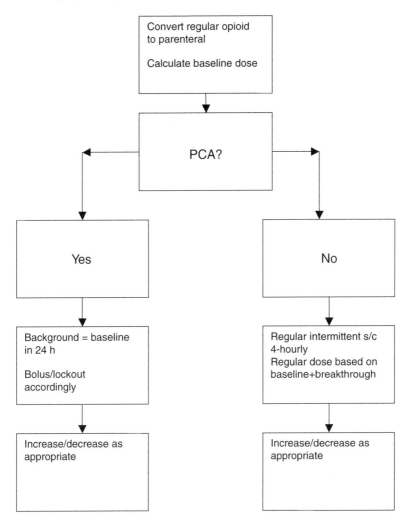

Figure 12.2 Conversion from a regular opioid to parenteral.

Withdrawal

The clinical syndrome is produced by withdrawal of an opioid drug from an opioid-dependent individual either by cessation of the drug or administration of an antagonist, such a naloxone, naltrexone or nalorphine. Initial signs and symptoms and signs may develop immediately after the administration of an opioid antagonist or up to 48 hr after cessation or reduction in dosage of the opioid, the time depends on the half-life of the opioid. These are listed in Table 12.6.

The management of withdrawal in the acute pain setting is mainly pharmacological either with substitution of the drug or with a long-acting opioid

Table 12.6 Signs and symptoms of withdrawal.

Mild to moderate	Severe
Restlessness	Muscle spasms
Mydriasis	Back ache
Lacrimation	Abdominal cramps
Rhinorrhea	Hot and cold flashes
Sneezing	Insomnia
Piloerection	Nausea
Yawning	Vomiting
Perspiration	Diarrhoea
Restless sleep	Tachypnoea
Aggressive behaviour	Hypertension
	Hypotension
	Tachycardia, bradycardia and cardiac dysrhythmias
	Seizures may be observed in neonates

such as methadone. Agents such as clonidine and sedatives mitigate signs and symptoms of withdrawal. The duration and severity of opioid withdrawal depends on the opioid involved and the drug history of the patient. Withdrawal of morphine has an onset at about 12 hr after the last dose, peaks within 48–72 hr and resolves over a period of days. Withdrawal of longer acting opioids such as methadone produced a withdrawal syndrome with a slower onset, milder severity and prolonged duration. The withdrawal syndrome produced by administration of naloxone is intense, occurs within 5 min, peaks at approximately 30 min and subsides within 2 hr.

Psychological support

There is little in the literature on the needed support for this patient group. However, depression and anxiety with a background of uncontrolled pain can be very distressing. Liaison psychiatric input can be very helpful, particularly in the 'suicidal' patient. Integrating psychological support into the inpatient setting is rare; however, in paediatric and adolescent wards, it is more common and their use in this situation is to be evaluated.

References

American Pain Society (1999) *Principles of Analgesic Use in the Treatment of Acute Pain and Cancer Pain*, 4th edn. American Pain Society, Chicago, IL.

Ayonrinde, O.T. & Bridge, D.T. (2000) The rediscovery of methadone for cancer pain management. *The Medical Journal of Australia*, **173** (10), 536–540.

Brandner, B., Seth Ward, M., Hall, C., Ashwell, M. & Baranowski, A. (2001) Managing the acute pain in patients with prior opioid consumption: PCA with continuous background. In: *11th European Congress of Anaesthesiology (CENSA) 2001: Presentation*, Florence, Italy.

British Pain Society (2005) *Recommendations for the Appropriate Use of Opioids in Persistent Non-Cancer Pain 2005*. British Pain Society, London. http://www.britishpainsociety.org. Accessed 15 November 2007.

Guignard, B., Bossa, A.E., Coste, C., *et al.* (2000) Acute opioid tolerance: intraoperative remifentanil increases postoperative pain and morphine requirement. *Anesthesiology*, **93** (2), 409–417.

Haller, G., Waeber, J.-L., Infante, N.K. & Clergue, F. (2002) Ketamine combined with morphine for the management of pain in an opioid addict. *Anesthesiology*, **96** (5), 1265–1266.

Rapp, S.E., Ready, L.B. & Nessly, M.L. (1995) Acute pain management in patients with prior opioid consumption: a case-controlled retrospective review. *Pain*, **61** (2), 195–201.

Woodhouse, A., Ward, M.E., Mather, L.E., *et al.* (1999) Intra subject variability in postoperative patient controlled analgesia (PCA): is the patient equally satisfied with morphine, pethidine and fentanyl? *Pain*, **80**, 545–553.

World Health Organization (1996) *Cancer Pain Relief*, 2nd edn. World Health Organization, Geneva.

ACUTE NEUROPATHIC PAIN

Ian McGovern

Key Messages

- Acute neuropathic pain is common after surgery.
- Patients with acute neuropathic pain may develop chronic post-surgical pain.
- Treatment of neuropathic pain may require a combination of pharmacological, psychological and physical therapies.

Introduction

Neuropathic pain is defined by the International Association for the Study of Pain (IASP) as pain initiated or caused by a primary lesion or dysfunction in the nervous system (Merskey & Bogduk 1994).

Traditional approaches to postoperative analgesia have concentrated on the treatment of nociceptive pain after surgery. In the immediate postoperative setting, neuropathic pain is often overlooked in the presence of 'normal' nociceptive pain resulting from tissue damage and inflammation. Some investigators suggest that neuropathic pain may be experienced in 1–2% of patients undergoing surgery (Hayes & Molloy 1997).

The incidence of chronic pain after surgery is becoming more widely recognised, with as many as two-thirds of patients undergoing surgery reporting persistent postoperative pain (Macrae 2001, Perkins & Kehlet 2000). In some cases, patients with acute neuropathic pain may go on to develop persistent or chronic pain. Treating this pain may be very difficult. The impact on quality of life and requirement for support is considerable.

Any comprehensive postoperative pain management programme must address both nociceptive and neuropathic pain modalities.

Pathophysiology

The mechanisms contributing to the production of neuropathic pain in the postoperative setting are complex and not fully understood. The relative importance of different mechanisms may vary between patients and with time.

The mechanisms resulting from nerve injury involve changes in the peripheral and central nervous systems. These changes involving alterations in neurotransmitter release, neuronal activity and intracellular events including gene expression and even anatomical changes may take place in a very short time.

In the peripheral nervous system, nerve injury results in structural and functional changes in the damaged neurone. Alterations in ion channels, receptor density and activity result in reduced activation threshold and ectopic discharge, both spontaneous and evoked. The neurotransmitter glutamate is thought to play an important role in the development of neuropathic pain. The *N*-methyl-D-aspartate (NMDA) receptor is rapidly activated after neuronal injury, may be involved in central sensitisation and is the target for a number of pharmacological agents that have been used with success in the treatment of neuropathic pain.

Microneuroanatomical changes include axonal sprouting and cross connections forming between efferent sympathetic fibres and nociceptors (sympathetic sensory coupling).

Phenotypical changes can occur, resulting in touch fibres actually becoming pain fibres.

In the spinal cord neuroplasticity, the alterations that occur in synaptic processing as a result of neuronal activity, can cause central sensitisation to develop, resulting in pain hypersensitivity or amplification. The loss of large fibre inhibition, deafferentation hyperactivity, anatomical reorganisation and reactive changes by glial cells may also be involved.

Re-organisation of the somatosensory cortex may be involved in the development of some chronic neuropathic pain states such as phantom limb pain and complex regional pain syndrome. Further reading on the physiology of pain can be found in Chapter 1.

Box 12.1   Features of neuropathic pain.

- Pain often burning or shooting in nature
- Pain in the absence of ongoing tissue damage
- Pain may be spontaneous or evoked by mechanical or thermal stimulation

    Allodynia – Pain following a normally innocuous stimulus
    Hyperalgesia – Pain disproportionate to a noxious stimulus
- Alteration of skin sensitivity

    Dysaesthesia – Unpleasant abnormal sensations (spontaneous or evoked)
- In established cases there may be physical or sympathetic manifestations

    Skin changes
    Motor weakness
    Changes in vasomotor tone

Clinical features

The symptoms described by a patient with neuropathic pain differ from 'normal' postoperative or wound pain. Neuropathic pain (see Box 12.1) is often described as 'strange', 'numb', 'burning', 'shooting' or 'tingling' in nature. It may present in an area not obviously related to the site of injury or may be provoked by stimuli not usually associated with discomfort (allodynia).

The pain may seem to be more severe than is normally experienced and often proves to be resistant to conventional analgesic approaches. Indeed, the clinician may first become suspicious because of an increasing analgesic requirement in a patient who seems to derive little relief.

In some cases the pain may persist for longer than would be expected following otherwise uncomplicated surgery.

Chronic post-surgical pain

Acute postoperative pain may progress to persistent or chronic post-surgical pain with serious long-term consequences for the patient and their carers.

Some operations (all with a notably high risk of nerve damage) are more commonly associated with the development of chronic pain following surgery. They and other predictive factors for the development of chronic post-surgical pain are outlined in Box 12.2.

Box 12.2   Predictive factors for chronic post-surgical pain.

Type of operation
Limb amputation
Thoracotomy
Mastectomy
Cholecystectomy
Inguinal hernia repair
Vasectomy

Preoperative factors
Duration and intensity of pain before surgery
Psychosocial factors (patient vulnerability, compensation)
Pre-treatment with opioids
Female gender
Young age
Radiotherapy to operative site
Chemotherapy

Postoperative factors
Severity of acute pain
Psychosocial factors (depression, vulnerability, anxiety, neuroticism)

Other
Genetic predisposition

Post-surgical neuropathic pain syndromes

Post-amputation pain syndromes

Traumatic or surgical removal of a limb invariably involves nerve injury and can result in a number of sequelae.

Stump pain

- Pain is experienced in the stump and may be of nociceptive or neuropathic origin.
- Usually it is short lived but may become persistent.

Phantom sensations

- Any sensation arising from or attributed to the missing body part. Sensations may range from the very vague to complete sensation in all sensory modalities.

- Usually decreases in both intensity and the size over time – a phenomena known as telescoping, where the phantom limb shrinks towards the stump.

Phantom pain

- Any noxious sensation of the missing body part.
- Risk of developing phantom pain is increased with the incidence of severe pain prior to the amputation as well as severe postoperative stump pain.

Complex regional pain syndromes

Neuropathic pain associated with abnormalities of the sympathetic nervous system.

- Symptoms develop after an injury or trauma that may appear to have been only minor.
- Duration and severity of pain exceed those expected for the incident.

The term *complex regional pain syndrome* (CRPS) *Type I* (previously termed *reflex sympathetic dystrophy*) is used when the features listed in Box 12.3 develop in the absence of a detectable nerve injury.

The term *CRPS Type II* (previously termed *causalgia*) is used when the above features develop following nerve injury:

Box 12.3   Clinical features of complex regional pain syndromes.

Pain
Spontaneous and/or burning in nature
Allodynia
Hyperalgesia

Changes in sensory function
Decreased sensation in a quadrant or hemibody distribution

Changes in motor function
Reduction in motor range and strength
Tremor
Dystonia

Sympathetic nervous system changes
Changes in skin blood flow and temperature
Oedema
Excessive sweating
Atrophy of skin, hair and nails

Treatment

Despite the obvious association of preoperative factors and the development of chronic post-surgical pain, there is little evidence to support the use of pre-emptive analgesic techniques in the prevention of acute neuropathic pain after surgery.

Any successful strategy must take into account not only preoperative factors but also the influence of ongoing postoperative inflammatory processes and peripheral sensitisation that continue to produce pain after surgery.

Preventive strategies should involve pharmacological, psychological and physical treatment modalities from an early stage.

Pharmacological treatments

It is important to note that until recently, there was little published evidence to support any particular treatment in acute neuropathic pain. Much of the cited evidence is based on treatment of established neuropathic pain states, and caution must be exercised when extrapolating this evidence to acute postoperative pain.

The evidence for the basis of pharmacological treatment of neuropathic pain has been assessed by a number of systematic reviews (Table 12.7).

Table 12.7 Systematic reviews for treatment of neuropathic pain.

Reference	Level of evidence	Title
McQuay *et al.* (1996)	I	A systematic review of antidepressants in neuropathic pain
Kingery (1997)	I	A critical review of controlled clinical trials for peripheral neuropathic pain and complex regional pain syndromes
McQuay (2002)	I	Neuropathic pain: evidence matters
Wiffen *et al.* (2005b)	I	Gabapentin for acute and chronic pain
Wiffen *et al.* (2005a)	I	Anticonvulsant drugs for acute and chronic pain
Wiffen *et al.* (2005c)	I	Carbamazepine for acute and chronic pain
Dworkin *et al.* (2007)	I	Pharmacologic management of neuropathic pain: evidence-based recommendations
Kong & Irwin (2007)	I	Gabapentin: a multimodal perioperative drug?

Opioids

Opioid medications are used widely for the treatment of postoperative nociceptive pain and their potential role for the treatment of postoperative neuropathic pain has, until recently, received little attention.

Oxycodone
Mechanism of action:

- μ-Opioid and κ-opioid receptor agonist

Effective for post-herpetic neuralgia and painful diabetic neuropathy.

Tramadol
Mechanism of action:

- μ-Opioid receptor agonist
- Pre-synaptic inhibition of norepinephrine and serotonin reuptake

Effective for post-herpetic neuralgia.

Tricyclic antidepressants

Mechanisms of action:

- Pre-synaptic inhibition of norepinephrine and serotonin reuptake
- Possible NMDA antagonistic effect and weak μ-opioid action
- Membrane stabilisation (sodium- and calcium-channel blockade)
- Post-synaptic α-adrenergic, cholinergic and histaminergic effects

Tricyclic antidepressants are effective for the treatment of diabetic neuropathy and post-herpetic neuralgia. Side effects are common and include sedation, anticholinergic effects, arrhythmias and postural hypotension (Level I: McQuay *et al*. 1996).

Selective serotonin reuptake inhibitors
Mechanisms of action:

- Pre-synaptic inhibition of serotonin reuptake
- No effect on norepinephrine reuptake
- No membrane-stabilising effects
- No post-synaptic effects

Selective serotonin uptake inhibitors (SSRIs) have a better side effect profile but seem to be less efficacious than the tricyclic antidepressants (Level I: McQuay *et al*. 1996).

NMDA-receptor antagonists

NMDA antagonists are used in the early stages of treatment of neuropathic pain in an effort to limit or reverse the changes in the peripheral and central nervous system, thus preventing the development of chronic neuropathic pain.

Ketamine has been reviewed extensively in postoperative pain but not specifically in acute neuropathic pain. Small studies seem to suggest that it is effective in neuropathic pain but its usefulness is limited by hallucinations (Level I: Hocking & Cousins 2003).

Dextromethorphan, amantadine and *memantadine* have been evaluated for various types of established neuropathic pain, with mixed and mostly disappointing results (Nikolajsen *et al.* 2000).

Anticonvulsants

Anticonvulsants may reduce spontaneous and movement-evoked pain as well as decrease opioid requirements postoperatively. There is good evidence to support the use of carbamazepine and gabapentin in the treatment of neuropathic pain and some early evidence to suggest that they may reduce chronic post-surgical pain (Level I: Gilron 2006).

Carbamazepine
Mechanism of action:

- Blockade of ionic (sodium and calcium) conduction

Effective and established for the treatment of trigeminal neuralgia and diabetic neuropathy.

There is no evidence that carbamazepine is effective for acute pain (Level I: Wiffen *et al.* 2005c).

Gabapentin
Mechanism of action:

- Pre-synaptic calcium-channel blockade
- Reduced glutamate release

Although there is evidence to show that gabapentin is effective in neuropathic pain, the evidence to show that gabapentin is effective in acute pain is conflicting (Level I: Wiffen *et al.* 2005b, Level II: Paech *et al.* 2007, Level I: Tiippana *et al.* 2007).

There is no evidence to support the use of gabapentin for the prevention of chronic post-surgical pain (Level I: Kong & Irwin 2007), and the side-effect profile (especially somnolence and dizziness) may limit patient compliance.

Phenytoin
Mechanism of action:

- Sodium-channel blockade

IV phenytoin infusion is effective in neuropathic pain.

244

Sodium-channel blockers/membrane stabilisers

Mechanisms of action:

- Reduce spontaneous activity in peripheral nerves and dorsal root ganglia
- Block glutamate-evoked activity in dorsal horn of spinal cord

Acute perioperative neuropathic pain may respond to parenteral (intravenous) lidocaine (lignocaine). Lidocaine undergoes extensive first-pass metabolism but mexilitine is available for oral administration. Use is limited by reported dizziness and gastrointestinal side effects (Kalso 2005).

α_2-Adrenergic agonists

There is limited support for the use of oral, topical and epidural *clonidine* for the treatment of peripheral neuropathic pain and complex regional pain syndromes (Level I: Kingery 1997).

Calcitonin

There is little firm evidence for the use of intranasal *calcitonin* in peripheral neuropathic pain and complex regional pain syndromes (Level I: Kingery 1997).

Topical agents

Lidocaine plasters have been used extensively in the treatment of post-herpetic neuralgia, with very few side effects.

Capsaicin

Mechanism of action:

- Causes release and thus depletion of substance P (a neurotransmitter) from unmyelinated sensory nerves

Capsaicin creams are used for the treatment of post-herpetic neuralgia and diabetic neuropathy. Efficacy is limited and the release of substance P caused by the initial application of capsaicin can produce an unpleasant burning sensation and hyperalgesia (Level I: Mason *et al.* 2004).

Other treatment options

Regional neural blockade

Regional and sympathetic blocks may be used peri- and postoperatively for the treatment of neuropathic pain. Examples of widely utilised techniques include lumbar epidural analgesia for lower limb amputation and continuous brachial plexus blockade for upper limb amputation. There may be a place for thoracic epidural or paravertebral analgesia in the prevention or reduction of incidence and severity of post-thoracotomy neuropathic pain.

Transcutaneous electrical nerve stimulation

It is widely used in both acute and chronic pain settings with a high degree of patient satisfaction. There is, however, little robust evidence to support the use of transcutaneous electrical nerve stimulation (TENS) in the treatment of acute neuropathic pain largely due to the difficulties in designing properly randomised and blinded trials. Chapter 13 describes the use of TENS in the perioperative setting.

Prevention

Changes in surgical approach avoiding repeated and unnecessary surgery and the increased utilisation of minimally invasive and nerve-sparing techniques should be sought in an effort to prevent the development of acute neuropathic pain and the risk of this progressing to a chronic post-surgical pain syndrome.

Summary

Acute postoperative neuropathic pain is an important and relatively frequent occurrence. It remains underdiagnosed and undertreated, with patients undergoing surgical procedures with a high incidence of nerve injury most at risk. While the pathophysiology is poorly understood, it is clear that the risks of the patient with acute neuropathic pain developing a chronic post-surgical neuropathic pain syndrome are significant. Many of the currently used treatments are established therapies in chronic neuropathic pain states. Further work is needed to establish their role in the treatment of acute neuropathic pain.

References

Dworkin, R.H., O'Connor, A.B., Backonja, M., *et al.* (2007) Pharmacologic management of neuropathic pain: evidence-based recommendations. *Pain*, **132** (3), 237–251.

Gilron, I. (2006) Review article: the role of anticonvulsant drugs in postoperative pain management: a bench-to-bedside perspective. *Canadian Journal of Anaesthesia*, **53** (6), 562–751.

Hayes, C. & Molloy, A.R. (1997) Neuropathic pain in the perioperative period. *International Anesthesiology Clinics*, **35** (2), 67–81.

Hocking, G. & Cousins, M.J. (2003) Ketamine in chronic pain management: an evidence-based review. *Anesthesia and Analgesia*, **97** (6), 1730–1739.

Kalso, E. (2005) Sodium channel blockers in neuropathic pain. *Current Pharmaceutical Design*, **11** (23), 3005–3011.

Kingery, W.S. (1997) A critical review of controlled clinical trials for peripheral neuropathic pain and complex regional pain syndromes. *Pain*, **73** (2), 123–139.

Kong, V.K. & Irwin, M.G. (2007) Gabapentin: a multimodal perioperative drug? *British Journal of Anaesthesia*, **99** (6), 775–786.

Macrae, W.A. (2001) Chronic pain after surgery. *British Journal of Anaesthesia*, **87** (1), 88–98.

Mason, L., Moore, R.A., Derry, S., Edwards, J.E. & McQuay, H.J. (2004) Systematic review of topical capsaicin for the treatment of chronic pain. *British Medical Journal*, **328** (7446), 991.

McQuay, H.J. (2002) Neuropathic pain: evidence matters. *European Journal of Pain*, **6** (Suppl A), 11–18.

McQuay, H.J., Tramèr, M., Nye, B.A., *et al.* (1996) A systematic review of antidepressants in neuropathic pain. *Pain* **68** (2–3), 217–227.

Merskey, H. & Bogduk, N. (1994) Part III: pain terms, a current list with definitions and notes on usage. In: *Classification of Chronic Pain Syndromes and Definitions of Pain Terms*, 2nd edn (eds H. Merskey & N. Bogduk). IASP Press, Seattle, pp. 209–214.

Nikolajsen, L., Gottrup, H., Kristensen, A.G. & Jensen, T.S. (2000) Memantine (a *N*-methyl-D-aspartate receptor antagonist) in the treatment of neuropathic pain after amputation or surgery: a randomized, double-blinded, cross-over study. *Anesthesia and Analgesia*, **91** (4), 960–966.

Paech, M.J., Goy, R., Chua, S., *et al.* (2007) A randomized, placebo-controlled trial of preoperative oral pregabalin for postoperative pain relief after minor gynecological surgery. *Anesthesia and Analgesia*, **105** (5), 1449–1453.

Perkins, F.M. & Kehlet, H. (2000) Chronic pain as an outcome of surgery. A review of predictive factors. *Anesthesiology*, **93** (4), 1123–1133.

Tiippana, E.M., Hamunen, K., Kontinen, V.K. & Kalso, E. (2007) Do surgical patients benefit from perioperative gabapentin/pregabalin? A systematic review of efficacy and safety. *Anesthesia and Analgesia*, **104** (6), 1545–1556.

Wiffen, P.J., Collins, S. & McQuay, H., *et al.* (2005a) Anticonvulsant drugs for acute and chronic pain. *Cochrane Database of Systematic Reviews*, Issue 3, Art No CD001133.

Wiffen, P.J., McQuay, H.J., Edwards, J.E. & Moore, R.A. (2005b) Gabapentin for acute and chronic pain. *Cochrane Database of Systematic Reviews*, Issue 3, Art No CD005452.

Wiffen, P.J., McQuay, H.J. & Moore, R.A. (2005c) Carbamazepine for acute and chronic pain. *Cochrane Database of Systematic Reviews*, Issue 3, Art No CD005451.

Further reading

Bennett, M. (ed.) (2006) *Neuropathic Pain*. Oxford University Press, Oxford.

Holdcroft, A. & Jaggar, S. (2005) *Core Topics in Pain*. Cambridge University Press, Cambridge.

Useful websites

Neuropathic Pain Network: *http://www.neuropathicpainnetwork.org/english/index.asp*.

Pain topics (European guidelines): *http://pain-topics.org/guidelines_reports/current_guidelines.php#neuropathicpain*.

13 Transcutaneous Electrical Nerve Stimulation in Perioperative Settings

Mark I. Johnson and Joanne Bagley

Key Messages

- Transcutaneous electrical nerve stimulation (TENS) has been used as an adjunct to pharmacotherapy in the perioperative setting for over 30 years.
- TENS is popular because it is safe, inexpensive and non-invasive, and patients can themselves administer treatment.
- TENS is likely to provide pain relief or reductions in analgesic intake for some patients, provided that it is administered appropriately. It may also be useful for postoperative nausea and vomiting and other post-surgical symptoms.
- In most instances, electrodes are positioned at dermatomes related to the painful area and TENS intensity increased to generate a strong non-painful electrical paraesthesia around the pain.
- Early systematic reviews on TENS for postoperative pain were negative, but recent reviews are more positive.

Introduction

Pain is a biopsychosocial phenomenon and effective pain management strategies use a multidisciplinary approach to address sensory, affective and cognitive dimensions of a person's pain experience. For this reason multimodal treatment approaches that combine pharmacological and non-pharmacological interventions are often more successful than either intervention on their own. In the acute or surgical settings, sensory components of pain predominate and primary analgesic drugs, which target the nociceptive system, are effective as first-line treatments. Non-pharmacological interventions can be used alongside pharmacotherapy to help reduce drug consumption and associated side effects.

Peripheral nerve stimulation techniques such as transcutaneous electrical nerve stimulation (TENS) and acupuncture are widely used in pain management. TENS is popular with patients and health care professionals because it is non-invasive and patients can themselves administer treatment. TENS has been used in perioperative settings for over 30 years to reduce postoperative pain, especially for patients who are reluctant to take medication or where medication fails to provide adequate analgesia or produces unwanted side effects. TENS is also used to promote mobilisation and healing, reduce analgesic consumption, and lessen postoperative nausea and vomiting (PONV), atelectasis and ileus. There has been debate about the usefulness of TENS for postoperative pain, with some respected authorities claiming that TENS provides no benefit (Bandolier 1999, Royal College of Surgeons of England and the Faculty of Anaesthetists 1990), whereas others claim that it does (Agency for Health Care Policy and Research (AHCPR) Acute Pain Management Guideline Panel 1992, Australian and New Zealand College of Anaesthetists and Faculty of Pain Medicine (ANZCA) 2005). Whether TENS is offered in perioperative settings depends on local policy and practice.

The purpose of this chapter is to outline the principles and practice of TENS in the perioperative setting and to review clinical research on its effectiveness.

Background

TENS is a non-invasive technique that is used for a wide range of pain conditions of nociceptive and neuropathic origin. TENS is useful as a stand-alone treatment for mild pain and in combination with other treatments, including pharmacotherapy, for moderate-to-severe pain (Barlas & Lundeberg 2006). TENS is administered using a hand-held battery-operated electrical pulse generator called a TENS device or stimulator. Currents are delivered across the intact surface of the skin via self-adhering conducting pads called electrodes (Figure 13.1). The purpose of TENS is to activate nerve fibres in tissue underneath the electrodes in order to produce physiological actions leading to pain relief. The mechanism of action of TENS when administered in its conventional form, termed conventional TENS, is akin to 'rubbing skin for pain relief'.

TENS is available throughout the world and can be purchased over the counter in the UK. TENS is safe and there is no potential for toxicity or overdose, so patients can adjust dosage according to need. Patients using TENS for the first time should be assessed for suitability and should be given instructions by a health care professional experienced in the principles and practice of TENS. In general, pain relief occurs when the user experiences a 'strong non-painful TENS paraesthesia' beneath the electrodes, so the patient should be told that it may be necessary to keep TENS switched on for long periods of time to achieve prolonged pain relief.

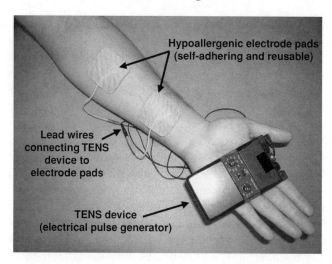

Figure 13.1 Electrode pad placement and connection to electrical pulse generator (TENS machine).

Historical context

Using electricity to produce pain relief is an age-old technique dating back to the ancient Egyptians (2500 BC), Greeks (400 BC) and Romans (AD 46) who treated headache and gout with electric catfish (*Malapterurus electricus*) and electric rays (*Torpedo marmorata*). This practice continued until the development of electrostatic generators in the eighteenth century, which led to a raft of electrotherapeutic devices appearing in mainstream medicine (Gildenberg 2006, Kane & Taub 1975). However, the emergence of pharmacological agents meant that the use of medical electricity had declined by the end of the nineteenth century. Modern medicine attributes the use of electrotherapy to Melzack & Wall (1965), who provided a physiological rationale for the effectiveness of electrical stimulation of nerves for pain relief in their seminal paper 'Pain Mechanisms: A New Theory'. Melzack & Wall suggested that the transmission of noxious information to the brain could be prevented by generating activity in:

1. Descending pain inhibitory nerve pathways which start in the brain and descend to the spinal cord
2. Large diameter non-noxious transmitting peripheral afferents that normally convey information related to mechanical stimuli such as touch and pressure

Reynolds stimulated descending pain inhibitory structures in rats and found that it eliminated their response to aversive stimuli (Reynolds 1969). Wall & Sweet used percutaneous electrical nerve stimulation to activate large-diameter fibres and found that it reduced chronic neuropathic pain (Wall & Sweet 1967).

Shealy *et al.* (1967) stimulated the dorsal columns which are the pathways that transmit non-noxious mechanical stimuli in the spinal cord and found that it relieved chronic pain. Initially, TENS was used to predict the success of dorsal column stimulation implants until it was realised that TENS itself was effective as a stand-alone treatment (Long 1973, Shealy 1974).

Definition of TENS

The standard TENS device

Health care professionals use the term 'TENS' to describe a 'standard TENS device' (Figures 13.1 and 13.2). Most standard TENS devices deliver biphasic pulsed currents and allow the user to adjust pulse amplitude (1–60 mA), pulse frequency (1–200 pulses per second, pps) and pulse duration (50–200 μs). Often devices have a variety of pulse patterns, including continuous, intermittent trains (bursts) and modulated amplitude, modulated frequency and modulated duration. There are minor differences in the technical output specifications of standard TENS devices between manufacturers which are

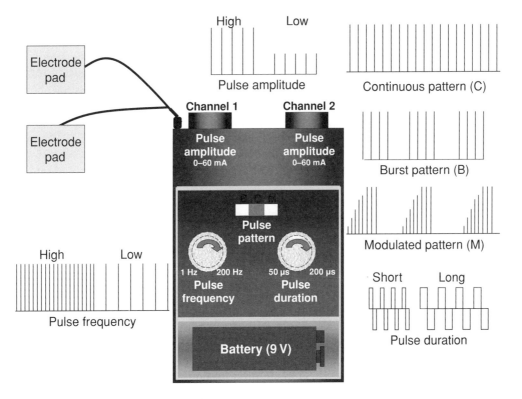

Figure 13.2 A standard TENS device.

mostly cosmetic and have limited impact on physiological and clinical outcome.

TENS-like devices

TENS-like devices are stimulators with markedly different technical output specifications from a standard TENS device (Johnson 2001). Electronic technology, rather than proven physiological outcome, has driven the development of many TENS-like devices, with most claims about effectiveness being overambitious (Table 13.1). Two TENS-like devices have been specifically marketed for use in perioperative settings and are worthy of further comment.

Transcutaneous cranial electrical stimulation using Limoge's current

Transcutaneous cranial electrical stimulation using Limoge's current (TCES-LC) delivers high-frequency (166-kHz) pulses interrupted with a repetitive low frequency (100 Hz) using a negative electrode placed between the eyebrows and two positive electrodes in the retromastoid region. TCES-LC is initiated a few hours prior to anaesthetic induction and continued throughout surgery and 48 hr postoperatively (Stanley *et al.* 1982). It is claimed that TCES-LC potentiates some drug effects, especially opioids and neuroleptics, during anaesthetic clinical procedures, including cardiac, thoracic, abdominal, urological and microsurgery (Level III-2: Limoge *et al.* 1999). Clinical trials have reported that TCES-LC decreases epidural anaesthetic dose requirement during intra- and postoperative phases during cardiac, thoracic, abdominal, urological and microsurgery (Level III-3: Stinus *et al.* 1990), urologic operations (Level III-1: Stanley *et al.* 1982), cancer surgery (Level IV: Limoge & Dixmerias-Iskandar 2005) and sigmoidoscopy (Level III-3: Limoges & Rickabaugh 2004). Although promising, much of the available evidence arises from the inventors of the TENS-like technique and needs to be conformed by independent investigators.

Transcutaneous electrical acupoint stimulation (ReliefBand)

TENS of the pericardium 6 (P6, Neiguan) acupuncture point has been used to reduce PONV. Dundee *et al.* (1989) pioneered early research and reported that stimulation of P6 helped women pre-medicated with nalbuphine 10 mg undergoing minor gynaecological operations under methohexitone–nitrous oxide–oxygen anaesthesia (Level III-1: Dundee *et al.* 1989). Similar effects were noted for invasive (manual or electroacupuncture) and non-invasive stimulation (conducting stud or pressure) during the early postoperative period, but invasive stimulation seemed to perform better in the 6-h postoperative period.

Transcutaneous electrical acupoint stimulation (TEAS) is a TENS-like device that is worn like a watch but on the underside of the wrist and over P6. Patients alter pulse amplitude to produce a mild tingling sensation beneath the

Table 13.1 Summary of TENS-like devices and their effectiveness.

	Transcranial electrical stimulation (e.g. Limoge's currents, TCES-LC)	Transcutaneous electrical acupoint stimulation (TEAS)	Transcutaneous spinal electroanalgesia (TSE)	Interferential therapy (IFT)	Microcurrent electrical therapy (MET)
Uniqueness	Claimed to deliver currents directly to brain tissue	Claimed to deliver currents to P6 (Neiguan) acupoint	Claimed to deliver currents directly to spinal cord tissue	Claimed to deliver currents to deep-seated tissue	Claimed to deliver currents which mimic currents that arise following tissue injury
Scientific rationale	Unclear – claims to alter brain neurotransmitter systems	P6 (Neguian) is a known anti-emetic acupuncture point	Claimed to reduce central sensitisation	Unclear – some claim that activation of deep-seated afferents more effective than TENS	Unclear – claimed that currents accelerate tissue healing
Clinical effectiveness	Some evidence that TCES-LC reduces postoperative analgesic consumption	Good evidence that stimulation of P6 by TEAS reduces PONV	Evidence limited and conflicting that TSE may reduce pain	Some evidence that IFT reduces pain to similar amount as TENS	Evidence conflicting that MET can promote healing and/or reduce pain

electrodes. Randomised controlled clinical trials (RCTs) suggest that TEAS reduces PONV especially when combined with ondansetron (Level II: Zarate *et al.* 2001) (Level II: Coloma *et al.* 2002), see the section on 'TENS for post-surgical nausea and vomiting' (p. 267).

Practitioners should use a standard TENS device to reduce postoperative pain in the first instance and this will be the focus of this chapter. The term *TENS* will refer to treatment using a standard TENS device.

The principles of TENS

TENS techniques

The goal of TENS is to activate different types of nerve fibres, leading to pain modulation. The following TENS techniques are used:

- Conventional TENS (low-intensity, high-frequency currents) to elicit segmental analgesia
- Acupuncture-like TENS (high-intensity, low-frequency currents) to elicit extrasegmental analgesia
- Intense TENS (high-intensity, high-frequency currents) to elicit peripheral nerve blockade, segmental and extrasegmental analgesia

In general, conventional TENS is used in first instance and AL-TENS for patients who do not response to conventional TENS. Intense TENS is used as a counterirritant and may be useful intraoperatively for surgical or medical procedures of short duration. An understanding of the physiological intention (purpose) of each TENS technique will underpin good clinical practice (Table 13.2).

Conventional TENS (low intensity, high frequency)

The International Association for the Study of Pain (IASP) definition for conventional TENS is 'high frequency (50–100 Hz), low intensity (paraesthesia, not painful), small pulse width (50–200 µs)' (Charlton 2005, p. 94). The intention of conventional TENS is to selectively activate low-threshold, large-diameter, myelinated, non-noxious transmitting afferent fibres (Aβ) to inhibit onward transmission of nociceptive information at synapses in the central nervous system (see the section on 'Mechanism of analgesic action'). High-threshold, small-diameter, noxious transmitting afferent fibres (Aδ and C) should not be activated during conventional TENS, as this would cause pain. In clinical practice, users increase TENS amplitude until they experience a strong, comfortable, non-painful electrical paraesthesia beneath the electrodes. Increasing TENS amplitude above this point leads to painful electrical paraesthesia indicative of Aδ activity, which is not appropriate during conventional TENS. Theoretically, selective activation is best achieved using currents that are high frequency (~10–200 pps) with pulse durations of 50–200 µs. High-frequency

Table 13.2 Summary of TENS devices and their mode of action.

	TENS experience	Nerve fibres activated	Electrode position	TENS settings	Analgesic profile	Regimen	Predominant action
Conventional TENS	Strong, non-painful TENS paraesthesia with minimal muscle activity	Large-diameter non-noxious afferents (Aβ)	Dermatomes Site of pain	Low intensity (amplitude), high frequency (10–200 pps)	Usually rapid onset and offset	Use TENS whenever in pain	Segmental
AL-TENS	Strong, comfortable muscle twitching	Small-diameter cutaneous and motor afferents (Aδ)	Myotomes Site of pain Muscles Motor nerves Acupuncture points	High intensity (amplitude), low frequency (1–5 bursts of 100 pps)	May be delayed onset and offset	Use TENS for 20–30 min at a time	Extrasegmental
Intense TENS	Uncomfortable (painful) electrical paraesthesia	Small-diameter cutaneous afferents (Aδ)	Dermatomes Site of pain Nerves proximal to pain	High amplitude (uncomfortable/noxious), high frequency (50–200 pps)	Rapid onset and delayed offset	Short periods only 5–15 min at a time	Peripheral

TENS also creates more impulses in afferent fibres, leading to greater inhibition of nociceptive transmission.

Acupuncture-like TENS (high intensity, low frequency)

The IASP define AL-TENS as hyperstimulation using currents that are 'low frequency (2–4 Hz), higher intensity (to tolerance threshold), [and] longer pulse width (100–400 μs)' (Charlton 2005, p. 94). AL-TENS was developed in the 1970s in an attempt to harness the mechanisms of action of TENS and acupuncture (Andersson *et al.* 1973, Eriksson & Sjölund 1976). The effects of acupuncture were believed to be mediated by small-diameter muscle afferents using low-frequency stimuli generated by twirling an acupuncture needle. AL-TENS offered a non-invasive method to activate small-diameter afferents and was used for patients resistant to conventional TENS (Level III-3: Eriksson & Sjölund 1976). Intermittent trains or bursts (2–4 Hz) of high-frequency pulses (~100 pps) were used in clinical practice to reduce discomfort experienced using high-intensity single pulses. Thus, the intention of AL-TENS is to generate activity in small-diameter afferents (Aδ) to activate descending pain inhibitory pathways (i.e. extrasegmental modulation) and endogenous opioid peptide release (see the section on 'Mechanism of analgesic action'). Many opinion leaders claiming that a non-painful muscle twitching produces the best effect (Johnson 1998, Meyerson 1983, Sjölund *et al.* 1990) (Table 13.2). AL-TENS is delivered at the site of pain and over muscles, motor points, acupuncture points and trigger points, although it is not known whether this changes outcome (Walsh 1996).

Intense TENS

Brief, intense TENS is a counterirritant delivered for short periods of time for short painful procedures, such as wound-dressing changes, suture removal and venepuncture. The intention of intense TENS is to activate small-diameter noxious Aδ afferents to block transmission of nociceptive information in peripheral nerves and to activate descending pain inhibitory pathways and diffuse noxious inhibitory controls (Ignelzi & Nyquist 1976, 1979, Le Bars *et al.* 1979). In clinical practice, intense TENS is administered over peripheral nerves arising form the site of pain using high frequencies and high intensities that are 'just tolerable' to the patient (Jeans 1979, Melzack *et al.* 1983) (Table 13.2).

Mechanism of analgesic action

TENS techniques overlap in their mechanism of action. From a physiological perspective, non-noxious TENS paraesthesiae (conventional TENS) cause segmental analgesia and higher TENS intensities cause extrasegmental analgesia. Antidromic activation of peripheral nerve fibres blocks incoming afferent impulses from areas of tissue damage.

Segmental mechanisms

Animal studies confirm that TENS inhibits central transmission of nociceptive information in the spinal cord (Garrison & Foreman 1994, 1996, Leem *et al.* 1995) (Level II: Chung 1985). Impulses generated by conventional TENS enter the spinal cord and ascend to the ipsilateral brainstem nuclei (nucleus gracilis and nucleus cuneatus) and onwards to the somatosensory cortex where they are processed and a sensation of TENS paraesthesia produced. On entering the spinal cord, TENS impulses also travel along collaterals of the Aβ afferents which synapse with inhibitory interneurones in the dorsal horn. Activation of these inhibitory interneurones results in the release neurotransmitters that inhibit peripheral C-fibre afferents (pre-synaptic inhibition) and second-order central nociceptive transmission cells (post-synaptic inhibition). Gamma-amino butyric acid (GABA) and met-enkaphalin are two key inhibitory neurotransmitters involved in this process (Figure 13.3). This mechanism is rapid

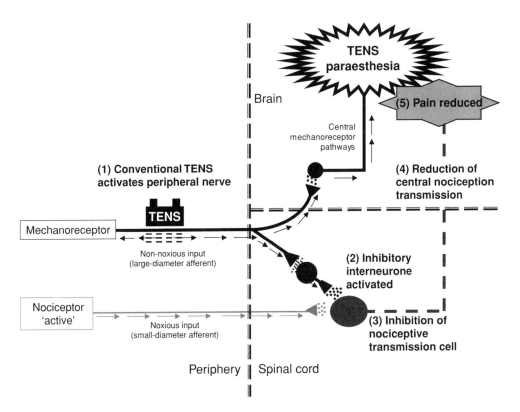

Figure 13.3 TENS activates peripheral, large-diameter, non-noxious afferents, causing inhibitory neurotransmitters to be released in the spinal cord. This reduces activity in second-order nociceptive transmission cells and nociceptive input to the brain, resulting in pain relief. TENS activates mechanoreceptor (non-noxious) transmitting pathways in the central nervous system, resulting in a sensation of TENS paraesthesia.

in onset and offset and maximal when TENS is applied to somatic receptive fields of the central nociceptive transmission cells (Level II: Garrison & Foreman 1994). Recently, TENS has also been shown to reduce inflammation-induced sensitisation of dorsal horn neurons in anaesthetised rats (Level II: Ma & Sluka 2001).

Extrasegmental mechanisms

At higher intensities, TENS activates Aδ afferents and produces a long-term depression (LTD) of central nociceptor cells lasting up to 2 hr after stimulation (Sandkühler 2000, Level II: Sandkühler *et al.* 1997). High-intensity TENS activates ascending pathways that activate extrasegmental structures on the descending pain inhibitory pathways, including the periaqueductal grey and ventromedial medulla. High-intensity TENS also inhibits descending pain facilitatory pathways, which normally amplify incoming nociceptive information. Larger effects have been observed when deep somatic rather than skin afferents were activated (Duranti *et al.* 1988, Level II: Radhakrishnan & Sluka 2005). When TENS itself causes pain (i.e. intense TENS), it is likely that diffuse noxious inhibitory controls become active (Le Bars *et al.* 1979).

Peripheral mechanisms

TENS leads to impulses travelling in both directions along peripheral nerve fibres. Impulses travelling towards the periphery will collide and extinguish afferent impulses arising from peripheral receptors that have activated by natural stimuli. TENS will block impulses arising from peripheral Aβ afferents and at higher intensities, will block afferent activity in peripheral Aδ afferents (Level II: Ignelzi *et al.* 1981, Ignelzi & Nyquist 1975, 1979). Conventional TENS has been shown to increase the latency of early somatosensory-evoked potentials (SEPs) in healthy subjects, confirming a 'busy-line effect' on large afferent fibres (Level II: Nardone & Schieppati 1989).

Neuropharmacology

Early evidence suggested that AL-TENS, but not conventional TENS, was mediated by endorphins (Eriksson *et al.* 1979, Sjölund *et al.* 1977). Recent research suggests a more complex process. Animal experiments have shown that low-frequency TENS involves μ-opioid receptors, whereas high-frequency TENS involves δ-opioid receptors (Kalra *et al.* 2001, Sluka *et al.* 1999, 2000, Level II: 2001, Sluka & Walsh 2003). The inhibitory neurotransmitter GABA is a critical mediator of the effects of conventional TENS (Duggan & Foong 1985, Maeda *et al.* 2007). Cholinergic, adrenergic and serotinergic systems also seem to be involved (Sluka & Walsh 2003) (Ainsworth *et al.* 2006, Chandran & Sluka 2003, Kalra *et al.* 2001, King *et al.* 2005, Radhakrishnan *et al.* 2003, Radhakrishnan & Sluka 2003, Level II: Sluka & Chandran 2002).

Principles of clinical technique

Electrode positions

TENS activates nerve fibres directly beneath the electrodes, so it is important that electrodes are placed on healthy sensate skin. A brief sharp–blunt skin test should be performed prior to electrode placement. For conventional TENS, electrodes are positioned at dermatomes related to the painful area. In most cases electrodes are placed around the site of pain and TENS paraesthesiae are directed to cover the pain (Figure 13.4). Electrodes are usually placed a minimum of a few centimetres apart.

For postoperative pain, 'strip-like' electrodes are placed either side of the incision scar in the first instance. It is important that electrodes are positioned at least 5 cm away from the scar to prevent mechanical damage of the incision site when removing electrodes. Often it is not the incision itself that causes the pain, but soft tissue injury resulting from surgical trauma and retraction.

If the patient cannot tolerate TENS at that site because dysaesthesia and/or tactile allodynia is present, as seen with post-thoracotomy pain, then

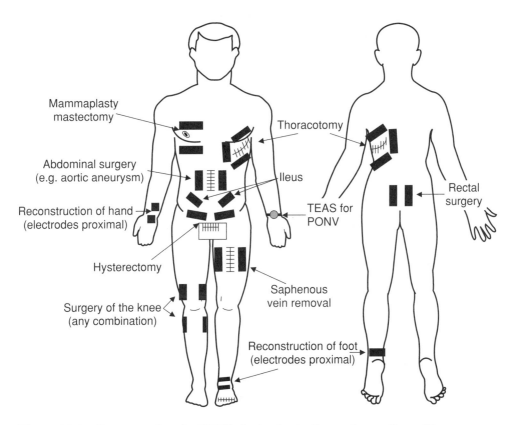

Figure 13.4 Common sites for TENS electrodes in the perioperative setting.

stimulation is given along peripheral nerves proximal to the pain. Applying TENS over allodynic skin may exacerbate the pain, although this is not always the case. Placing electrodes along the main nerves proximal to the site of pain is the practical alternative when patients cannot generate TENS paraesthesia due to nerve damage. Other instances where it is not possible to site electrodes close to the pain are the absence of the body part following limb or breast amputation; if skin is damaged due to a wound; if skin is frail due to eczema; and if tissue is fragile due to reconstructive surgery of the hand or foot. Electrodes can be positioned along the main nerves proximal to the site of pain in these instances. For example electrodes can be positioned over the median, ulnar or radial nerves to generate paraesthesia in the hand following hand surgery.

Dual-channel TENS devices with four electrodes can be used for large areas of pain following major surgery of the thorax, abdomen or spine. The electrodes of one channel are placed at the site of pain and the electrodes of the other channel over proximal nerves or paravertebrally at the relevant spinal segment. Dual-channel stimulators are also useful for multiple pains and for the simultaneous management of pain and ileus or pain and nausea.

Electrodes can also be positioned paravertebrally at spinal segments or on specific dermatomes related to the pain. For example during the pain of child-birth, electrodes are positioned on the back at spinal segments related to peripheral structures involved in the first and second stages of labour. Electrodes can also be placed at contralateral 'mirror' sites, as has been used in phantom limb pain. TENS has also been used on acupuncture and points in the perioperative setting with some success.

Electrodes should not be positioned:

- Over the anterior neck because stimulation of baroreceptors at the carotid sinus may cause a hypotensive response. Furthermore, stimulation of laryngeal nerves may cause a laryngeal spasm and compromise breathing
- Over the eyes because it may increase intraocular pressure
- Through the chest using anterior and posterior positions because it interferes with intercostal muscle activity leading to severely compromised breathing (Mann 1996)
- Internally except in specific circumstances, such as dental analgesia, using a specifically designed TENS device or to treatment incontinence using vaginal and anal stimulation devices

Electrode polarity

Nerve fibres are depolarised under the cathode electrode (usually the black lead), so the cathode is placed proximal to prevent blockade of impulses as they pass over the anode. However, positing of the red and black leads often has little effect, as biphasic waveforms with zero net current flow are used.

260

Electrical characteristics of TENS

Pulse amplitude (intensity) is the key determinant of TENS outcome, so users titrate pulse amplitude to the desired effect (Table 13.2). The search for specific settings for TENS for different pain conditions has in the main been unsuccessful. Animal studies suggest that pulse frequencies affect neuropharmacology of TENS (see the section on 'Mechanism of analgesic action'), although a systematic review of experimental studies in healthy human volunteers concluded that TENS pulse frequencies do not influence hypoalgesia when TENS intensity, pulse pattern and pulse duration are kept constant (Level I: Chen *et al.* 2008). For this reason, practitioners should be cautious of claims about differential TENS based on the selection of pulse frequencies, durations and patterns of TENS. In clinical practice, practitioners select electrode location and pulse intensity according to the principles described and select other parameters using a trial and error according to 'personal comfort' for the pain at that moment in time.

Timing and dosage

Pain relief with conventional TENS is usually rapid in onset and offset and is maximal in the presence of TENS paraesthesia. Hence, TENS needs to be switched on whenever the patient requires pain relief. Electrodes can be left in situ so that patients can deliver TENS intermittently throughout the day on an as-needed basis. Patients can leave TENS switched on for long periods of time if necessary, provided the condition of the skin beneath the electrodes is frequently monitored. The intensity of TENS is likely to fade during individual treatment sessions, so patients should be instructed to adjust the intensity dial to maintain a strong, but comfortable, paraesthesia. Longer post-TENS effects occur with higher intensities of TENS (Level II: Sandkühler 2000). Repeated use of TENS may cause TENS tolerance due to nervous system habituation (Fargas-Babjak *et al.* 1992). Experimenting with TENS settings and/or electrode placement may overcome the problem. Temporarily withdrawing TENS treatment can help patients to establish whether TENS is providing meaningful benefit.

Contraindications

Cardiac pacemakers, pregnancy and epilepsy are often listed as contraindications by manufacturers because it may be difficult to exclude TENS as a potential cause of a problem from a legal perspective. TENS has been used in these patient groups under the guidance of appropriate medical specialists. In these circumstances electrodes are not applied locally (e.g. over the chest, abdomen and head or neck respectively) and decisions are left to the discretion of the medical practitioner with patients monitored carefully throughout. In cardiothoracic surgery, TENS should not be used in patients with internal cardiac defibrillators or ventricular assist devices, also known as artificial hearts. The

UK Chartered Society for Physiotherapy, *Guidance for the Clinical Use of Electrophysical Agents*, lists bleeding tissue as an additional contraindication (Chartered Society of Physiotherapy 2006). They also suggest that electrodes should not be positioned over an active tumour for a patient whose tumour is treatable or over active epiphysis.

Precautions and adverse events

Serious adverse events from TENS appear to be rare, although there has been no systematic review to confirm. Patients should be warned that TENS worsens pain in some patients and that this is not possible to predict. Contact dermatitis, causing redness, and minor skin irritation, such as itch, beneath the electrodes may occur. It is important to monitor the extent of this. Nausea and feeling faint may occur in some patients.

There is no known evidence to suggest that adverse events occur when TENS is used with metal implants, stents, percutaneous central catheters or drainage systems. In these instances, practitioners should be alert to muscle contractions caused by TENS, resulting in mechanical stresses that may affect the implant. TENS may interfere with monitoring equipment, including fetal monitoring equipment and cardiac monitoring equipment (Bundsen & Ericson 1982, Pyatt *et al.* 2003). It is important that medical staff are able to identify a TENS artefact. Interface units that filter TENS interference can be useful under the guidance of the hospital medical physics department. TENS should not be delivered close to transdermal drug delivery systems in case they affect the dosage of drugs delivered across the skin by the process of iontophoresis. TENS should be used with caution for patients on an anticoagulant treatment. TENS should not be used while operating hazardous equipment, including motor vehicles.

TENS in the perioperative setting

Clinical indications

TENS has been used postoperatively to reduce incision and soft-tissue pain resulting from surgical procedures and retractions during major thoracic, abdominal and orthopaedic surgery. There have been clinical trials evaluating TENS for postoperative pain following thoracotomy, post–open heart surgery, coronary artery bypass graft (CABG) surgery, cholecystectomy, appendicectomy, myomectomy, haemorrhoidectomy, tonsillectomy, hernia, surgery for retroperitoneal lymph node dissection, gynaecological surgery, post-caesarean pain and pain associated with dental procedures.

TENS is also used to reduce postoperative analgesic consumption, pulmonary atelectasis, ileus and PONV. A survey of pain management after thoracotomy in 24 Australian hospitals found that TENS was used infrequently, which may be a reflection of concern about effectiveness (Cook & Riley 1997) (see the section on 'TENS efficacy: clinical research evidence').

TENS is also used for intraoperative pain relief during short-stay surgical procedures, including endoscopies, and painful laser and dental surgery. TENS also has a role in managing painful medical procedures such as drain management and removal and wound-dressing changes. TENS has been used in the perioperative setting for adolescents (Level IV: Finley & Steward 1983) and children as young as 4 years (Level IV: Carman & Roach 1988, Level II: Lander & Fowler-Kerry 1993, Level IV: Merkel *et al.* 1999).

Merits of TENS

TENS does not produce many of the side effects associated with drugs, including sedation, dizziness, nausea and disorientation. TENS does not interact with other drugs and therefore can be used in conjunction with other analgesics and techniques including patient-controlled analgesia. TENS can help to reduce the dosage of drug medication, which will reduce the incidence of drug-related side effects. The excellent safety and toxicity profile of TENS means that it can be used for long periods of time without the fear of overdose or adverse effects.

In the perioperative setting, treatment needs to be dynamic and TENS serves this purpose well. TENS has a rapid onset of action, with many patients experiencing pain relief as soon as TENS paraesthesiae begin. Patients can administer TENS whenever they need and can increase TENS intensity to manage severe breakthrough or incident pain without the need to call a nurse for rescue medication. Patients can increase the intensity of TENS just prior to coughing to pre-empt pain.

Perioperative TENS protocol

It is important that the patient is provided with sufficient information to ensure informed consent for TENS as part of their overall surgical consent.

Preoperative TENS trial

A preoperative assessment is necessary for potential TENS patients so that they can be screened for suitability, educated about TENS principles, instructed on how to operate TENS and given an opportunity to try TENS on themselves (Mannheimer & Lampe 1988, *Recommended Best Practice*).

Patients should be screened against contraindications. Patients who are not able to comprehend principles of TENS or operational instructions (e.g. learning difficulties, mental illness or phobias to electricity) should not be given TENS. Anxieties about surgery, post-surgical pain and TENS should be addressed and the reason for using TENS made clear. Patients need to be aware that they have to take an active role in TENS treatment and that they are in control of TENS dosage, which often empowers the patient. It should be emphasised that TENS may not remove all pain and discomfort and that it should be used in conjunction with other pain management treatments.

A preoperative TENS trial enables patients to familiarise themselves with TENS. A skin sensation test should be performed and TENS applied on a convenient body part such as the arm. It is important that patients are confident about experimenting with all TENS settings as different settings may provide better relief at different times. Ideally, TENS should also be tried at the site to be used postoperatively.

Care should be taken when using TENS on a patient for the first time. Patients should provide verbal feedback about TENS sensations when titrating pulse amplitude. If possible, patients should turn up intensity to generate a tingling that is uncomfortable (possibly painful) and then they can be told that this level, although relatively safe, is too high. It is important that the patient is aware that the intensity of TENS should be maintained at a 'strong, but comfortable, non-painful, intensity' but that experimenting with all other settings is necessary. It may be useful to get the patient to pinch the skin between electrodes, so they can appreciate the nature of the TENS analgesic effects. It is also useful to demonstrate the sensations associated with TENS-induced muscle twitching by applying TENS over a muscle or the median nerve. It should be emphasised that they should *not* produce muscle twitching near the incision site because this may hinder healing and even cause further damage in underlying tissue.

Settings preferred during the preoperative TENS trial should be recorded so that TENS can be set up with these settings for the patient to use in the early postoperative stages. However, the settings preferred during the preoperative trial may differ from those preferred in the presence of post-surgical pain. Patients should be warned that a successful preoperative trial does not necessitate success postoperatively and that TENS may worsen their pain following surgery.

TENS procedures in the operating room

Sterile electrodes and aseptic procedures should always be used when placing electrodes along the incision site in the operating theatre. In some instances, electrodes may have to be applied when the patient is still under general anaesthesia. It is important to recheck the condition of the patient's skin and whenever an iodine-based surgical preparation is used, the site should be rinsed and dried before electrodes are applied. Once the outer packaging is open, the scrub nurse can remove the electrodes and apply them to the patient's skin parallel to the incision and usually at least 5 cm away from any sutures. It is important that all parts of the electrodes adhere to the skin. The wound dressing can then be applied, remembering to protrude the electrode's lead wire connection from under the dressing so that it can be connected to the electrode leads and TENS device at a later time. If the surgical procedure does not require a dressing, electrodes can be applied in the recovery room or ward. However, infection-control process must be carefully adhered to and care must be taken as the incision site may be tender.

TENS procedures in the hospital ward or recovery room

The earlier that TENS treatment is started the better, although the patient needs to be fully conscious to control the device. When the patient is sufficiently alert and able to provide verbal feedback, the TENS device can be attached to the electrode lead wires. TENS should be preset to parameters established in the preoperative TENS trial and the device can be switched on. The patient, if able, or the nurse can increase the intensity of TENS so that the patient can report the first TENS tingling sensation and then a strong, but comfortable, stimulation. The patient can take control of their treatment and encouraged to keep TENS on as long as they need, provided it is comfortable and providing relief. TENS devices with timers that automatically switch TENS off can be used by patients who require pain relief to help to go to sleep.

It is crucial that the patient is checked frequently in the early stages of post-operative TENS treatment to ensure that there are no adverse effects. TENS should be discontinued if there are any postoperative complications or the pain worsens. Whenever possible it is important to monitor the skin under electrodes and close to the incision by lifting the corner of electrode. Itchiness may indicate that electrodes need to be replaced. All incidents related to TENS should be recorded.

TENS efficacy: clinical research evidence

TENS for pain

An in-depth study of long-term TENS users concluded that any type of pain may respond to TENS (Level IV: Johnson *et al.* 1991). *The Compendium of Audit Recipes* published by the Royal College of Anaesthetists identifies patient satisfaction as a key target of performance (Royal College of Anaesthetists 2006, pp. 244–245). Surveys suggest that patients are satisfied with TENS as a treatment, although reports of satisfaction do not necessarily reflect true clinical effectiveness. A study of 198 postoperative inpatients found that some patients reported high satisfaction with pain relief treatments, even though they remained in severe pain (Level III-2: Idvall 2002). Hence, systematic reviews of RCTs are necessary to establish true clinical effectiveness.

Many systematic reviews for non-surgical chronic pain are inconclusive, although authors are often positive in their reports, suggesting that TENS may be effective for low back pain (Level I: Khadilkar *et al.* 2005), knee osteoarthritis (Level I: Osiri *et al.* 2000), rheumatoid arthritis of the hand (Level I: Brosseau *et al.* 2003), whiplash and mechanical neck disorders (Level I: Kroeling *et al.* 2005), post-stroke shoulder pain (Level I: Price & Pandyan 2000), primary dysmenorrhoea (Level I: Proctor *et al.* 2003) and chronic recurrent headache (Level I: Bronfort *et al.* 2004). A meta-analysis of 38 studies on TENS and peripheral nerve stimulation for chronic musculoskeletal pain reported significant decreases in pain at rest and on movement (Level I: Johnson & Martinson 2007). TENS can be used in surgical wards for non-surgical pain.

Postoperative pain

Initial clinical trials reported that TENS was effective for postoperative pain (Level III-1: Hymes *et al.* 1974, Pike 1978, VanderArk & McGrath 1975) but a less positive picture has emerged over time. The Royal College of Surgeons of England and the then Faculty of Anaesthetists Working Party on Pain after surgery concluded that TENS was not effective as a stand-alone treatment for moderate-to-severe postoperative pain (Royal College of Surgeons of England and the Faculty of Anaesthetists 1990 – Expert Committee Report), whereas the acute pain management guideline panel of the Agency for Health Care Policy and Research in the USA concluded that TENS was effective in reducing postoperative pain and improving function (Agency for Health Care Policy and Research (AHCPR) Acute Pain Management Guideline Panel 1992 – Expert Committee Report). The Australian and New Zealand College of Anaesthetists and Faculty of Pain's *Medicine Acute Pain Management: Scientific Evidence* (second edition 2005) document states that 'there is limited evidence that physical therapies [such as TENS] help acute pain but some people find them helpful' (ANZCA and Faculty of Pain Medicine 2005 – Expert Committee Report, p. 18).

Systematic reviews of RCTs on TENS for postoperative pain are conflicting. A health technology assessment reported that TENS did not produce significant postoperative pain relief when compared to control in 12/20 RCTs (Level I: Reeve *et al.* 1996). A systematic review by Carroll *et al.* concluded that TENS did not produce significant postoperative pain relief based on the finding that TENS had a positive analgesic outcome in only 2 of 17 RCTs (Level I: Carroll *et al.* 1996). The two positive outcome RCTs reported reductions in pethidine injections and better treatment ratings on the first postoperative day (Level III-1: Pike 1978) and better pain reduction when TENS was administered for 20 min, three times a day (Level III-1: VanderArk & McGrath 1975). Carroll *et al.* judged that none of the 14 trials that compared TENS to sham TENS found any appreciable difference between groups. Five of the seven RCTs that compared TENS in combination with opioids reported no difference between groups. This has led Bandolier to conclude that 'TENS is not effective in the relief of postoperative pain. Patients should be offered effective methods of pain relief' (Bandolier 1999).

A subsequent meta-analysis has challenged these conclusions (Level I: Bjordal *et al.* 2003). This review did not use pain relief as the primary outcome measure because many RCTs had allowed patients in sham and active TENS groups to titrate analgesic consumption to achieve similar levels of pain relief. This review also used criteria for adequate TENS technique in its analysis. When TENS was administered using a strong, subnoxious electrical stimulation at the site of pain analgesic consumption was reduced by 35.5% (range 14–51%) when compared to placebo. Interestingly, only 11 (964 patients) of the

21 RCTs met this criteria for adequate technique. Inadequate TENS produced a 4.1% reduction in analgesic consumption (range −10 to +29%). It was concluded that TENS could reduce analgesic consumption during postoperative care, provided it is administered appropriately. Hence, at present it seems unwise to dismiss TENS as a potential treatment option for postoperative pain management.

Intraoperative pain

There is some evidence to support the use of TENS during minor surgical procedures. An RCT using 142 patients undergoing office hysteroscopy found that TENS on the abdomen lowered pelvic pain when compared to a no-TENS treatment control (Level II: De Angelis *et al.* 2003). An RCT using 45 patients undergoing microlaryngeal endoscopic surgery found that TENS given during surgery improved cardiovascular status and decreased the use of nicardipine when compared to controls (Level II: Toyota *et al.* 1999). Within this study, TENS was delivered to Hoku (LI4) and Tsusanli (ST36) acupoints using a modified device. In contrast, an RCT of 33 patients undergoing diagnostic colonoscopy found no differences in pain relief between TENS combined with midazolam when compared to sham TENS combined with midazolam (Level II: Robinson *et al.* 2001). Hruby *et al.* also failed to detect differences in pain in 148 patients receiving TENS or sham TENS for flexible cystoscopy (Level II: Hruby *et al.* 2006).

Evidence is equivocal for the use of TENS devices during dental surgery, although it is well tolerated and preferred to injections by adults and children. Clinical trials have reported positive outcome for dental hygiene procedures (Level III-1: Bruzek & Geistfeld 1996), intra-oral injections (Level III-1: Meechan *et al.* 1998, Level III-1: Meechan & Winter 1996), occlusal restoration (Level III-1: Cho *et al.* 1998, Level II: Modaresi *et al.* 1996). In an RCT of 100 women undergoing painful laser treatment of the cervix, TENS was found to generate considerable patient satisfaction but did not provide any additional pain-relieving effect when used in combination with direct infiltration of lignocaine (Level II: Crompton *et al.* 1992).

TENS has been used with success to manage painful medical procedures as adjunct to local anaesthesia during distension shoulder arthrography for 'frozen shoulder' (Level III-1: Morgan *et al.* 1996) or as a stand-alone treatment to aid wound pain accompanying dressing changes (Level IV: Merkel *et al.* 1999), lithotripsy (Level II: Kararmaz *et al.* 2004, Level III-1: Rawat *et al.* 1991) and venepuncture (Level II: Coyne *et al.* 1995, Lander & Fowler-Kerry 1993).

TENS for post-surgical nausea and vomiting

A Cochrane review of 24 RCTs concluded that non-pharmacologic techniques such as TENS, acupuncture and electroacupuncture were better than placebo in reducing nausea and vomiting within 6 hr of surgery in adults (Level I: Lee & Done 2004). A review of 26 trials (over 3000 patients) concluded that P6 stimulation was better than sham for both adults and children (Level I: Ezzo *et al.* 2006, Streitberger *et al.* 2006), which has been confirmed by a similar review by another group (Level I: Dune & Shiao 2006).

A multicentre RCT using 221 outpatients undergoing laparoscopic chole-cystectomy with a standardised general anaesthetic found that P6 TEAS (see the section on 'TENS-like devices') given for 9 hr postoperatively decreased moderate-to-severe nausea for up to 9 hr after surgery but did not reduce vomiting or need for rescue anti-emetic drugs (Level II: Zarate *et al.* 2001). An RCT investigating 90 patients with PONV found that ondansetron (4 mg IV) combined with TEAS reduced the incidence of emetic events to a greater extent than ondansetron with sham TEAS or placebo (2-mL IV sodium chloride) with TEAS (Level II: Coloma *et al.* 2002). Similar findings have been reported following breast surgery under general anaesthesia (Level II: Gan *et al.* 2004), laparoscopic procedures (Level II: Khan *et al.* 2004) and tonsillectomy under general anaesthesia on sedated children (Level II: Kabalak *et al.* 2005). One RCT on 94 patients following caesarean delivery with spinal anaesthesia found no difference between active and sham TEAS in PONV (Level II: Habib *et al.* 2006).

A recent sham-controlled RCT using 40 patients following laparoscopic cholecystectomy reported that TENS of the vestibular system may be useful for PONV. TENS was administered to the trapezoid area for 6 hr using one electrode applied to the neck and two electrodes applied to the mastoid area. Currents were delivered at 5 Hz, 50 ms, with a current density of 0.5–4 mA (Level II: Cekmen *et al.* 2007).

TENS for other post-surgical symptoms

Evidence is conflicting about the effectiveness of TENS to reduce postoperative pulmonary dysfunction (atelectasis) following chest and upper abdominal surgery (Level III-1: Ali *et al.* 1981). TENS reduced pain intensity during deep breathing postoperatively when used as a supplement to pharmacologic analgesia but did not alter pain at rest (Level III-1: Rakel & Frantz 2003). TENS improved peak expiratory flow rates (PEFRs) for the first two postoperative days and forced vital capacity (FVC) on the second postoperative day when compared to sham in 31 patients following cardiac surgery (Level II: Navarathnam *et al.* 1984). TENS improved FEV1, FVC, PaO_2 and $PaCO_2$ compared to sham TENS (Level II: Erdogan *et al.* 2005) and tolerance of chest physical therapy following thoracotomy (Level II: Warfield *et al.* 1985). In contrast, no significant differences were found between TENS and sham for pain with cough, FVC, FEV1 or PEFR in 45 CABG patients (Level II: Forster *et al.* 1994). Similarly PEFR and analgesic requirement did not differ between post-thoracotomy patients using TENS with intramuscular papaveretum when compared to intramuscular papaveretum alone (Level II: Stubbing & Jellicoe 1988).

There is very limited evidence on which to judge the ability of TENS to reduce postoperative ileus. Theron & Vermeulen investigated the effect of transcutaneous diadynamic currents on intestinal motility in 30 adult patients after laparotomy and reported that bowel sounds returned immediately following electrical stimulation and that more than 50% of the patients passed flatus within 24 hr (Level III-3: Theron & Vermeulen 1983).

TENS has been used to reduce disuse muscle atrophy following open meniscectomy (Level III-2: Gould *et al.* 1983). TENS was delivered as neuromuscular stimulator to generate 400, 5-s tetanising muscular contractions each day over a period of 2 weeks. The electrically stimulated group had less postoperative knee swelling, used significantly less pain medication and had smaller loss of muscle volume and strength and could walk earlier without crutches.

Summary

There appears to be a potential role for TENS as an adjunct to pharmacotherapy in the perioperative setting. Providing that it is administered appropriately it is likely to provide pain relief or reductions in analgesic intake for some, but not all, patients. It may also be useful for PONV and other post-surgical symptoms.

References

Agency for Health Care Policy and Research (AHCPR) Acute Pain Management Guideline Panel (1992) *Acute Pain Management: Operative or Medical Procedures and Trauma* (Clinical Practice Guideline No 1). AHCPR Publication No 92-0032. US Public Health Service, Rockville, MD, pp. 24–25.

Ainsworth, L., Budelier, K., Clinesmith, M., *et al.* (2006) Transcutaneous electrical nerve stimulation (TENS) reduces chronic hyperalgesia induced by muscle inflammation. *Pain*, **120** (1–2), 182–187.

Ali, J., Yaffe, C.S. & Serrette, C. (1981) The effect of transcutaneous electric nerve stimulation on postoperative pain and pulmonary function. *Surgery*, **89** (4), 507–512.

Andersson, S., Ericson, T., Holmgren, E. & Linquist, G. (7 December 1973) Electroacupuncture. Effect of pain threshold measured with electrical stimulation of teeth. *Brain Research*, **63**, 393–396.

Australian and New Zealand College of Anaesthetists and Faculty of Pain Medicine (ANZCA) (2005) *Acute Pain Management: Scientific Evidence*. Australian and New Zealand College of Anaesthetists. www.rcoa.ac.uk. Accessed 13 December 2007.

Bandolier (1999) *Transcutaneous Electrical Nerve Stimulation (TENS) in Postoperative Pain*. Bandolier. www.jr2.ox.ac.uk/bandolier/booth/painpag/Acutrev/Other/AP019. html. Accessed 13 December 2007.

Barlas, P. & Lundeberg, T. (2006) Transcutaneous electrical nerve stimulation and acupuncture. In: *Melzack and Wall's Textbook of Pain* (eds S. McMahon & M. Koltzenburg). Elsevier Churchill Livingstone, Philadelphia, pp. 583–590.

Bjordal, J.M., Johnson, M.I. & Ljunggreen, A.E. (2003) Transcutaneous electrical nerve stimulation (TENS) can reduce postoperative analgesic consumption. A meta-analysis with assessment of optimal treatment parameters for postoperative pain. *European Journal of Pain*, **7** (2), 181–188.

Bronfort, G., Nilsson, N., Haas, M., *et al.* (2004) Non-invasive physical treatments for chronic/recurrent headache. *Cochrane Database of Systematic Reviews*, Issue 3, Art No CD001878. DOI: 10.1002/14651858.CD001878.pub2.

Brosseau, L., Judd, M.G., Marchand, S., *et al.* (2003) Transcutaneous electrical nerve stimulation (TENS) for the treatment of rheumatoid arthritis in the hand. *Cochrane Database of Systematic Reviews*, Issue 2, Art No CD004377. DOI: 10.1002/14651858.CD004377.

Bruzek, D. & Geistfeld, N. (1996) Clinical study to evaluate the use of electronic anesthesia during dental hygiene procedures. *Northwest Dentistry*, **75** (3), 21–26.

Bundsen, P. & Ericson, K. (1982) Pain relief in labor by transcutaneous electrical nerve stimulation. Safety aspects. *Acta Obstetricia et Gynecologica Scandinavica*, **61** (1), 1–5.

Carman, D. & Roach, J.W. (1988) Transcutaneous electrical nerve stimulation for the relief of postoperative pain in children. *Spine*, **13**, 109–110.

Carroll, D., Tramer, M., McQuay, H., *et al.* (1996) Randomization is important in studies with pain outcomes: systematic review of transcutaneous electrical nerve stimulation in acute postoperative pain. *British Journal of Anaesthesia*, **77** (6), 798–803.

Cekmen, N., Salman, B., Keles, Z., *et al.* (2007) Transcutaneous electrical nerve stimulation in the prevention of postoperative nausea and vomiting after elective laparoscopic cholecystectomy. *Journal of Clinical Anesthesia*, **19** (1), 49–52.

Chandran, P. & Sluka, K.A. (2003) Development of opioid tolerance with repeated transcutaneous electrical nerve stimulation administration. *Pain*, **102** (1–2), 195–201.

Charlton, J. (2005) *Core Curriculum for Professional Education in Pain*, 3rd edn. IASP Press, Seattle, pp. 93–96.

Chartered Society of Physiotherapy (2006) *Guidance for the Clinical use of Electrophysical Agents.* Chartered Society of Physiotherapy, London.

Chen, C.C., Tabasam, G. & Johnson, M.I. (2008) Does the pulse frequency of transcutaneous electrical nerve stimulation (TENS) influence hypoalgesia? A systematic review of studies using experimental pain and healthy human participants. *Physiotherapy*, **94** (1), 11–20.

Cho, S.Y., Drummond, B.K., Anderson, M.H. & Williams, S. (1998) Effectiveness of electronic dental anesthesia for restorative care in children. *Pediatric Dentistry*, **20** (2), 105–111.

Chung, J.M. (1985) Antinociceptive effects of peripheral nerve stimulation. *Progress in Clinical and Biological Research*, **176**, 147–161.

Coloma, M., White, P.F., Ogunnaike, B.O., *et al.* (2002) Comparison of acustimulation and ondansetron for the treatment of established postoperative nausea and vomiting. *Anesthesiology*, **97** (6), 1387–1392.

Cook, T.M. & Riley, R.H. (1997) Analgesia following thoracotomy: a survey of Australian practice. *Anaesthesia and Intensive Care*, **25** (5), 520–524.

Coyne, P., MacMurren, M., Izzo, T. & Kramer, T. (1995) Transcutaneous electrical nerve stimulator for procedural pain associated with intravenous needlesticks. *Journal of Intravenous Nursing*, **18** (5), 263–267.

Crompton, A.C., Johnson, N., Dudek, U., *et al.* (1992) Is transcutaneous electrical nerve stimulation of any value during cervical laser treatment? *British Journal of Obstetrics and Gynaecology*, **99** (6), 492–494.

De Angelis, C., Perrone, G., Santoro, G., *et al.* (2003) Suppression of pelvic pain during hysteroscopy with a transcutaneous electrical nerve stimulation device. *Fertility and Sterility*, **79** (6), 1422–1427.

Duggan, A.W. & Foong, F.W. (1985) Bicuculline and spinal inhibition produced by dorsal column stimulation in the cat. *Pain*, **22** (3), 249–259.

Dundee, J.W., Ghaly, R.G., Bill, K.M., *et al.* (1989) Effect of stimulation of the P6 anti-emetic point on postoperative nausea and vomiting. *British Journal of Anaesthesia*, **63** (5), 612–618.

Dune, L.S. & Shiao, S.Y. (2006) Metaanalysis of acustimulation effects on postoperative nausea and vomiting in children. *Explore (NY)*, **2** (4), 314–320.

Duranti, R., Pantaleo, T. & Bellini, F. (1988) Increase in muscular pain threshold following low frequency-high intensity peripheral conditioning stimulation in humans. *Brain Research*, **452**, 66–72.

Erdogan, M., Erdogan, A., Erbil, N., *et al.* (2005) Prospective, randomized, placebo-controlled study of the Effect of TENS on postthoracotomy pain and pulmonary function. *World Journal of Surgery*, **29** (12), 1563–1570.

Eriksson, M.B. & Sjölund, B.H. (1976) Acupuncture-like electroanalgesia in TNS resistant chronic pain. In: *Sensory Functions of the Skin* (ed Y. Zotterman). Pergamon Press, Oxford/New York, pp. 575–581.

Eriksson, M.B., Sjolund, B.H. & Nielzen, S. (1979) Long term results of peripheral conditioning stimulation as an analgesic measure in chronic pain. *Pain*, **6** (3), 335–347.

Ezzo, J., Streitberger, K. & Schneider, A. (2006) Cochrane systematic reviews examine P6 acupuncture-point stimulation for nausea and vomiting. *Journal of Alternative and Complementary Medicine*, **12** (5), 489–495.

Fargas-Babjak, A.M., Pomeranz, B. & Rooney, P.J. (1992) Acupuncture-like stimulation with codetron for rehabilitation of patients with chronic pain syndrome and osteoarthritis. *Acupuncture and Electro-Therapeutics Research*, **17** (2), 95–105.

Finley, G.A. & Steward, D.J. (1983) Transcutaneous electrical nerve stimulation for control of postoperative pain following spinal fusion in adolescents. *Canadian Anesthetists Society Journal*, **30S**, 60.

Forster, E.L., Kramer, J.F., Lucy, S.D., *et al.* (1994) Effect of TENS on pain, medications, and pulmonary function following coronary artery bypass graft surgery. *Chest*, **106** (5), 1343–1348.

Gan, T.J., Jiao, K.R., Zenn, M. & Georgiade, G. (2004) A randomized controlled comparison of electro-acupoint stimulation or ondansetron versus placebo for the prevention of postoperative nausea and vomiting. *Anesthesia and Analgesia*, **99** (4), 1070–1075.

Garrison, D.W. & Foreman, R.D. (1994) Decreased activity of spontaneous and noxiously evoked dorsal horn cells during transcutaneous electrical nerve stimulation (TENS). *Pain*, **58** (3), 309–315.

Garrison, D.W. & Foreman, R.D. (1996) Effects of transcutaneous electrical nerve stimulation (TENS) on spontaneous and noxiously evoked dorsal horn cell activity in cats with transected spinal cords. *Neuroscience Letters*, **216** (2), 125–128.

Gildenberg, P.L. (2006) History of electrical neuromodulation for chronic pain. *Pain Medicine*, **7** (Suppl 1), S7–S13.

Gould, N., Donnermeyer, D., Gammon, G.G., *et al.* (September 1983) Transcutaneous muscle stimulation to retard disuse atrophy after open meniscectomy. *Clinical Orthopaedics and Related Research*, **178**, 190–197.

Habib, A.S., Itchon-Ramos, N., Phillips-Bute, B.G. & Gan, T.J. (2006) Transcutaneous acupoint electrical stimulation with the ReliefBand for the prevention of nausea and vomiting during and after cesarean delivery under spinal anesthesia. *Anesthesia & Analgesia*, **102** (2), 581–584.

Hruby, G., Ames, C., Chen, C., *et al.* (2006) Assessment of efficacy of transcutaneous electrical nerve stimulation for pain management during office-based flexible cystoscopy. *Urology*, **67** (5), 914–917.

Hymes, A., Raab, D., Yonchiro, E., Nelson, G. & Printy, A. (1974) Electrical surface stimulation for control of post operative pain and prevention of ileus. *Surgical Forum*, **65**, 1517–1520.

Idvall, E. (2002) Post-operative patients in severe pain but satisfied with pain relief. *Journal of Clinical Nursing*, **11** (6), 841–842.

Ignelzi, R.J. & Nyquist, J.K. (1975) Peripheral nerve stimulation for pain relief: effect on cutaneous peripheral nerve evoked activity. *Surgical Forum*, **26**, 474–476.

Ignelzi, R.J. & Nyquist, J.K. (1976) Direct effect of electrical stimulation on peripheral nerve evoked activity: implications in pain relief. *Journal of Neurosurgery*, **45** (2), 159–165.

Ignelzi, R.J. & Nyquist, J.K. (1979) Excitability changes in peripheral nerve fibers after repetitive electrical stimulation. Implications in pain modulation. *Journal of Neurosurgery*, **51** (6), 824–833.

Ignelzi, R.J., Nyquist, J.K. & Tighe, W.J. (1981) Repetitive electrical stimulation of peripheral nerve and spinal cord activity. *Neurological Research*, **3** (2), 195–209.

Jeans, M. (1979) Relief of chronic pain by brief, intense transcutaneous electrical stimulation – a double blind study. In: *Advances in Pain Research and Therapy*, Vol. 3 (eds J. Bonica, J. Liebeskind & D. Albe-Fessard). Raven Press, New York, pp. 601–606.

Johnson, M.I. (1998) The analgesic effects and clinical use of Acupuncture-like TENS (AL-TENS). *Physical Therapy Reviews*, **3** (2), 73–93.

Johnson, M.I. (2001) Transcutaneous electrical nerve stimulation (TENS) and TENS-like devices. Do they provide pain relief? *Pain Reviews*, **8** (3–4), 121–128.

Johnson, M. & Martinson, M. (2007) Efficacy of electrical nerve stimulation for chronic musculoskeletal pain: a meta-analysis of randomized controlled trials. *Pain*, **130** (1–2), 157–165.

Johnson, M.I., Ashton, C.H. & Thompson, J.W. (1991) An in-depth study of long-term users of transcutaneous electrical nerve stimulation (TENS). Implications for clinical use of TENS. *Pain*, **44** (3), 221–229.

Kabalak, A.A., Akcay, M., Akcay, F. & Gogus, N. (2005) Transcutaneous electrical acupoint stimulation versus ondansetron in the prevention of postoperative vomiting following pediatric tonsillectomy. *Journal of Alternative and Complementary Medicine*, **11** (3), 407–413.

Kalra, A., Urban, M.O. & Sluka, K.A. (2001) Blockade of opioid receptors in rostral ventral medulla prevents antihyperalgesia produced by transcutaneous electrical nerve stimulation (TENS). *The Journal of Pharmacology and Experimental Therapeutics*, **298** (1), 257–263.

Kane, K. & Taub, A. (1975) A history of local electrical analgesia. *Pain*, **1** (2), 125–138.

Kararmaz, A., Kaya, S., Karaman, H. & Turhanoglu, S. (2004) Effect of the frequency of transcutaneous electrical nerve stimulation on analgesia during extracorporeal shock wave lithotripsy. *Urological Research*, **32** (6), 411–415.

Khadilkar, A., Milne, S., Brosseau, L., *et al.* (2005) Transcutaneous electrical nerve stimulation (TENS) for chronic low-back pain. *Cochrane Database of Systematic Reviews*, Issue 3, Art No CD003008. DOI: 10.1002/14651858.CD003008.pub2.

Khan, R.M., Maroof, M., Hakim, S., *et al.* (2004) Intraoperative stimulation of the P6 point controls postoperative nausea and vomiting following laparoscopic surgery. *Canadian Journal of Anaesthesia*, **51** (7), 740–741.

King, E.W., Audette, K., Athman, G.A., *et al.* (2005) Transcutaneous electrical nerve stimulation activates peripherally located alpha-2A adrenergic receptors. *Pain*, **115** (3), 364–373.

Kroeling, P., Gross, A.R. & Goldsmith, C.H. (2005) A Cochrane review of electrotherapy for mechanical neck disorders. *Spine*, **30** (21), 641–648.

Lander, J. & Fowler-Kerry, S. (1993) TENS for children's procedural pain. *Pain*, **52** (2), 209–216.

Le Bars, D., Dickenson, A.H. & Besson, J.M. (1979) Diffuse noxious inhibitory controls (DNIC) 1. Effects on dorsal horn convergent neurones in the rat. *Pain*, **6** (3), 283–304.

Lee, A. & Done, M.L. (2004) Stimulation of the wrist acupuncture point P6 for preventing postoperative nausea and vomiting. *Cochrane Database of Systematic Reviews*, Issue 3, Art No CD003281. DOI: 10.1002/14651858.CD003281.pub2.

Leem, J., Park, E. & Paik, K. (1995) Electrophysiological evidence for the antinociceptive effect of transcutaneous electrical stimulation on mechanically evoked responsiveness of dorsal horn neurons in neuropathic rats. *Neuroscience Letters*, **192** (3), 197–200.

Limoge, A. & Dixmerias-Iskandar, F. (June 2005) Improvement of postoperative analgesia during cancer surgery with Limoge's current. *Journal of Alternative and Complementary Medicine*, **11** (3), 543–547.

Limoge, A., Robert, C. & Stanley, T.H. (1999) Transcutaneous cranial electrical stimulation (TCES): a review 1998. *Neuroscience and Biobehavioral Reviews*, **23** (4), 529–538.

Limoges, M.F. & Rickabaugh, B. (2004) Evaluation of TENS during screening flexible sigmoidoscopy. *Gastroenterology Nursing*, **27** (2), 61–68.

Long, D.M. (1973) Electrical stimulation for relief of pain from chronic nerve injury. *Journal of Neurosurgery*, **39** (6), 718–722.

Ma, Y.T. & Sluka, K.A. (2001) Reduction in inflammation-induced sensitization of dorsal horn neurons by transcutaneous electrical nerve stimulation in anesthetized rats. *Experimental Brain Research*, **137** (1), 94–102.

Maeda, Y., Lisi, T.L., Vance, C.G. & Sluka, K.A. (2007) Release of GABA and activation of GABA(A) in the spinal cord mediates the effects of TENS in rats. *Brain Research*, **1136** (1), 43–50.

Mann, C. (1996) Respiratory compromise: a rare complication of transcutaneous electrical nerve stimulation for angina pectoris. *Journal of Accident and Emergency Medicine*, **13** (1), 68.

Mannheimer, J. & Lampe, G. (1988) *Clinical Transcutaneous Electrical Nerve Stimulation*. F.A. Davis Company, Philadelphia.

Meechan, J. & Winter, R. (1996) A comparison of topical anaesthesia and electronic nerve stimulation for reducing the pain of intra-oral injections. *British Dental Journal*, **181** (9), 333–335.

Meechan, J.G., Gowans, A.J. & Welbury, R.R. (1998) The use of patient-controlled transcutaneous electronic nerve stimulation (TENS) to decrease the discomfort of regional anaesthesia in dentistry: a randomised controlled clinical trial. *Journal of Dentistry*, **26** (5–6), 417–420.

Melzack, R., Vetere, P. & Finch, L. (1983) Transcutaneous electrical nerve stimulation for low back pain. A comparison of TENS and massage for pain and range of motion. *Physical Therapy*, **63** (4), 489–493.

Melzack, R. & Wall, P.D. (1965) Pain mechanisms: a new theory. *Science*, **150** (699), 971–979.

Merkel, S.I., Gutstein, H.B. & Malviya, S. (1999) Use of transcutaneous electrical nerve stimulation in a young child with pain from open perineal lesions. *Journal of Pain and Symptom Management*, **18** (5), 376–381.

Meyerson, B. (1983) Electrostimulation procedures: effects presumed rationale, and possible mechanisms. In: *Advances in Pain Research and Therapy*, Vol. 5 (eds J.J. Bonica, U. Lindblom & A. Iggo). Raven Press, New York, pp. 495–534.

Modaresi, A., Lindsay, S., Gould, A. & Smith, P. (1996) A partial double-blind, placebo-controlled study of electronic dental anaesthesia in children. *International Journal of Paediatric Dentistry*, **6** (4), 245–251.

Morgan, B., Jones, A.R., Mulcahy, K.A., *et al.* (1996) Transcutaneous electric nerve stimulation (TENS) during distension shoulder arthrography: a controlled trial. *Pain*, **64** (2), 265–267.

Nardone, A. & Schieppati, M. (1989) Influences of transcutaneous electrical stimulation of cutaneous and mixed nerves on subcortical and cortical somatosensory evoked potentials. *Electroencephalography and Clinical Neurophysiology*, **74** (1), 24–35.

Navarathnam, R.G., Wang, I.Y., Thomas, D. & Klineberg, P.L. (1984) Evaluation of the transcutaneous electrical nerve stimulator for postoperative analgesia following cardiac surgery. *Anaesthesia and Intensive Care*, **12** (4), 345–350.

Osiri, M., Welch, V., Brosseau, L., *et al.* (2000) Transcutaneous electrical nerve stimulation for knee osteoarthritis. *Cochrane Database of Systematic Reviews*, Issue 4, Art No CD002823. DOI 10.1002/14651858.CD002823.

Pike, P.M. (1978) Transcutaneous electrical stimulation. Its use in the management of postoperative pain. *Anaesthesia*, **33** (2), 165–171.

Price, C.I. & Pandyan, A.D. (2000) Electrical stimulation for preventing and treating post-stroke shoulder pain. *Cochrane Database of Systematic Reviews*, Issue 4, Art No CD001698. DOI: 10.1002/14651858.CD001698.

Proctor, M.L., Smith, C.A., Farquhar, C.M. & Stones, R.W. (2003) Transcutaneous electrical nerve stimulation and acupuncture for primary dysmenorrhoea (Cochrane review). *Cochrane Database of Systematic Reviews Issue*, Issue 1, Art No CD002123. DOI: 10.1002/14651858.CD002123.

Pyatt, J.R., Trenbath, D., Chester, M. & Connelly, D.T. (2003) The simultaneous use of a biventricular implantable cardioverter defibrillator (ICD) and transcutaneous electrical nerve stimulation (TENS) unit: implications for device interaction. *Europace*, **5** (1), 91–53.

Radhakrishnan, R., King, E.W., Dickman, J.K., *et al.* (2003) Spinal 5-HT(2) and 5-HT(3) receptors mediate low, but not high, frequency TENS-induced antihyperalgesia in rats. *Pain*, **105** (1–2), 205–213.

Radhakrishnan, R. & Sluka, K.A. (2003) Spinal muscarinic receptors are activated during low or high frequency TENS-induced antihyperalgesia in rats. *Neuropharmacology*, **45** (8), 1111–1119.

Radhakrishnan, R. & Sluka, K.A. (2005) Deep tissue afferents, but not cutaneous afferents, mediate transcutaneous electrical nerve stimulation-Induced antihyperalgesia. *The Journal of Pain*, **6** (10), 673–680.

Rakel, B. & Frantz, R. (2003) Effectiveness of transcutaneous electrical nerve stimulation on postoperative pain with movement. *The Journal of Pain*, **4** (8), 455–464.

Rawat, B., Genz, A., Fache, J.S., *et al.* (1991) Effectiveness of transcutaneous electrical nerve stimulation (TENS) for analgesia during biliary lithotripsy. *Investigative Radiology*, **26** (10), 866–869.

Reeve, J., Menon, D. & Corabian, P. (1996) Transcutaneous electrical nerve stimulation (TENS): a technology assessment. *International Journal of Technology Assessment in Health Care*, **12** (2), 299–324.

Reynolds, D.V. (1969) Surgery in the rat during electrical analgesia induced by focal brain stimulation. *Science*, **164** (878), 444–445.

Robinson, R., Darlow, S., Wright, S.J., *et al.* (2001) Is transcutaneous electrical nerve stimulation an effective analgesia during colonoscopy? *Postgraduate Medical Journal*, **77** (909), 445–446.

Royal College of Anaesthetists (2006) *Compendium of Audit Recipes*. Royal College of Anaesthetists, London.

Royal College of Surgeons of England and the Faculty of Anaesthetists (1990) *Report of the Working Party on Pain after Surgery*. The Royal College of Surgeons of England and the College of Anaesthetists, London.

Sandkühler, J. (2000) Long-lasting analgesia following TENS and acupuncture: spinal mechanisms beyond gate control. In: *Progress in Pain Research and Management* (eds M. Devor, M.C. Rowbotham & Z. Wiesenfeld-Hallin). IASP Press, Seattle, pp. 359–369.

Sandkühler, J., Chen, J.G., Cheng, G. & Randic, M. (1997) Low-frequency stimulation of afferent Adelta-fibers induces long-term depression at primary afferent synapses with substantia gelatinosa neurons in the rat. *Journal of Neuroscience*, **17** (16), 6483–6491.

Shealy, C.N. (1974) Transcutaneous electrical stimulation for control of pain. *Clinical Neurosurgery*, **21**, 269–277.

Shealy, C.N., Mortimer, J.T. & Reswick, J.B. (1967) Electrical inhibition of pain by stimulation of the dorsal columns: preliminary clinical report. *Anesthesia and Analgesia*, **46** (4), 489–491.

Sjölund, B., Eriksson, M. & Loeser, J. (1990) Transcutaneous and implanted electric stimulation of peripheral nerves. In: *The Management of Pain*, Vol. 2 (ed. J. Bonica). Lea & Febiger, Philadelphia, pp. 1852–1861.

Sjölund, B.H., Terenius, L. & Eriksson, M. (1977) Increased cerebrospinal fluid levels of endorphins after electro-acupuncture. *Acta Physiologica Scandinavica*, **100**, 382–384.

Sluka, K.A. & Chandran, P. (2002) Enhanced reduction in hyperalgesia by combined administration of clonidine and TENS. *Pain*, **100** (1–2), 183–190.

Sluka, K.A., Deacon, M., Stibal, A., Strissel, S. & Terpstra, A. (1999) Spinal blockade of opioid receptors prevents the analgesia produced by TENS in arthritic rats. *Journal of Pharmacology and Experimental Therapeutics*, **289** (2), 840–846.

Sluka, K.A., Judge, M.A., McColley, M.M., Reveiz, P.M. & Taylor, B.M. (2000) Low frequency TENS is less effective than high frequency TENS at reducing inflammation-induced hyperalgesia in morphine-tolerant rats. *European Journal of Pain*, **4** (2), 185–193.

Sluka, K.A., Kalra, A. & Moore, S.A. (2001) Unilateral intramuscular injections of acidic saline produce a bilateral, long-lasting hyperalgesia. *Muscle Nerve*, **24** (1), 37–46.

Sluka, K.A. & Walsh, D.M. (2003) Transcutaneous electrical nerve stimulation: basic science mechanisms and clinical effectiveness. *Journal of Pain*, **4** (3), 109–121.

Stanley, T.H., Cazalaa, J.A., Atinault, A., *et al.* (1982) Transcutaneous cranial electrical stimulation decreases narcotic requirements during neurolept anesthesia and operation in man. *Anesthesia and Analgesia*, **61** (10), 863–866.

Stinus, L., Auriacombe, M., Tignol, J., *et al.* (1990) Transcranial electrical stimulation with high frequency intermittent current (Limoge's) potentiates opiate-induced analgesia: blind studies. *Pain*, **42** (3), 351–363.

Streitberger, K., Ezzo, J. & Schneider, A. (2006) Acupuncture for nausea and vomiting: an update of clinical and experimental studies. *Autonomic Neuroscience*, **129** (1–2), 107–117.

Stubbing, J.F. & Jellicoe, J.A. (1988) Transcutaneous electrical nerve stimulation after thoracotomy. Pain relief and peak expiratory flow rate – a trial of transcutaneous electrical nerve stimulation. *Anaesthesia*, **43** (4), 296–298.

Theron, E.J. & Vermeulen, A.M. (1983) The utilization of transcutaneous electric nerve stimulation in postoperative ileus. *South African Medical Journal*, **63** (25), 971–972.

Toyota, S., Satake, T. & Amaki, Y. (1999) Transcutaneous electrical nerve stimulation as an alternative therapy for microlaryngeal endoscopic surgery. *Anesthesia and Analgesia*, **89** (5), 1236–1238.

VanderArk, G.D. & McGrath, K.A. (1975) Transcutaneous electrical stimulation in treatment of postoperative pain. *American Journal of Surgery*, **130** (3), 338–340.

Wall, P.D. & Sweet, W.H. (1967) Temporary abolition of pain in man. *Science*, **155** (758), 108–109.

Walsh, D.M. (1996) Transcutaneous electrical nerve stimulation and acupuncture points. *Complementary Therapies in Medicine*, **4** (2), 133–137.

Warfield, C., Stein, J. & Frank, H. (1985) The effect of transcutaneous electrical nerve stimulation on pain after thoracotomy. *Annals of Thoracic Surgery*, **39** (5), 462–465.

Zarate, E., Mingus, M., White, P.F., *et al.* (2001) The use of transcutaneous acupoint electrical stimulation for preventing nausea and vomiting after laparoscopic surgery. *Anesthesia and Analgesia*, **92** (3), 629–635.

14 Risk Management in Perioperative Analgesia

Jeremy Mitchell

Key Messages

- Consent needs to be gained for any perioperative analgesia technique.
- Patients must be sufficiently informed about all significant risks and the benefits of the proposed procedure in the language they can understand.
- Patients must be made aware that there is a risk of neurological damage associated with neuraxial analgesic techniques including haematoma and abscess formation.
- Peripheral nerve blocks may result in direct trauma to the nerve.
- Each organisation must have a comprehensive approach to risk management including the active identification of potential risks associated with perioperative analgesia.

Introduction

This chapter focuses on aspects of patient-related risk management in perioperative analgesia, although there are other risks which may need to be considered by health care professionals and organisations (for example the risks of controlled drug dependency in anaesthetists and anaesthetic support practitioners). The chapter is written from the perspective of perioperative practice within the United Kingdom, although the issues are relevant across the world.

Inevitably, the provision of any form of perioperative analgesia increases the risks of mortality and morbidity to the patient, in addition to the risks associated with the operation or the pre-existing medical condition of the patient. In each case, the provider of the analgesia needs to consider the balance of risks and benefits in the proposed treatment. Usually this consideration is straightforward and the benefits of the intervention (such as reduction in pain and pulmonary complications) outweigh the potential risks of that intervention (for example unwanted drug effects). Sometimes the difference in benefits and risks between one analgesic intervention and another may be less clear-cut and the subject of considerable debate (such as the use of epidural analgesia or intravenous opioids following major surgery) (Level I: Dolin *et al.* 2002, Level I: Hansdottir *et al.* 2006, Rathmell *et al.* 2006).

Consent to treatment (Department of Health 2004)

Any treatment should only be provided with the consent of the patient or those with parental responsibility (if the patient is aged under 18 years). The position with the administration of perioperative analgesia is no different to any other proposed treatment. In order for a patient or person with parental responsibility to give their consent to the treatment, the patient or the person with parental responsibility should:

- Be competent to take the particular decision
- Have received sufficient information to take it
- Not be acting under duress

Consent may be given orally by the patient or in writing. It is usual practice for written consent to be obtained for procedures which require general or regional anaesthesia and analgesia. For major procedures, consent should be regarded as a process involving several steps, culminating in the formal documentation in writing rather than the immediate process of completing a consent form.

The General Medical Council (GMC) has revised its guidelines for medical practitioners on obtaining consent for treatment or investigation (General Medical Council 2008), taking into account changes in United Kingdom law relating to decision making and consent, particularly in patients who lack capacity. The revised guidelines emphasise the importance of the partnership between patients and doctors, based on openness, trust and good communication, in ensuring good care. The revised guidelines state that doctors must:

(a) Listen to patients and respect their views about their health
(b) Discuss with patients what their diagnosis, prognosis, treatment and care involve
(c) Share with patients the information they want or need in order to make decisions
(d) Maximise patients' opportunities, and their ability, to make decisions for themselves
(e) Respect patients' decisions

Throughout the United Kingdom there should be a presumption that adult patients have the capacity to make decisions about their care and treatment. A mentally competent patient may refuse treatment for any reason, rational or otherwise, even if such a decision is fatal for the patient. Capacity issues are dealt with by different legislation in different parts of the United Kingdom. In

England, the Mental Capacity Act 2005 introduced a single test for assessing whether a person lacks capacity to take a particular decision at a particular time.[1] The test, set out in Section 3 (1), of the act is:

> A person is unable to make a decision for himself if he is unable; to understand the information relevant to the decision, to retain the information, to use or weigh the information as part of the process of making the decision, or to communicate the decision (whether by talking, using sign language or any other means).

In England and Wales, the Mental Capacity Act 2005[2] sets out who can make treatment decisions in patients who lack capacity (including individuals with lasting powers of attorney) and introduces the role of the Independent Mental Capacity Advocate in the case of patients without anyone else to take an interest in their welfare. Treatment decisions should be made in the patient's 'best interests', as long as the treatment has not been refused in advance in a valid and applicable advance directive.

It is obvious that if an adult patient has been given a general anaesthetic or sedation, the patient temporarily lacks capacity. It is important that, wherever possible, there has been a proper discussion and agreement with the patient about relevant perioperative analgesic techniques before general anaesthesia or sedation is commenced. This is particularly important when a regional anaesthetic technique is being proposed as an adjunct to general anaesthesia or sedation.

Not infrequently, the surgical plan may change during the course of an operation – for example changing from an endoscopic to an open approach to a body cavity – and the preoperative discussion about analgesic techniques should take into account reasonably foreseeable changes in the surgical plan. For example a discussion with a patient about the analgesic options prior to a video-assisted thoracoscopy may need to include the consequences of the possibility of conversion to a thoracotomy (for example placement of an epidural catheter). It would be unwise for the anaesthetist to rely on an assertion that he or she was acting in the 'best interests' of the patient by placing an epidural catheter once the patient has lost the capacity to consent, without discussing this in advance.

Consent for perioperative analgesia

The situation regarding informed consent for perioperative analgesia should be no different to that for any other treatment. However, the provision of perioperative analgesia is inevitably related to the procedure being proposed and there may be some information given to the patient about perioperative analgesia by the surgeon (for example on the possibility of regional anaesthesia and analgesia) before the patient comes into contact with an anaesthetist.

The provision of an appropriate patient information leaflet in advance of the patient's admission may be helpful, particularly for elective surgery.

The anaesthetist should wherever possible visit the patient before the operation to discuss relevant issues about perioperative analgesia. Patients should be given the opportunity to ask questions during this discussion. It is usual for the anaesthetist to rely on the verbal consent of the patient to relevant analgesic techniques. However, the salient aspects of that discussion should be documented in the medical records. It is not considered necessary in the United Kingdom at present to have a separate written consent for anaesthesia or analgesia (AAGBI 2006).

Adequate patient information

The anaesthetist needs to ensure that patients have been sufficiently informed about the risks and benefits of the proposed procedure. The Association of Anaesthetists advises (AAGBI 2006):

> In broad terms, patients must understand what they are consenting to. Therefore, anaesthetists should tell the patient: what procedures they intend to do, and why they intend to do them; what the significant, foreseeable risks of these procedures are, and what the significant, foreseeable consequences of these risks might be.

Patients should be informed about all significant risks as a result of their treatment (General Medical Council 2008). A small, but well-established, risk of serious injury should be considered as 'significant' (Chester v Afshar 2004). If a neuraxial analgesic technique is being proposed, then there should be an adequate discussion about the risks of epidural haematoma and abscess formation and the potential for permanent neurological damage.

A recent study in North America showed that there continue to be significant inconsistencies in the way in which serious risks are discussed with patients (Brull *et al.* 2007). There has been a considerable change in practice over the past 10 years in the United Kingdom about the information given to patients prior to thoracic epidural analgesia, with a significant increase in the proportion of anaesthetists discussing complications such as dural tap and neurological injury (Pennefather *et al.* 2006). It is likely that there have been similar changes in practice in other areas of perioperative analgesia.

It is important to ensure that the patient's expectations are not raised unduly. Patients should be given some indication of the likely success of the proposed analgesic technique, particularly in reference to control of postoperative pain, and the risk of inadequate analgesia should be clearly explained prior to the procedure.

It can become difficult to ensure that there is a balanced discussion about the principal risks and benefits of the proposed procedure, yet at the same time, ensure that sufficient information has been given about all significant risks, in a fashion suited to each patient, without taking an unreasonable amount of time.

The anaesthetist should be careful to ensure that the discussion about perioperative analgesia is balanced so that if there is more than one option, information about each option is given. The anaesthetist may recommend a particular option, but should not put pressure on the patient to accept the anaesthetist's advice (General Medical Council 2008).

A suitable patient information leaflet may help explain the issues and allow for more focus in the discussion between the anaesthetist and the patient about issues important to the individual patient. Patient information leaflets cannot replace an individual discussion between anaesthetist and patient. Careful consideration should be given to the needs of non-English readers and those with impaired vision, and suitable versions in Braille and other languages may be appropriate.

The Royal College of Anaesthetists has produced several patient information leaflets on perioperative analgesia. An example is shown in Figures 14.1. and 14.2 illustrates a method of presenting complications in order of frequency (RCoA & AAGBI 2004). It may be helpful to have locally produced leaflets

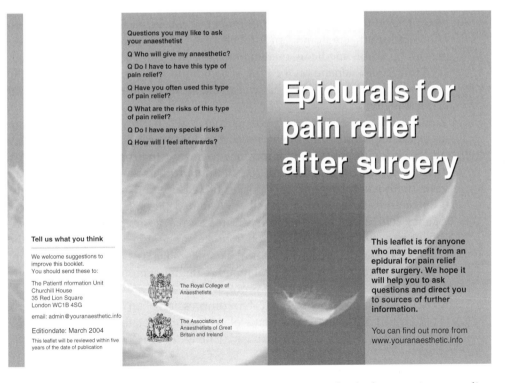

Figure 14.1 Patient information leaflet, illustrating a method of presenting complications in order of frequency. (© The Royal College of Anaesthetists and the Association of Anaesthetists of Great Britain & Ireland (2004), reproduced with permission.)

Very common	Common	Uncommon	Rare	Very rare
1 in 10	1 in 100	1 in 1 000	1 in 10 000	1 in 100 000

Figure 14.2   A method of presenting complications in order of frequency for a patient information leaflet. (© The Royal College of Anaesthetists and the Association of Anaesthetists of Great Britain & Ireland (2004), reproduced with permission.)

setting out the issues associated with specific procedures, particularly when there are significant risks and concerns, for example where thoracic epidural analgesia is planned in relation to cardiac surgery and where there is considerable concern about the risks of developing an epidural haematoma, which may lead to permanent neurological damage.

Neurological damage associated with neuraxial analgesic techniques

Neurological damage may have a number of causes, including the formation of an epidural haematoma, epidural abscess, needle- and catheter-related injury and possibly medicine-related neurotoxicity. The potential for neurological damage will depend on the type of technique and the site chosen, with the greatest risk occurring with epidural analgesia techniques in the thoracic and cervical regions.

Successful management of these neurological complications requires a high index of suspicion, rapid diagnosis and early surgical decompression of any space-occupying mass. It is important to ensure that patients are regularly monitored following institution (or attempted institution) of epidural analgesia, with careful regular monitoring of sensory and motor nerve deficits. (This requires an appropriate number of trained staff (National Patient Safety Agency 2007).) Prolonged recovery from a local anaesthetic block or an extension of an existing block without obvious cause should prompt a review of the cause. Once the diagnosis of epidural haematoma is suspected, it is important to obtain appropriate neurological imaging (either computerised tomography or magnetic resonance imaging) promptly and refer the patient immediately for neurosurgical review. If surgical decompression of an epidural haematoma is not carried out within a few hours of symptom onset, the likelihood of a full neurological recovery is much reduced (Cheney *et al.* 1999, Vandermeulin *et al.* 1994).

Epidural abscesses typically present several days after the placement of an epidural catheter, sometimes with back pain, raised erythrocyte sedimentation rate and peripheral leukocyte count (Rigamonti *et al.* 1999). The neurological examination may be normal until the epidural abscess starts to expand, when there may be rapid changes in sensation and motor power deficits. There may be localised tenderness and discharge of pus around the catheter insertion site indicating a superficial infection, but this does not necessarily indicate the presence of infection within the epidural space. Appropriate neurological imaging should be performed promptly. Treatment will include intravenous antibiotics and possible neurosurgical intervention. Rarely meningitis may occur in association with neuraxial analgesia. There needs to be ready access to appropriate neurological imaging and prompt neurosurgical review.

The risk of neurological infection may be reduced by avoiding neuraxial analgesic techniques in patients who have untreated systemic infection. A survey of anaesthetists in England revealed that 68% of centres would not site an epidural in a patient with positive blood cultures (Low 2002). It is appropriate to avoid local infections when siting an epidural or spinal needle. Several studies have shown greater likelihood of infection in patients with epidural catheters in place for prolonged periods, including Ruppen *et al.* (Level I: 2007), who calculated that the infection rates associated with epidural indwelling catheters was 0.4/1000 catheter treatment days.

Direct nerve injury may occur at the time of siting the neuraxial block, either to the spinal cord or to a nerve root. This may be related to injury either from the needle or from the catheter (if used). It may be associated with paraesthesia or pain on injection. It is suggested that if insertion of an epidural catheter is planned in conjunction with general anaesthesia, the catheter insertion should be performed with the patient awake prior to commencement of general anaesthesia, so that the patient can inform the anaesthetist about such symptoms during the epidural catheter insertion.

A recent survey of anaesthetists who regularly place thoracic epidural catheters in the United Kingdom showed that 84% of those who responded to the survey place the epidural catheter with the patient awake (Pennefather *et al.* 2006). A 'small' additional risk was identified in anaesthetised patients undergoing lumbar epidural catheter placement, although the relative risk compared with awake patients was not quantified (Level IV: Horlocker *et al.* 2003).

Likelihood of neurological damage from neuraxial analgesic techniques

There are a considerable number of publications on this subject. The likelihood of neurological damage is low, and this means that it is difficult to accurately quantify the risk.

The risk of epidural haematoma formation in patients undergoing cardiac surgery was estimated in 1994 (Level II: Vandermeulin *et al.* 1994) as being 1:150000 after an epidural analgesic technique and 1:220000 following an intrathecal technique. It was noted that the haematoma can develop following catheter removal as well as following catheter insertion. In addition, spontaneous epidural haematoma can form in the absence of either technique. It was felt that the risk of haematoma formation is greater in patients with a coagulopathy (including drug induced) and in those where the neuraxial technique is difficult or traumatic.

The risk of haematoma formation following intrathecal analgesic techniques in patients undergoing cardiac surgery may be as great as 1:3600 using a mathematical model (using 95% confidence intervals) (Ho *et al.* 2000). This was based on the evidence available in the literature at that time, with over 10000 cases documented (but with no cases where an epidural haematoma was reported). For patients undergoing cardiac surgery who have had an epidural analgesic technique, the risk of epidural haematoma formation might be as high as 1:1500 (95% confidence intervals, over 4500 documented cases, no reported epidural haematoma).

A meta-analysis reviewed 12 studies reporting the use of epidural analgesia in over 14000 patients undergoing cardiothoracic or vascular surgery (Level I: Ruppen *et al.* 2006). There were no reported cases of epidural haematoma, eight cases of transient neurological injury (1:1700) and no cases of persistent neurological injury. The maximum expected rate of epidural haematoma was 1:4700 across all the patient groups studied.

It has been suggested that there are a number of cases of permanent neurological damage in the United States, following the use of epidural analgesia, where the details have not been published (Chaney 2006). Chaney suggested that the analysis of the risk–benefit ratio of neuraxial analgesic techniques in cardiac surgery was difficult without well-designed studies with adequate numbers of patients.

Timing of insertion and removal of epidural catheters in relation to administration of anticoagulants

Concern has been raised that the risk of epidural haematoma formation is likely to be greater in those who receive anticoagulation either before or shortly after the epidural catheter insertion or removal. The American Society for Regional Anesthesia has produced consensus guidelines for regional analgesia techniques in anticoagulated patients (Level IV: Horlocker *et al.* 2002). The society emphasised that these guidelines were based on clinical experience and the consensus of expert opinion and that individual physicians still need to make an assessment of the risks and benefits of intervention in each individual patient based on their clinical judgement.

These guidelines obviously reflect medical opinion in 2002 in the United States; however, they do provide a useful reference for current practice in the United Kingdom. There are differences between the guidelines produced by American Society of Regional Anesthesia (ASRA) (outlined in Table 14.1) and a number of national societies in Europe (Gogarten 2006).

Table 14.1 Main recommendations from second consensus conference on neuraxial anesthesia.

Issue	Main recommendations
Patient receiving thrombolytic therapy	• No data available on minimum period between discontinuation of thrombolytic drug and time of neuraxial block or catheter removal • Careful monitoring of neuraxial block if instituted in patient receiving thrombolytic drug • Measurement of plasma fibrinogen level may help in decision about whether to remove catheter
Patient receiving unfractionated heparin	• Subcutaneous prophylaxis not a contraindication; delay heparin dose until after neuraxial block • Monitor platelet count prior to neuraxial block if patient receiving heparin for more than 4 days • In vascular surgery, delay heparin administration until 1 hr after needle placement; remove catheter 2–4 hr after last heparin dose; re-heparinisation should occur 1 hr after catheter removal • Caution if traumatic needle insertion, but no data to support mandatory cancellation of operation if blood in needle • Careful monitoring of neuraxial block postoperatively, use minimal concentrations of local anaesthetic agents to enhance early detection of epidural haematoma • Insufficient data to determine whether risk of epidural haematoma increased with full systemic anticoagulation for cardiac surgery
Patient receiving low-molecular-weight heparin (LMWH)	• Monitoring of factor Xa not recommended • Antiplatelet or oral anticoagulants increase risk of neuraxial haematoma • LMWH therapy should be delayed for 24 hr if blood in needle or catheter • Needle placement should occur at least 10–12 hr following last LMWH dose • Catheter should be removed at least 10–12 hr after last dose of LMWH, and next dose of LMWH should occur at least 2 hr after catheter removal

(continued)

Table 14.1 Main recommendations from second consensus conference on neuraxial anesthesia. *(Cont.)*

Issue	Main recommendations
Patient receiving oral anticoagulants	• Caution with any neuraxial technique • Adequate levels of factors II and X may be present only when prothrombin time/INR within normal limits • Catheter should be removed when INR ≤1.5 • If INR >3, consider withholding anticoagulant
Patient receiving antiplatelet medication	• Difficult to monitor platelet function reliably • Use of other medications may increase risk of bleeding complications • NSAIDs do not add significant risk for development of epidural haematoma in patients having epidural or spinal analgesia techniques • Suggested interval of 7 days between discontinuation of clopidogrel and neuraxial blockade • Neuraxial techniques should be avoided until platelet function has recovered following cessation of platelet IIb/IIIa antagonists (e.g. 24–48 hr for abciximab)

INR, international normalised ratio; NSAIDS, non-steroidal anti-inflammatory drugs.
Adapted and reprinted with permission from Horlocker *et al.* (2002) and American Society of Regional Anesthesia and Pain Medicine (ASRA).

Complications associated with peripheral nerve blocks

Toxic reactions to local anaesthetic drugs

There are several causes for toxic reaction. Anaphylaxis is associated with the use of amino-ester-linked local anaesthetic drugs. Methaemoglobinaemia may occur with some local anaesthetic drugs, particularly prilocaine. Localised toxicity includes myotoxicity and neurotoxicity. The risk of neurotoxicity is associated with increased concentration of local anaesthetic and the type of drug used (Heavner 2007).

Systemic toxicity may occur due to accidental intravascular injection or systemic absorption. It may present some time after the initial injection of local anaesthetic. There may be a sudden loss of consciousness, which may be associated with seizure activity, and acute cardiovascular collapse. The relative central nervous system and cardiovascular toxicity of local anaesthetic drugs is variable. Bupivacaine has been shown to cause less central nervous system symptoms than ropivacaine (Level II: Scott *et al.* 1989) or levobupivacaine (Level II: Bardsley *et al.* 1998).

There has been considerable debate about the maximum recommended doses of local anaesthetic drugs, which may be affected by the site of injection and patient-related factors (Rosenberg *et al.* 2004). Systemic toxicity will be related to the likelihood of systemic absorption of the drug, which is associated with the vascularity of the injection site. It is well established that injection of local anaesthetic into the brachial plexus will lead to greater systemic absorption than a sciatic nerve block.

Peripheral nerve blocks should only be performed in a place where full patient monitoring is available (and used) (AAGBI 2007a) and there are facilities for the acute treatment of systemic toxicity. The dose of local anaesthetic drug used should be tailored to the nerve block being performed and inadvertent intravascular injection avoided.

Recent guidelines have been published in the United Kingdom for the management of severe local anaesthetic toxicity (AAGBI 2007b). These refer to the treatment of severe cardiotoxicity with lipid emulsion and to consider the use of cardiopulmonary bypass (if available). The management of this patient group is outlined in Chapter 8.

Neurological injury following peripheral nerve blocks

Neurological injury may result from direct trauma to the nerve from the needle (or a catheter if used) or intraneural injection. The use of a peripheral nerve stimulator will assist in determining whether the needle is close to the relevant nerve, but will not prevent neurological injury. A short bevelled needle may help the operator detect passage of the needle through tissue layers, but again will not prevent neurological injury. The incidence of neurological injury following peripheral nerve blockade remains uncertain (Watts & Sharma 2007). The use of ultrasound-guided nerve blocks in adults and children is expanding.

The operator should monitor the patient for persistent paraesthesia during the placement of the block or pain on injection. Pain on injection of the local anaesthetic solution implies intraneural injection (Hartle & Jaggar 2005). It will be difficult to monitor these symptoms in patients who have been given general anaesthesia or sedation.

Perioperative pain management and organisational risk management

Acute health care organisations need to ensure that they provide a safe and effective perioperative analgesia service. There should be adequate physical facilities and appropriately trained staff. There should be an appropriate analysis of the risks and benefits of the options for perioperative analgesia in each individual patient.

The Royal College of Anaesthetists and Department of Health recommend that each acute hospital within the United Kingdom should have a multidisciplinary acute pain service, with appropriate input from specialist nurses, pharmacists and others.

The Royal College of Anaesthetists sets out guidelines for the provision of the acute pain service (RCoA 2004), which included guidance on:

- Staffing requirements
- Equipment, support services and facilities
- Training and education
- Research and audit
- Patient information

A number of professional bodies within the United Kingdom have jointly set out advice on good practice in the safe management of epidural analgesia (RCoA *et al.* 2004). The recommendations include appropriate supervision of patients with continuous epidural infusions in ward areas, the need for comprehensive 24-h access to anaesthetic advice and the need for appropriate documentation, local guidelines and protocols.

Each health care organisation should have a system for the reporting of adverse incidents in relation to patient treatment (including perioperative pain management issues). Local review of incident reports should generate action to change systems, ideally based on trends in reported incidents rather than in response to isolated issues. It may be difficult to ensure effective reporting of all types of relevant incidents (for example infection in relation to analgesic techniques), whereas other areas (such as medication-related issues) may be easier to identify and report.

A system has been set up by the National Patient Safety Agency (NPSA) in England and Wales, which enables the central collation of suitably anonymised data from incident reports from all National Health Service (NHS) trusts. This quantity of data allows for more effective analysis of trends and feedback of information in the form of guidance to individual trusts. Several issues have been highlighted by the NPSA recently, including the need to prevent inadvertent intravascular injection of drug infusions intended for epidural infusion (NPSA 2007). This has been prompted by several reported deaths and several other incidents in the United Kingdom in the period between 2000 and 2004 due to the inadvertent intravenous injection of bupivacaine. The main recommendations are listed in Box 14.1.

Risk assessment

Each health care organisation should ensure that there is a system in place to actively look for risks to prevent patient injury rather than merely act on

Box 14.1 Main recommendations from NPSA patient safety alert 21: safer practice with epidural injections and infusions (2007).

- Clearly label infusion bags and syringes for epidural therapy with 'for epidural use only'
- Minimise the likelihood of confusion between different types and strengths of epidural injections
- Reduce the risk of the wrong medicine being selected by storing epidural infusions in separate storage areas
- Use clearly labelled epidural administration sets and catheters which distinguish them from those used for intravenous and other routes
- Use infusion pumps and syringe drivers that are clearly distinguishable from those used for intravenous and other routes
- Ensure that all relevant staff receive adequate training

---

incident reports in a retrospective manner (Vincent 2001). There are a number of risk assessment models described, which may be suitable for use by health care organisations (National Patient Safety Agency 2006). The process of risk assessment may involve:

- The systematic identification of hazards
- The identification of the consequences of each hazard
- The estimation of the risks involved with each hazard
- An assessment of the current control measures
- An evaluation of the current risks
- An assessment of measures to reduce risks to a tolerable level

It is usual to refer to some form of matrix to determine a level of risk as a product of the likelihood of recurrence of a risk and the likely frequency of recurrence (National Patient Safety Agency 2008). The level of risk should allow comparison with other risks within the organisation and enable a rank order of risks to be constructed. The process should be used to inform decision making within the organisation and be used to prioritise funding to mitigate those risks that are considered to be 'intolerable' or significant.

The process of risk assessment should be considered an issue for the whole pain management team. Risk assessments should be carried out in a systematic fashion and the process reviewed on a regular basis. Difficulty may occur because of the subjective method of assessing risks and ensuring consistency across the organisation in the scope of each risk considered. (For example should medication issues be viewed on a ward-by-ward basis with a different risk assessment in each location, or should risks be assessed across the whole organisation?)

Box 14.2 NHS Litigation Authority (2007) risk management standards for acute trusts.

Risk management standards are designed to:

- Provide a structured framework within which to focus effective risk management activities in order to deliver quality improvements in organisational governance, patient care and the safety of patients, staff, contractors, volunteers and visitors
- Increase awareness and encourage implementation of the national agenda for the NHS
- Encourage and support organisations in taking a proactive approach to improvement
- Reflect risk exposure and empower organisations to determine how to manage their own risks
- Contribute to embedding risk management into the organisation's culture
- Reduce the level of claims by reducing the number of incidents and the likelihood of recurrence
- Assist in the management of adverse incidents and claims
- Provide assurance to the organisation, other inspecting bodies and stakeholders, including patients

---

Risk management standards

Most health care organisations within the NHS in England are members of the Clinical Negligence Scheme for Trusts, which is a scheme operated by the National Health Service Litigation Authority (NHSLA) in order to fund clinical negligence claims made against the NHS. Similar schemes are in operation in Scotland (Clinical Negligence and Other Risks Indemnity Scheme) and Wales (Welsh Risk Pool). The NHSLA (and similar bodies) promote good risk management by setting standards (see Box 14.2). These standards are also intended to be applicable to private-sector providers of NHS care, and a similar level of risk management should be expected in all other health care organisations.

Summary

Risk management in perioperative analgesia should be seen as the responsibility of all health care practitioners across all the relevant specialties and disciplines. The issues relating to perioperative analgesia are closely linked to the accompanying surgical intervention. Patients need to be fully informed about treatment decisions, with effective communication about the risks and benefits, and good documentation is essential. Health care organisations should ensure that there is effective clinical leadership in all aspects of perioperative analgesia and good teamworking between clinical staff and those supporting them in the organisation.

References

AAGBI (2006) *Consent for Anaesthesia.* AAGBI, London. http://www.aagbi.org/publications/guidelines/docs/consent06.pdf. Accessed 7 December 2007.

AAGBI (2007a) *Guidelines for the Management of Severe Local Anaesthetic Toxicity.* AAGBI, London. http://www.aagbi.org/publications/guidelines/docs/latoxicity07.pdf. Accessed 7 December 2007.

AAGBI (2007b) *Recommendations for Standards of Monitoring During Anaesthesia and Recovery.* AAGBI, London. http://www.aagbi.org. Accessed 7 December 2007.

Bardsley, H., Gristwood, R., Baker, H., *et al.* (1998) A comparison of the cardiovascular effects of levobupivacaine and rac-bupivacaine following intravenous administration to healthy volunteers. *British Journal of Clinical Pharmacology,* **46** (3), 245–249.

Brull, R., McCartney, C., Chan, V., *et al.* (2007) Disclosure of risks associated with regional anesthesia: a survey of academic regional anesthesiologists. *Regional Anesthesia and Pain Medicine,* **32** (1), 7–11.

Chaney, M. (2006) Intrathecal and epidural anesthesia and analgesia for cardiac surgery. *Anesthesia and Analgesia,* **102** (1), 45–64.

Cheney, F.W., Domino, K.B., Caplan, R.A. & Posner, K.L. (1999) Nerve injury associated with anesthesia: a closed claims analysis. *Anesthesiology,* **90** (4), 1062–1069.

Chester v Afshar (2004) UKHL, 41, Pt 2.

Department of Health (2004) *Reference Guide to Consent for Examination or Treatment.* Department of Health, London. http://www.dh.gov.uk/consent. Accessed 7 December 2007.

Dolin, S.J., Cashman, J.N. & Bland, J.M. (2002) Effectiveness of acute postoperative pain management: I. Evidence from published data. *British Journal of Anaesthesia,* **89** (3), 409–423.

General Medical Council (1998) *Seeking Patients' Consent: The Ethical Considerations.* General Medical Council, London.

General Medical Council (2007) *Consent: Patients and Doctors making Decisions Together' – A Draft for Consultation.* General Medical Council, London. https://gmc.e-consultation.net/making_decisions/index_https.asp. Accessed 7 December 2007.

General Medical Council (2008) *Consent: Patients and Doctors Making Decisions Together.* http://www.gmc-uk.org/guidance/ethical_guidance/consent_guidance/Consent_guidance.pdf. Accessed 12 June 2008.

Gogarten, W. (2006) The influence of new antithrombotic drugs on regional anesthesia. *Current Opinion in Anaesthesiology,* **19** (5), 545–550.

Hansdottir, V., Philip, J., Olsen, M., *et al.* (2006) Thoracic epidural versus intravenous patient-controlled analgesia after cardiac surgery. *Anesthesiology,* **104** (1), 142–151.

Hartle, A. & Jaggar, S. (2005) Regional nerve blocks. In: *Core Topics in Pain* (eds A. Holdcroft & S. Jaggar). Cambridge University Press, Cambridge, pp. 235–240.

Heavner, J. (2007) Local anesthetics. *Current Opinion in Anaesthesiology,* **20** (4), 336–342.

Ho, A.M., Chung, D. & Joynt, G. (2000) Neuraxial blockade and hematoma in cardiac surgery. *Chest,* **117** (2), 551–555.

Horlocker, T., Abel, M., Messick, J. & Schroeder, D. (2003) Small risk of serious neurologic complications related to lumbar epidural catheter placement in anesthetised patients. *Anesthesia & Analgesia*, **96** (6), 1547–1552.

Horlocker, T., Benzon, H.T., Brown, D.L., *et al.* (2002) *ASRA Second Consensus Conference on Neuraxial Anesthesia in the Anticoagulated patient: Defining the Risks.* ASRA, Park Ridge, IL. http://www.asra.com/consensus-statements/2.html.Accessed 7 December 2007.

Low, J.H. (2002) Survey of epidural analgesic management in general intensive care units in England. *Acta Anaesthesiologica Scandinavica*, **46** (7), 799–805.

NHS Litigation Authority (2007) *NHSLA Risk Management Standards for Acute Trusts.* NHS Litigation Authority, London, p. 5. http://www.nhsla.com/RiskManagement/CnstStandards/. Accessed 22 November 2007.

National Patient Safety Agency (2006) *Risk Assessment Programme.* National Patient Safety Agency, London. http://www.npsa.nhs.uk/patientsafety/improvingpatient safety/patient-safety-tools-and-guidance/risk-assessment-guides/. Accessed 12 June 2008.

National Patient Safety Agency (2007) *Patient Safety Alert 21: Safer Practice with Epidural Injections and Infusions.* National Patient Safety Agency, London. http://www.npsa.nhs.uk/patientsafety/alerts-and-directives/alerts/epidural-injections-and-infusions/. Accessed 7 December 2007.

National Patient Safety Agency (2008) *A Risk Matrix for Risk Managers.* National Patient Safety Agency, London. http://www.npsa.nhs.uk/patientsafety/improvingpatientsafety/patient-safety-tools-and-guidance/risk-assessment-guides/risk-matrix-for-risk-managers/. Accessed 12 June 2008.

Pennefather, S., Gilby, S., Danecki, A. & Russell, G. (2006) The changing practice of thoracic epidural analgesia in the United Kingdom: 1997–2004. *Anaesthesia*, **61** (4), 363–369.

Rathmell, J., Wu, C., Sinatra, R., *et al.* (2006) Acute post-surgical pain management: a critical appraisal of current practice. *Regional Anesthesia and Pain Medicine*, **31** (4 Suppl 1), 1–42.

Rigamonti, D., Liem, L., Sampath, P., *et al.* (1999) Spinal epidural abscess: contemporary trends in etiology, evaluation, and management. *Surgical Neurology*, **52** (2), 189–196.

RCoA (2004) *Guidelines for the Provision of Anaesthetic Services.* Royal College of Anaesthetists, London. http://www.rcoa.ac.uk. Accessed 7 December 2007.

RCoA & AAGBI (2004) *Epidurals for Pain Relief after Surgery.* Royal College of Anaesthetists, Association of Anaesthetists of Great Britain & Ireland, London. http://www.rcoa.ac.uk. Accessed 7 December 2007.

RCoA, RCN, AAGBI, BPS & ESRA (November 2004) *Good Practice in the Management of Continuous Epidural Analgesia in the Hospital Setting.* Royal College of Anaesthetists, London. http://www.rcoa.ac.uk. Accessed 7 December 2007.

Rosenberg, P., Veering, B. & Urmey, W. (2004) Maximum recommended doses of local anesthetics: a multifactorial concept. *Regional Anesthesia and Pain Medicine*, **29** (6), 564–575.

Ruppen, W., Derry, S., McQuay, H. & Moore, A. (2006) Incidence of epidural haematoma and neurological injury in cardiovascular patients with epidural analgesia/anaesthesia: systematic review and meta-analysis. *BMC Anesthesiology*, **12** (6), 10–16.

Ruppen, W., Derry, S., McQuay, H. & Moore, A. (2007) Infection rates associated with epidural indwelling catheters for 7 days or longer: systematic review and meta-analysis. *BMC Palliative Care*, **6**, 3.

Scott, D.B., Lee, A., Fagan, D., *et al.* (1989) Acute toxicity of ropivacaine compared with that of bupivacaine. *Anesthesia & Analgesia*, **69** (5), 563–569.

Vandermeulin, E., Van Aken, H. & Vermylen, J. (1994) Anticoagulants and spinal-epidural anesthesia. *Anesthesia and Analgesia*, **79** (6), 1165–1177.

Vincent, C. (2001) *Clinical Risk Management*, 2nd edn. BMJ Books, London.

Watts, S. & Sharma, D. (2007) Long-term neurological complications associated with surgery and peripheral nerve blockade: outcomes after 1065 consecutive blocks. *Anaesthesia and Intensive Care*, **35** (1), 24–31.

Further reading

Bould, M.D., Hunter, D. & Haxby, E.J. (2006) Clinical risk management in anaesthesia. *Continuing Education in Anaesthesia Critical Care and Pain*, **6** (6), 240–243.

Contractor, S. & Hardman, J.G. (1996) Injury during anaesthesia. *Continuing Education in Anaesthesia Critical Care and Pain*, **6** (2), 67–70.

Useful websites

National Health Service Litigation Authority: *http://www.nhsla.com.*

Welsh Risk Pool: *http://www.walesconcordat.org.uk.*

Clinical Negligence and Other Risks Indemnity Scheme (Scotland): *http://www.cnoris.com.*

Healthcare Commission: *http://www.healthcarecommission.org.uk.*

The Health & Safety Executive: *http://www.hse.gov.uk/.*

The Medicines and Healthcare Products Regulatory Authority: *http://www.hse.gov.uk/.*

The National Patient Safety Agency: *http://www.npsa.nhs.uk/.*

Notes

1. In Scotland, the Adults with Incapacity (Scotland) Act 2000 applies to those aged 16 years and over who lack capacity, and in Northern Ireland, there is no primary legislation, and decisions about treatment should be made in the best interests of patients in accordance with common law.
2. In Scotland, the Adults with Incapacity (Scotland) Act 2000.

15 Education

Angela Cousins

Key Messages

- Patient education is fundamental to improving the patient experience of acute postoperative pain.
- Patients have greater access to information regarding pain management issues than ever before; therefore, we must ensure that this information is accurate and comprehensible.
- Staff education must be targeted towards all members of the health care profession involved in caring for patients with pain.
- Ongoing educational programmes constitute a major part of the workload for the acute pain service.
- Education may be undertaken in many different forms and all available resources should be utilised to improve staff knowledge and patient outcomes.

Introduction

Despite the introduction of acute pain services (APSs) and educational pro- grammes in the public and independent sectors, many staff still fail to treat acute pain effectively. Although clinical ward staff are on the 'frontline' of acute pain management, Coulling (2005) suggests that many staff gain different levels of knowledge and experience depending on their basic level of education. They may even have already developed their own beliefs and attitudes towards pain and its management. In a survey of nurses' and doctors' knowledge of pain af- ter surgery, Coulling (2005) found that nursing staff were more knowledgeable in assessing patient's pain and were often more confident in managing pain than their medical colleagues, despite their lack of understanding of analgesic pharmacology. Although this is not an unusual finding, given the different roles of medical and nursing staff, it does highlight the fact that basic education in each profession is failing to focus on all aspects of pain management.

Health care professionals are now able to access a range of educational tools to source information regarding pain management. Increasingly popular is the use of the internet and networks designed for specialists in this chosen field. Membership of the British Pain Society (BPS) is open to all health care professionals and the society has specialist interest groups that provide the opportunity for networking. The BPS is the British Chapter of the International Association for the Study of Pain (IASP), a non-profit organisation dedicated to pain research and the provision of services for patients in pain. Further information can be found at http://www.iasp-pain.org.

The Royal College of Nursing (RCN) has a national pain forum that has local chapters that are specifically aimed at pain nurse specialists within regional areas. Regular meetings are held and topics for discussion are e-mailed to all members on a regular basis. This form of networking is particularly useful for the newly appointed clinical nurse specialist (CNS) in pain as it can be a great source of support and information. Network chat rooms are also available, such as 'pain-talk', which offers discussion forums for health care professionals who are interested in acute, chronic or palliative pain and are targeted at national rather than local level.

This chapter aims to explore the provision of education for health care professionals who have an active involvement in managing pain in the perioperative patient; the role of the APS to provide education to nursing, medical and allied health care professionals and the variety of educational resources available to them; education of members of the multidisciplinary team (MDT) on when to refer patients to the APS; areas of relevant safety with regard to prescribing and, most importantly, the role of patient education in acute pain management.

Health professionals' education

Undergraduate education

The inclusion of pain management in undergraduate education for all multi-professional disciplines appears to be lacking, as previously discussed in Chapter 3. As a result, it would appear that the majority of staff rely on professional journals and attendance at study days to attain postgraduate information regarding pain management. Surely, if this is the case, then what importance is given to acute pain within the clinical setting to undergraduates? How are we able to improve undergraduate education in pain if the curricula do not value its importance or must we simply continue to rely on individuals to seek training for themselves? Currently, these questions remain unanswered, but it is clearly the role of the APS within the hospital environment to keep the profile of pain management high on the educational agenda.

Postgraduate education for members of the APS

Nursing staff who choose a career in pain management usually possess experience within an acute setting, such as post-anaesthetic care units, theatres or intensive care units. However, it would not be unreasonable to expect a nurse from a less acute background to become interested in acute pain management and be very successful given the appropriate training, support and desire to fulfil the role. Specialist posts are not restricted to individuals with a nursing background and can include operating department practitioners, physiotherapists and pharmacists.

Clinical nurse specialists in pain management are required to be educated to a reasonable level and have the necessary experience to support their qualifications. Essential basic qualifications required are as a Level 1 registered nurse but may also include being educated to degree level (or willing to undertake further education), a teaching qualification, such as the SLICE or equivalent (formerly ENB 998), as well as a postgraduate qualification in a chosen subject relevant to the nature of their work (such as a cardiac certificate in those working in a cardiothoracic speciality). Desirable qualifications may include relevant experience in acute or chronic pain management and possibly being educated to masters' level.

Another desirable quality may be to possess appropriate skills in information technology (IT). Data collection and analysis for audit and research purposes form an important part of the job specification for specialist pain nurses and practitioners and data can be utilised as an excellent educational resource.

Clinical nurse specialists are also required to ensure that their practice is based on the best available evidence. Attendance at a multiprofessional Evidence-Based Healthcare Course should be highly recommended to any nurse specialist as it teaches them not only how to gather relevant evidence but also how to critically appraise its content. These courses are available at postgraduate level for all health care professionals and are designed to develop an understanding of the role of evidence-based health care within the clinical setting.

Continuing education may take the form of attendance and participation at forums and conferences at local, regional and national level. Conferences may be specifically related to pain management and its associated topics or may include allied conferences, for example those designed for anaesthetists or critical care staff.

Dissemination of knowledge regarding pain management may be delegated to pain link nurses at ward level. The pain link nurse has an important role as they are ideally positioned to provide support and education to staff at ward level whilst keeping the pain team informed of any arising issues. The link nurse should be given the opportunity to undertake simple audit and data collection as an extended member of the pain service. As part of their continuing education they should also be encouraged to attend pain conferences to maintain interest and morale in the role.

Postgraduate tertiary education

A new subsection of the Nursing and Midwifery Council (NMC) is currently under review to allow the inclusion of advanced nurse practitioners (APN) onto the nurse's register. APNs are post-registration nurses who have completed an additional educational qualification, such as a masters' degree programme, and who have gained the relevant clinical training to undertake services that were once regarded to fall within the scope of the medical profession (Nursing and Midwifery Council 2007). In the light of this change, it is felt that more specialist practitioners will be required to complete advanced education.

Masters' level qualifications in pain are offered by a number of higher educational institutions, which follow the core curricula outlined by the IASP and are open to all health care disciplines involved in pain management. Applicants may have very different experiences of pain management, as the degree programme is suitable for medical and nursing staff, physiotherapists and occupational therapists, pharmacists and dentists. The degree programme is usually of 2 years' duration, involving compulsory and elective modules. If less elective modules are completed, a diploma may be awarded, and if only the compulsory modules are undertaken, a certificate is awarded. This allows for greater flexibility for students who may not wish to complete the degree course within the specified timeframe. Distance-learning packages are also available for those students who wish to complete the course in their own home. This mode of education has become increasingly popular due to time constraints at work and offers more options in choice of institutional courses available to students.

Information on advanced training in pain management for medical staff is now available from the Faculty of Pain Medicine website. Since its formation, in August 2007, the faculty has been inundated with applications to join the Foundation Fellowship of the faculty. This training is competency based and members are encouraged to keep evidence of practice via a logbook throughout their training placements. More information is available on the Royal College of Anaesthetists (RCoA) website (www.rcoa.ac.uk).

Postgraduate institutional education

A major role of the CNS is to disseminate knowledge to other members of the MDT and provide any new or innovative information in relation to their chosen speciality. This may be achieved via in-house study days, poster presentations or simply through informal teaching sessions at clinical level. Study days need to be targeted towards a particular target group, for example junior medical staff or physiotherapists, and therefore should provide relevant information appropriate to the participant's area of clinical practice.

As part of the continuing professional development of medical staff, organisers of well-designed and evidence-based courses or seminars are able to apply to the regulating bodies (for example the RCoA) for ratification of training, which allows them to award continuing professional development points to attendees.

There are a number of postgraduate professional societies that offer further education in the management of pain and pain-related topics. These include the BPS, the RCoA, the RCN and the IASP, to name but a few. The BPS and IASP are targeted at all health care professionals with an interest in pain and their role is to organise conferences and meetings, provide reviews and publications for all members and disseminate knowledge based on the best available evidence. The RCoA and the RCN are specifically tailored to anaesthetists and nursing staff working within the field of pain but also organise conferences and meetings for those with an interest in the topic.

Certification and accreditation

Before any health professional interacts with a patient or compiles a pain management plan, most health care organisations require that competency is demonstrable. At ward level this implies nursing and medical education followed by certification. Those that perform this routine education and provide certification must also be educated and, ideally, accredited for that role. Examples include attendance at an organised institutional study day in pain followed by an assessment of competency before certification. An introduction to basic pain management should be available to all nursing and allied health care professionals who regularly come in contact with patients in pain. Attendance at an institutional epidural study day should be an essential part of caring for patients receiving regional analgesia, and competency should involve a practical assessment of clinical skills, for example the removal of an epidural catheter before certification is given. Examples of pain and epidural study day programmes, demonstrating suggested topics and speakers, are shown in Boxes 15.1 and 15.2.

Box 15.1   Example of acute pain study day programme.

0900–0915	Introduction and learning objectives	Pain CNS
0915–0945	Physiology of acute pain	Anaesthetist
0945–1030	Pain assessment and management	Pain CNS
	Break	
1045–1115	Pharmacology of acute pain	Pharmacist
1115–1200	Regional anaesthesia and analgesia, including epidural, intrathecal and paravertebral techniques	Anaesthetist
	Lunch	
1300–1345	Management of analgesia side effects including nausea and vomiting, pruritus, sedation, urinary retention and constipation	Anaesthetist
1345–1430	The psychology of acute pain	Psychologist
	Break	
1445–1515	Pain infusion device training workshop	Pain CNS
1515–1600	TENS workshop	Physiotherapist
1600–1630	Summary and evaluation	
CNS, clinical nurse specialist; TENS, transcutaneous electrical nerve stimulation.		

Box 15.2 Example of an epidural study day programme.

0900–0915	Introduction and learning objectives	Pain CNS
0915–1030	History	Anaesthetist
	Patient-selection criteria	
	Anatomy and physiology	
	Epidural insertion techniques	
	Break	
1045–1120	Epidural medicines	Pharmacist
	• Pharmacokinetics	
	• Pharmacodynamics	
1120–1200	Patient monitoring and troubleshooting	Anaesthetist
	Lunch	
1300–1445	**Workshops (each 30-min duration)**	
	Assessment and monitoring of patients with epidurals in the clinical area	Anaesthetist
	Care and removal of the epidural catheter	Pain CNS
	Changing infusions, drug concentrations and calculations	Pharmacist
	Break	
1500–1545	Theoretical assessment, practice and answers	Pain CNS
1500–1615	Pain infusion device training	Pain CNS
	Summary, feedback and close	

CNS, clinical nurse specialist.

As junior medical staff rotate in relatively large groups at predictable times it is easy to set a programme of APS education for this group. Areas that must be covered include the routine and emergency protocols of the APS, as well as higher levels of APS pump device operation where appropriate (for example the training of anaesthetists in PCA pump programme alteration). In 2006, the RCoA published a document that aimed at improving standards within anaesthesia. The compendium of audit recipes include targets for best practice for APSs in relation to pain education by the acute pain team. It suggests that at all pre-registration junior doctors attend an induction tutorial in pain management and that all junior surgical staff be given the opportunity to attend a pain management tutorial at least every 3 years. However, it also recognised that standards were not always met as a result of lack of study time, low staffing levels and poor communication of educational resources available (The Royal College of Anaesthetists 2006).

Specialised education can be performed locally or regionally or nationally. An example of local level is to arrange a live demonstration of the insertion of an epidural to a lead member of ward staff. This promotes good working relations between members of the MDT.

Aside from individual patient reviews, education of clinical nursing staff represents the second largest proportion of APS staff workload. The recent introduction of Agenda for Change (AfC) and subsequent Knowledge and Skills Framework (KSF) competencies has allowed staff to focus on their own professional development in order to further their career appropriately. The fundamental principle of KSF is to provide 'lifelong learning' and allow development of all staff (Department of Health 2004). The emphasis has been placed on learning and development within the workplace as opposed to how many study days have been attended within a specified period of time. Examples of this may take the form of 'on-job learning', such as reflective practice or learning from and development of others (mentorship and coaching); 'off-job learning with self', such as private study, electronic or distance learning; or 'off-job learning with others', such as formal courses, inductions and conferences (Department of Health 2004). Fulfilling competencies in relation to pain allows staff to recognise the important aspects of pain assessment, management and documentation, as well as ensures that they are adhering to trust policies and guidelines.

As time is often a constraint in the modern National Health Service (NHS), staff are more inclined to indulge in private study as a means of furthering their education. Websites to enable online learning have been developed with this purpose in mind. E-learning is spreading and is an excellent way to deliver training. Accessible from any computer with internet connection, e-learning solves the problem of clinical staff becoming too busy to engage in organised study. It allows solo learning in own time, providing flexible and cost-effective education. Managers are able to monitor progress and modules may even be tailored to individual trusts and different staff groups. An example of e-learning is www.thelearningclinic.co.uk.

Educational resources

Educational resources are the cornerstone of a good APS. They allow effective education of all staff, including medical and surgical teams. This in turn allows traditional hierarchical barriers to a team approach to pain management to be removed. Although ongoing education should be provided by the APS, printed information should also be available to ward staff in the form of a resource file as outlined in Table 15.1.

Criteria for referral to pain management service

Acute pain services have been established since the early 1990s, following the report published by the Royal College of Surgeons and Faculty of Anaesthetists,

Table 15.1 Educational resources for clinical staff.

General pain information	• Acute pain pathways and physiology • Acute-pain-scoring systems (including those in different languages) • Pharmacology of agents used and current formulary to check posology/dosage • Acute pain review articles from general journals (e.g. *Journal of Clinical Nursing* or *British Medical Journal*) • Original source references that have been used to formulate trust protocols and policies • Information on paediatric and elderly variations of all above categories as necessary
Protocols/ guidelines/ policies	**Patient-controlled analgesia protocols** • Prescription guidelines relating to different opioids • Bolus dose and lockout parameters • Infusion device instructions (including any locking codes and troubleshooting issues) • Contact details of daytime and on-call support • Management of side effects including overdose and respiratory depression **Epidural protocols** • Prescription guidelines (for anaesthetic staff only) • Device instructions (including any locking codes and bolus administration) • Contact details of daytime and on-call support (pain team/pharmacists/anaesthetists and site managers) • Care and removal instructions including observations post-catheter removal Advice documents for overdose of opioids, local anaesthetic toxicity and other potential adverse effects

Handover documents	The following should be available (at least in summary) at all times and be part of a documented handover to the out-of-hour APS representatives who may consist of senior nurses, anaesthetists or site managers
	• Current APS patients detailing the following:
	  (1) Agreed pain management plan and its efficacy
	  (2) Individualised 24-h action plan
	  (3) Recent pain management service (PMS) issues
	  (4) Surgical or medical planning
	  (5) Any patient-specific contraindications or allergies
	  (6) Recent PMS failures (e.g. a failed epidural insertion)
	  (7) Details of any chronic pain elements noted in acute cases, such as development of neuropathic pain
	• Likely issues/plans for the next 24-h period
	• Recent patient discharges from the APS in case of re-presentation
	• Potential inpatient or expected admissions with known acute or chronic pain issues, including those with chronic opioid use

entitled 'Pain after Surgery' (1990). The role of the APS is to provide advice, education, audit and research in the management of any pain that can be classified as acute in nature. The APS should be based on a team approach and include an anaesthetist (with an interest in pain management), specialist nurses and a pharmacist. To improve the holistic approach of pain management liaison with other members of the multidisciplinary team, such as physiotherapists, psychologists and occupational therapists, may be required. The Royal College of Anaesthetists and The Pain Society (2003) published guidelines for the provision of APSs and stated recommendations for practice within the hospital setting. These guidelines highlight the importance of education to ensure the safe and effective treatment of acute pain in both the surgical and non-surgical patient.

An effective APS will issue criteria for referral at local level but there are several categories which cover the majority of referrals to an APS. Before considering the criteria, it is wise to empower the relevant groups of referring health professionals. Examples of these are dietitians who detect subtle signs of nausea or constipation or physiotherapists who note acute pain limits their therapeutic interventions. Referral criteria for the APS are listed in Table 15.2.

Safer prescribing

Patient safety is high on the agenda within the NHS and forms a part of clinical governance. Medication errors were the second largest incidents, after patient accident, reported to the National Reporting and Learning System (NRLS) between January 2005 and June 2006. Opioid overdose was found to be the most commonly reported medication incident (13%) resulting in serious harm, i.e. death. The NRLS has issued an action plan to ensure that medication errors are minimised. The action plan states that the education of staff must be improved through staff competencies and the reporting of medication incidents must be increased to enable learning to take place using reflective practice (National Patient Safety Agency 2007). To ensure safety the prescribing of certain medicines should be limited to those with adequate knowledge and training; for example epidural infusions should only be prescribed by an anaesthetist.

As part of the initiative to improve medication safety, the National Patient Safety Agency (NPSA) published a patient-safety alert regarding epidural injection and infusions (National Patient Safety Agency 2007). This alert was a result of incidents reported involving the incorrect administration of epidural infusions and suggested action of how to improve the safety of patient care. One of the main points includes the training and competency of staff involved in the administration, assessment and monitoring of patients requiring epidural therapy. Recommendations include staff formal training to include protocols, drugs and pump devices with regular updates. Senior staff should be able to supervise and complete the work competencies of recently trained staff to ensure safer practice.

Table 15.2 Acute pain services patient-referral criteria.

Criteria	
(1) A new acute pain	A patient may report new acute pain to the nurse responsible for their care. After scoring the pain using a valid assessment tool, such as a visual analogue scale (VAS), the acute pain services (APS) should be notified and review the patient accordingly. All new or unexpected changes in the nature of pain should also be referred to the medical team, as a diagnosis should not be delayed. For example a patient complaining of new-onset abdominal pain, which is unrelated to their type of surgery, may require further investigations to rule out bowel obstruction
(2) A failing pain management system	**Epidural** – An inadequate epidural block, device failure, connection or delivery set issues, new-onset pain, abnormal neurology or adverse effects such as low blood pressure. Many issues arising in those receiving epidural therapy should be referred to the pain management nurse or anaesthetist before the decision to discontinue its use is made **PCA** – Dose or interval either too great or too small, device failure, connection or delivery set issues, side effects such as nausea, vomiting, constipation or adverse effects, e.g. overdose or respiratory depression **Oral** – Patient may need to be 'nil by mouth' as a result of a particular type of surgery (such as gastrointestinal)
(3) Weaning of existing pain management plan	**Epidural** – Issues related to weaning techniques when converting to oral or parenteral cover, catheter removal regarding anticoagulation and appropriate removal of the epidural catheter in accordance to trust policy and guidelines **PCA** – Dose and interval alterations, conversion to oral medication using the previous 24-h opioid usage and ensuring that a multimodal pain management plan is adopted
(4) Abnormal observations	These may include new-onset neurology, respiratory depression or chronic pain symptoms in an acute pain setting
(5) Education	**Patient** – This may include information relating to the mode of analgesia chosen in individual patients, e.g. how to use PCA or what effects to expect from a local anaesthetic block **Staff** – Support and education for an unfamiliar mode of analgesia, e.g. a continuous regional anaesthetic block such as a paravertebral block or a rarely used technique in that setting, such as epidural analgesia or a pump device to deliver subcutaneous medications more often seen in palliative care

An e-learning package has also been developed by the National Infusion Device Training Programme, which enables staff to gain confidence and achieve competency in the safe use of medical devices designed for infusions.

Prescribing may be improved with the use of pre-printed, multifaceted prescription charts that combine the prescription, assessment documentation and any recommendations for practice within one complete chart (Coulling 2005). Examples of such documents in acute pain include high-tech modes of analgesia, such as epidural therapy and patient-controlled analgesia (PCA).

Safer analgesia administration

- Pain infusion device training and competency covering the need for distinct infusion devices, delivery sets and labelling. Standardisation of infusion devices has been encouraged to reduce the incidence of error.
- The NPSA PSA 20 *Safer use of injectable medicines* was published in March 2007. As part of the alert, the training, assessment and supervision of all staff responsible for injectable medicines were highlighted. Competencies focused on prescribing, preparation and administration of medicines as well as monitoring of patients. These competencies are directed at medical, pharmacy and nursing staff respectively.

Patients

The role of the patient in the NHS has changed over the years and is no longer a passive one. Their involvement in their own care has taken great steps forward. Since the Department of Health outlined its 'vision of the health service' in the NHS Plan (Department of Health 2000), emphasis has been placed on a patient-centred approach of health care. Information has empowered patients to make decisions and has allowed them to have more control of their own treatment. With easy access to medical information available on the world wide web, patients are more likely to understand a great deal more about their disease, treatment and prognosis than ever before. It would seem prudent to ensure that all patients are given adequate knowledge and support to enable them to make informed choices about their health care.

Patient education should be a fundamental process at all levels along the patient's journey, from primary care to discharge from hospital and subsequent follow-up. There has been much debate on the value of preoperative education within the hospital setting, as well as the impact and importance of advice given in the form of verbal and written material.

Patient education and its effect on postoperative outcomes have been scrutinised in recent years. The evidence on the impact of preoperative education in patients is divided and doubts remain as to its beneficial effect in relation to postoperative pain. However, several studies suggest that there are some positive outcomes to be gained, which include the active involvement of patients and an increase in overall patient satisfaction in their postoperative pain management (Level III: Sjöling *et al.* 2003, Walker 2007).

Interestingly, a review of the literature by the Cochrane Collaboration (Level I: McDonald *et al.* 2004) suggests that preoperative education has little or no effect on the length of hospital stay, postoperative complications and pain. Indeed, the only positive benefit of preoperative education appeared to be in the reduction of anxiety. However, the anxious patient is more likely to describe increased pain and therefore their understanding and retention of knowledge in the preoperative period is of paramount importance. Other outcome measures, such as satisfaction, may demonstrate this in future work.

Fear of pain

Admission to hospital is an enormously stressful situation and anxiety is a normal response to stress. Anxiety has a huge impact on the psychological and emotional stability of the hospitalised patient. One of the greatest anxieties is that of fear and in particular the fear of pain. Royston & Cox (2003) explored the concerns of patients awaiting surgery. They found that patients in several studies rated fear of postoperative pain almost as high as the fear of death or awareness during anaesthesia. Although the risk of death under anaesthetic is a rare event, the possibility of experiencing moderate-to-severe pain following surgery is still a real threat and patients may believe that this fear is justified.

Patients may also fear the choice of analgesia employed postoperatively and this may be a barrier to effective pain management. Greer *et al.* (2001) postulate that this fear is irrational and often due to a lack of knowledge, the result of which may lead to the underuse of opioids in the management of pain. The fear of addiction to strong opioids, and in particular morphine, has concerned not only patients but many health care professionals. In reality, only a small minority (1%) of patients will develop an addiction to strong opioids, without pre-existing psychological addiction (Acello 2000). Physical dependence or tolerance to an opioid is often mistaken for addiction as the patient may begin demanding the drug, as its effect wears off, before it is due to be administered again. This behaviour is known as 'clock watching' and may predispose the patient to being labelled as an addict. Patients who require long-term use of opioids should be made aware that physical dependence always occurs and that there is often a need to increase the opioid dose as they become more tolerant to its analgesic effect.

The use of focus groups to improve educational material intended for patient use has increased in popularity within medicine and is in keeping with the NHS Plan (Department of Health 2000) as it involves the patient. Chumbley *et al.* (Level II: 2002) demonstrated that patients are better informed in the use of PCA following their involvement in the redesign of a patient information leaflet. Focus groups and patient questionnaires were used in the study to establish what information patients already knew about this mode of analgesia and what they considered important to know. It was found that patients wanted to understand more about PCA in relation to safety, side effects, addiction and the type of drug used. Common misconceptions regarding pain and analgesia were identified and new educational material was designed to improve patient knowledge. Involvement of the patient in this way improves the readability of educational material.

Treatment options

There are various modes of analgesia available to patients in the management of acute pain. The choice of analgesia is often dependent on the type of pain/surgery, patient suitability and medical preference. Patients rely on the knowledge and expertise of medical and nursing staff before making a decision on which mode of analgesia they would prefer. Patient consent to treatment and risk is outlined in Chapter 14. Table 15.3 reviews the pharmacological

Table 15.3 Analgesia-related patient information and outcomes.

Mode of analgesia	Patient information	Patient outcomes
Regional blockade: epidural analgesia (including spinal/caudal)	• Risks and complications • Insertion technique • Drugs used in infusion • Duration of action • Removal procedure • Discharge advice	Less likely to lead to chronic pain Improved pulmonary function May avoid need for general anaesthesia (GA)
Patient-controlled analgesia (PCA)	• Drug used in infusion • How to use the device • Common side effects • Minimal risk of addiction/overdose	Patient satisfaction and autonomy
Neural blockade (including plexus block, peripheral nerve block, paravertebral block and infiltration)	• Insertion technique • Duration of action • Safety aspects (e.g. loss of sensation and proprioception)	May avoid need for GA Multimodal approach to pain management and may reduce use of opioids
Intramuscular (IM) Subcutaneous (SC) injection	• Drugs used • Insertion technique • Duration of action • Common side effects	May be used in patients with an ileus IM injection likely to be painful, therefore unpopular
Oral analgesia	• Drugs used • Common side effects • Duration of action • Breakthrough analgesia	May be commenced early in patients without ileus

treatment options available, the information patients need to know about each technique and the impact on patient outcomes.

Patient-related educational material

The introduction of IT has been a revolution in terms of consumer education. The use of the internet to access information on all aspects of disease and medical management has increased the patient's awareness and understanding of the disease process. As a result of the NHS Plan (Department of Health 2000), patients have been given a greater understanding of the level of treatment they can expect from the NHS. The National Institute for Health and Clinical Evidence has published 'patient-friendly' guidelines available on the internet. Patients are also able to access the NHS Direct online, providing them with a website which is officially recognised in comparison to the use of global search engines which cite information from a variety of unrecognised sources.

A survey of patients' use of the internet, in The Netherlands, by de Boer *et al.* (2007) established that many patients increasingly use the internet to search for medical information in relation to pain. Although 50% of all respondents used the internet, the authors acknowledge that it should not be assumed that all the information provided is accurate and recommend that medical staff encourage patients to ask questions about any information that may cause concern or require further questioning.

Printed educational material in the form of patient information leaflets has long been established within the health care setting. Such information should be readily available to patients and easy to understand (including other commonly used languages). The information itself should reflect current evidence-based practice within the hospital and correspond with trust guidelines and policies. Review of the information should be undertaken at regular intervals and ideally involve patient focus groups to ascertain readability, comprehension and reflect any frequently asked questions relating to the patient population (for example information on sickle cell crisis should be reviewed by those who experience it). Multimedia educational tools are commercially available from a variety of sources or can be developed locally to meet specific patient group's needs.

Summary

A truly modern APS will have moved away from the traditional role of simply assisting medical staff in the delivery of drugs into a whole new arena. The model APS sees the patient at its very centre and organises its services to re-duce pain and enhance recovery through many methods. By maintaining high standards of internal education, the APS is able to update the evidence base for protocols, guidelines and policies that are used by the entire MDT. Man-agement structures need to ensure that funding is continuous and adequate to maintain a high-quality APS. As a major role is educational, this area can appear to be a soft target for cost control but, clearly, is a very important aspect of the patient's journey.

It is evident that there are a variety of educational tools available to the APS within the hospital setting; however, there is also a wealth of information outside of the clinical environment, which can be utilised to improve pain management. Surprisingly, undergraduate pain education remains poor, with perhaps too much reliance on postgraduate education to improve staff knowledge and skills in this subject. As a result, the onus is placed on individuals, pain management teams and pain societies.

A proactive APS embraces its educational role and targets the learning needs of not only patients and nursing staff but also its colleagues within medicine, surgery, pharmacy and other allied health care professions to achieve these high standards of care.

References

Acello, B. (2000) Facing fears about opioid addiction.*Nursing*, **30** (5), 72.

Coulling, S. (2005) Doctor's and nurse's knowledge of pain after surgery. *Nursing Standard*, **19** (34), 41–49.

Chumbley, G.M., Hall, G.M. & Salmon, P. (2002) Patient-controlled analgesia: what information does the patient want? *Journal of Advanced Nursing*, **39** (5), 459–471.

de Boer, M.J., Versteegen, G.J. & van Wijhe, M. (2007) Patients' use of the Internet for pain-related medical information. *Patient Education and Counseling*. Epub: 22 June 2007. ISSN: 0738-3991.

Department of Health (2000) *The NHS Plan*. HMSO, London. http://www.dh.gov.uk/en/Publicationsandstatistics/Publications/PublicationsPolicyAndGuidance/DH_4002960. Accessed 13 September 2007.

Department of Health (2004) *The NHS Knowledge and Skills Framework (NHS KSF) and the Development Review Process*. HMSO, London. http://www.dh.gov.uk/prod_consum_dh/idcplg?IdcService=GET_FILE&dID=18018&Rendition=Web. Accessed 13 December 2007.

Greer, S.M., Dalton, J.A., Carlson, J. & Youngblood, R. (2001) Surgical patient's fear of addiction to pain medication: the effect of an educational program for clinicians. *The Clinical Journal of Pain*, **17** (2), 157–164.

McDonald, S., Hetrick, S. & Green, S. (2004) Pre-operative education for hip and knee replacement. *Cochrane Database of Systematic Reviews*, Issue 1, Art No CD003526.

National Patient Safety Agency (2007) *PSA 21 Safer Practice with Epidural Injections and Infusions*. National Patient Safety Agency, London. www.npsa.nhs.uk. Accessed 13 December 2007.

Nursing and Midwifery Council (2007) *Advanced Nursing Practice*. Update 19 June 2007. www.nmc-uk.org. Accessed 13 December 2007.

Royal College of Surgeons of England and College of Anaesthetists (1990) *Commission on the Provision of Surgical Services. Report of the working party on Pain after Surgery*. Royal College of Surgeons, London.

Royston, D. & Cox, F. (2003) Anaesthesia: the patient's point of view. *The Lancet*, **362** (9396), 1648–1658.

Sjöling, M., Nordahl, G., Olofsson, N. & Asplund, K. (2003) The impact of preoperative information on state anxiety, postoperative pain and satisfaction with pain management. *Patient Education and Counseling*, **51** (2), 169–176.

The Royal College of Anaesthetists (2006) *Raising the Standard – A Compendium of Audit Recipes for Continuous Quality Improvement in Anaesthesia*, 2nd edn. The Royal College of Anaesthetists, London. www.rcoa.ac.uk. Accessed 13 December 2007.

The Royal College of Anaesthetists and The Pain Society (2003) *Pain Management Services Good Practice*. The Royal College of Anaesthetists, London. www.rcoa.ac.uk. Accessed 13 December 2007.

Walker, J.A. (2007) What is the effect of preoperative information on patient satisfaction? *British Journal of Nursing*, **16** (1), 27–32.

Useful websites

International Association for the Study of Pain: *http://www.iasp-pain.org/*.
Royal College of Anaesthetists: *http://www.rcoa.ac.uk/*.
British Pain Society: *http://www.britishpainsociety.org/*.
Chronic Pain Coalition: *http://www.paincoalition.org.uk/*.
American Pain Society: *http://www.ampainsoc.org/*.
Canadian Pain Society: *http://www.canadianpainsociety.ca/*.
Australian and New Zealand College of Anaesthetists: *http://www.anzca.edu.au/*.
Pain Talk: *http://www.pain-talk.co.uk/*.
National Infusion Device Training Programme: *http://www.clpu.nhs.uk/*.

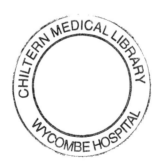

Index

Index